Surgery:
an Oxford Core Text

Oxford Core Texts

Clinical Dermatology

Clinical Pathology

Clinical Skills

Endocrinology

Human Physiology

Medical Genetics

Neurology

Oncology

Psychiatry

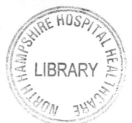
Surgery: an Oxford Core Text

Edited by

Peter Stonebridge
David Smith
Lesley Duncan
and
Alastair Thompson

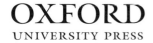
OXFORD
UNIVERSITY PRESS

OXFORD
UNIVERSITY PRESS

Great Clarendon Street, Oxford OX2 6DP

Oxford University Press is a department of the University of Oxford.
It furthers the University's objective of excellence in research, scholarship,
and education by publishing worldwide in

Oxford New York

Auckland Cape Town Dar es Salaam Hong Kong Karachi
Kuala Lumpur Madrid Melbourne Mexico City Nairobi
New Delhi Shanghai Taipei Toronto

With offices in

Argentina Austria Brazil Chile Czech Republic France Greece
Guatemala Hungary Italy Japan South-Korea Poland Portugal
Singapore Switzerland Thailand Turkey Ukraine Vietnam

Oxford is a registered trade mark of Oxford University Press
in the UK and in certain other countries

Published in the United States
by Oxford University Press Inc., New York

British Library Cataloguing in Publication Data

Data available

Library of Congress Cataloguing in Publication Data

Data available

Typeset by EXPO Holdings Sdn Bhd., Malaysia
Printed in Great Britain on acid-free paper
by Ashford Colour Press Limited, Gosport, Hampshire

ISBN 0-19-262990-5 (Pbk.)   978-0-19-262990-6 (Pbk.)

10 9 8 7 6 5 4 3 2 1

Preface

Medicine has been described as the practical application of scientific knowledge; this is particularly true of surgery. Yet knowledge requires understanding, which is the step before safe practice.

The requirements of a medical student are very different than for a newly qualified doctor. Certain core knowledge is required, yet an understanding of practical aspects of the care of a patient is necessary to function as a doctor.

How to put across the necessary knowledge in a way that will promote understanding? When I was a medical student I was advised to read up about a condition when I had seen a patient with it on the ward as it would fix some of the knowledge in my mind. This book uses this principle and takes 'typical' case scenarios and explains the whys and the wherefores.

This book is meant to be read. It does contain lists and summaries to aid revision and allow dipping into it, but understanding does not come with brief encounters.

It is better to understand than to simply remember and it is easier to remember when you understand.

Acknowledgements

Many thanks to Sam Chakraverty, Consultant Radiologist, Ian Zealley, Consultant Radiologist, and Mohamad Thaha, Lecturer in Surgery, for a number of the figures used in this book.

Dundee
Spring 2005

Peter Stonebridge

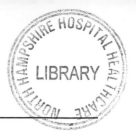

Contents

Editors and contributors *ix*

PART ONE

1.1 Oesophagus, stomach, and duodenum *1*
Conditions of the oesophagus *1*
Conditions of stomach and duodenum *8*

1.2 Small bowel *17*

1.3 Colorectal and perianal disorders *31*
Colorectal conditions *31*
Perianal conditions *46*

1.4 Disorders of the pancreas, biliary tree, liver, and jaundice *53*
Pancreatic disorders *53*
Disorders of the biliary system *61*
Jaundice *64*

1.5 Lumps in the scrotum and hernias *73*
Lumps in the scrotum *73*
Groin hernia *75*

1.6 Breast lumps *81*

1.7 Lumps in the neck and thyroid gland *87*
Lumps in the neck *87*
Thyroid *91*

1.8 Vascular conditions *97*
Chronic arterial occlusive disease *97*
Abdominal aortic aneurysm *110*
Venous disorders *112*

PART TWO

2.1 Perioperative care *121*
Preoperative assessment, investigation, and premedication *122*
Issues of consent *132*
Anaesthesia and sedation *133*
Fluid management *145*
Transfusion and blood products *148*
Nutrition *152*

2.2 Postoperative problems *157*
ABC, Patient assessment and resuscitation *158*
Assessment of the critically ill surgical patient *164*
Postoperative complications: hypoxia *167*
Postoperative complications: hypotension and cardiac ischaemia *173*
Postoperative complications: oliguria and electrolyte disturbance *179*
Postoperative sepsis *184*
Deep vein thrombosis and pulmonary embolism *189*

Index *197*

Editors and contributors

Editors

Peter Stonebridge
Professor of Vascular Surgery
Dundee University and Ninewells Hospital, Dundee,
Tayside

David Smith
Consultant Surgeon
Ninewells Hospital, Dundee, Tayside

Lesley Duncan
Consultant Anaesthetist
Ninewells Hospital, Dundee, Tayside

Alastair Thompson
Professor of Surgical Oncology
Dundee University and Ninewells Hospital, Dundee,
Tayside

Contributors

In addition to material written by the editors the following have made contributions to the text.

Matthew Checketts
Consultant Anaesthetist
Ninewells Hospital, Dundee, Tayside

Michael Fried
Consultant Anaesthetist
St John's Hospital, Livingston, West Lothian

Michael Lavelle-Jones
Consultant Surgeon
Ninewells Hospital, Dundee, Tayside

William McClymont
Consultant Anaesthetist
Ninewells Hospital, Dundee, Tayside

Carol McMillan
Consultant Anaesthetist
Ninewells Hospital, Dundee, Tayside

Sami Shimi
Senior Lecturer and Consultant Surgeon
Dundee University and Ninewells Hospital, Dundee,
Tayside

Robert Steele
Professor of Surgery
Dundee University and Ninewells Hospital, Dundee,
Tayside

Oesophagus, stomach, and duodenum

Chapter contents

Conditions of the oesophagus *1*

    Scenario 1: heartburn *1*

    Scenario 2: difficulty with swallowing *2*

    Background: oesophagus *2*

Conditions of stomach and duodenum *8*

    Scenario 1: acute upper abdominal pain *8*

    Scenario 2: vomiting and weight loss *10*

    Scenario 3: haematemesis *11*

    Background: stomach and duodenum *11*

Conditions of the oesophagus

Scenario 1: heartburn

> A 45-year-old male presents with a history of recurrent heartburn with occasional central chest pain. He also complains of regurgitation of acid into his mouth (waterbrash).

Heartburn is a very common complaint. Regurgitation of acid into the mouth is part of the same spectrum. The gastro-oesophageal sphincter fails to prevent stomach acid into the lower oesophagus giving rise to the burning retrosternal pain. A boring back pain would indicate that the patient may have developed an ulcer at the lower end of the oesophagus.

> There is no history of difficulty in swallowing (dysphagia).

Dysphagia is an important symptom as it may indicate the development of a benign stricture or the presence of oesophageal cancer.

> The patient smokes 20 cigarettes per day, is a heavy social alcohol drinker, and is overweight.

Obesity, smoking, alcohol, and coffee drinking all predispose to the development of oesophageal reflux. Stopping smoking, avoiding alcohol and coffee, and losing weight are all things the patient can do to help himself.

> There was nothing abnormal found on examination.

A physical examination should be carried out. **In a case of reflux oesophagitis no abnormal findings will be evident.**

Young patients (aged <55) with dyspepsia and no worrying symptoms can be treated symptomatically. Older patients (aged >55) or any patient with worrying symptoms (dysphagia or weight loss) should be investigated.

To evaluate the condition an upper GI endoscopy should be performed to identify a stricture and allow a biopsy to be taken. A barium swallow is useful to assess the length and nature of any identified stricture (Fig. 1.1a).

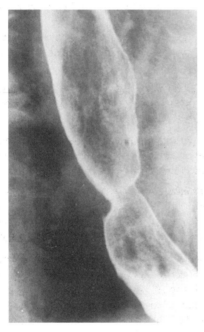

Fig 1.1a Barium swallow study of a benign oesophageal stricture secondary to reflux oesphagitis.

Scenario 2: difficulty with swallowing

> A 65-year-old male presents with a history of increasing difficulty with swallowing solid food (dysphagia). He is finding he either has to chew everything excessively or eat sloppy food. If he tries to eat solid food it merely comes back up.

Dysphagia is a worrying complaint. The cause of dysphagia should *always* be investigated. As a tumour of the oesophagus grows it gradually closes off the oesophagus.

> He drinks large amounts of alcohol and smokes 40 cigarettes per day.

As with many conditions, cigarettes and alcohol predispose to oesophageal cancer.

> He has lost a lot of weight (10 kilos).

Dysphagia and weight loss are the two worrying symptoms, suggestive of malignancy. As less food gets into the patient, a large amount of weight is lost.

> On examination the patient is found to have supraclavicular lymphadenopathy and hepatomegaly.

Evidence of weight loss, supraclavicular lymphadenopathy or hepatomegaly may point to an underlying neoplasm. Supraclavicular lymphadenopathy is due to lymphatic spread and hepatomegaly is due to blood borne metastases.

To evaluate the condition an endoscopy is performed to identify a narrowed oesophageal lumen with a shouldered appearance (Fig. 1.1b) and would allow a biopsy to be taken.

Clinical key points in oesophageal reflux

- Ask about heartburn (retrosternal burning pain): this is the commonest symptom and is usually worse lying flat
- Dysphagia (difficulty in swallowing) is an **important** symptom and may indicate the presence of an oesophageal cancer or the development of a benign stricture
- In a case of reflux oesophagitis no abnormal findings will be evident
- Young patients (aged <55) with dyspepsia and no worrying symptoms can be treated symptomatically. Older patients (aged >55) or any patient with worrying symptoms (dysphagia or weight loss) should have an upper gastrointestinal endoscopy

---

Background: oesophagus

The oesophagus is a muscular tube that transports food boluses and fluid down from the pharynx to the stomach, aided by peristalsis. At the lower end of the oeso-

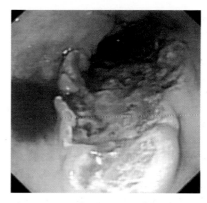

Fig 1.1b Endoscopic view of a carcinoma of the lower oesophagus with rolled edges and an irregular surface.

Clinical key points in oesophageal cancer

- Dysphagia is a worrying complaint

- Ask the patient about weight loss—as the patient eats less they lose weight. Dysphagia and weight loss are the two worrying symptoms, suggestive of malignancy

- Examination of a patient with dysphagia should include checking for supraclavicular lymph nodes

- Upper gastrointestinal endoscopy will establish the diagnosis

---

phagus is the gastro-oesophageal sphincter, which serves to stop gastric acid from going up into the oesophagus. Disorders of the oesophagus relate to problems with the gastro-oesophageal sphincter, leading to gastro-oesophageal reflux, problems with peristalsis, leading to motility disorders, or problems with narrowing of the oesophagus, caused by either benign or malignant strictures.

Conditions:

- reflux, oesophagitis, and hiatus hernia
- motility disorders
- cancer of the oesophagus.

Reflux, oesophagitis, and hiatus hernia

Gastro-oesophageal reflux describes reflux of gastric contents back up to the lower oesophagus. It is a physiologically normal phenomenon especially in the post-prandial period. It occurs in the majority of people and is not pathological. In some individuals, excessive reflux of gastric contents (which may be acid or contain bile) to the lower oesophagus increases the exposure of the lower oesophagus, leading to symptoms which include:

- *heartburn*: a gnawing burning sensation in the retrosternal area

- *regurgitation* of sour acid or green bile into the pharynx or mouth with occasional overspill of these noxious substances on to the bed clothes at night

- *dysphagia*: difficulty in swallowing or a sensation of food sticking

- *chest pain*: a dull or severe pain in the chest, which may radiate up to the jaw and down the arms, imitating cardiac origin pain.

These patients are said to have *gastro-oesophageal reflux disease* (GORD). The majority of symptoms are controlled by antacids. A number of patients continue to experience troublesome symptoms and they are referred for investigations. If over 55 years the investigation of choice in these patients is upper gastrointestinal endoscopy. The complications of gastro-oesophageal reflux include:

- *oesophagitis*: inflammation of the oesophagus, which can be mild or severe. Some patients may have erosions, which may be linear or form an ulcer

- *stricture formation*: stenosis of the lower oesophagus as a result of repetitive peptic injury and fibrous tissue formation in attempts at healing

- *Barrett's metaplasia*: transformation from the normal squamous epithelium to columnar epithelium. Its importance lies in the malignant potential (40 times greater than normal) of this columnar epithelium.

In addition, patients may have a hiatus hernia—this occurs when the hiatal opening is enlarged to allow a portion of the stomach into the chest. There are two types of hiatus hernia: sliding and rolling.

In a sliding hiatus hernia the gastro-oesophageal junction is above the hiatus and in the chest (Fig. 1.1c)—this is the commonest type and is associated with obesity and smoking. In a rolling hiatus hernia the gastro-oesophageal junction is below the hiatus but a portion of the fundus of the stomach is able to slip up into the chest. This type of hernia is potentially more dangerous as the fundal portion can get stuck and become ischaemic.

Treatment of gastro-oesophageal reflux disease

1. *General measures*:

- avoid factors that encourage reflux: such as obesity, tight abdominal garments; reduce reflux

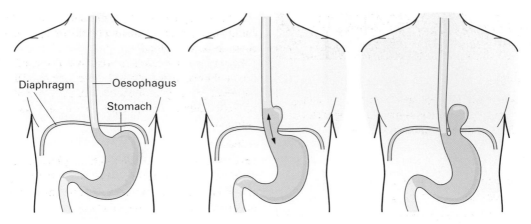

Fig 1.1c Diagram of (a) normal anatomy; (b) sliding hiatus hernia (in which the gastro-oesophageal junction is above the diaphragm and the upper portion of the stomach is abnormally placed in the chest); (c) rolling hiatus hernia (in which the gastro-oesophageal junction is below the diaphragm but the upper portion of the stomach has entered the chest alongside the oesophagus).

by raising the head of the bed, or lying on extra pillows, in order to keep the head above the stomach

- avoid factors that relax the lower oesophageal sphincter: such as coffee, alcohol, smoking, and fat rich food.

2. *Medical treatment.* The following categories of drugs can be given as single agents or in combination depending on the severity of symptoms and complications:

- drugs that neutralize acid; such as antacids with or without alginates, or that suppress acid output H$_2$ receptor blockers, such as ranitidine, or proton pump inhibitors, e.g. omeprazole

- drugs that encourage peristalsis to clear the reflux-ate; such as prokinetic agents, e.g. metoclopramide, domperidone

- mucosal protective agents such as sucralfate or misoprostil.

3. *Surgical treatment.* This is reserved for two categories of patient:

- young patients with severe symptoms who are expected to take maintenance medical therapy for the rest of their life

- patients in whom medical therapy has failed due to lack of compliance, development of side-effects to medication, or poor response to medication.

The surgical procedure has three components: to tighten the hiatus if it is lax; to place the oesophagogastric junction in the abdominal cavity and to strengthen the lower oesophageal sphincter by wrapping part of the gastric fundus around it (fundoplication).

Side-effects of surgery such as dysphagia (due to a tight wrap) and gas bloat (inability to belch due to tightness of wrap) are mainly temporary.

Surgery controls reflux symptoms without untoward side-effects in up to 85% of patients.

Peptic strictures of the oesophagus are treated by a combination of dilatation and long-term acid suppression to prevent recurrence. In young patients, antireflux surgery may be appropriate to prevent recurrence following dilation. In resistant strictures (those that recur after a short period), particularly in young patients, resection of the fibrous lower oesophagus is indicated. The resected segment of oesophagus is replaced by an iso-peristaltic segment of small bowel.

Motility disorders

The oesophagus functions as a muscular tube, which transfers food from the pharynx to the stomach. Abnormalities of the nerves or muscles of the oesophagus give rise to problems in moving a bolus of food and subsequent difficulty in swallowing (dysphagia).

In some patients, swallowing may be accompanied by a painful burning sensation in the retrosternal region. This is called odynophagia. It usually occurs as a consequence of erosive mucosal lesions within the oesophagus such as peptic, viral, or candidal oesophagitis.

Fast facts—Gastro-oesophageal reflux (passage of stomach contents into the oesophagus with resulting inflammation)

Aetiology

- Failure of lower oesophageal sphincter, allowing reflux of gastric contents—predisposing factors: obesity, smoking, alcohol, and coffee

Pathology

- Inflammation in the lower end of the oesophagus (reflux oesophagitis)
- Scarring leading to stricture
- Mucosal metaplastic change (Barrett's oesophagus)—40× greater malignant potential

Clinical features

- Burning retrosternal chest pain
- Regurgitation of acid into the mouth (waterbrash)
- Dysphagia is a WORRYING symptom

Investigations

- Upper GI endoscopy
  —biopsy areas of oesophagitis, metaplasia
  —assesses ulceration
- 24-hour pH monitoring—to assess degree of reflux
- Barium swallow
  —assesses the anatomy of the hiatus
  —assesses oesophageal strictures

Management

- Lose weight, stop cigarettes, alcohol, and coffee
- Antacids for symptomatic relief
- Control acid secretion—H_2 antagonists, proton pump inhibitors
- Protect the oesophagus—alginates
- Antireflux surgery

into the oesophagus, which measures the swallowing contraction pressures created by the oesophageal muscle in response to food.

Primary motility disorders arise as a result of a functional abnormality within the oesophagus. The three common primary oesophageal motility disorders are achalasia, diffuse oesophageal spasm, and 'nutcracker oesophagus'.

Achalasia

This is a disease of unknown aetiology characterized by the absence of peristalsis in the body of the oesophagus and failure of the gastro-oesophageal sphincter to relax normally in response to swallowing.

- *Clinical features*: dysphagia is present in all patients, its intensity varying from day to day. The dysphagia is for both solids and liquids from the beginning of the disease, but is more pronounced for solids. Regurgitation at meal times occurs in most patients but can also happen during sleep. Cramp-like chest pain occurs in some patients during the course of their disease. The majority of patients will lose weight due to the inability to eat comfortably.

- *Radiology*: on barium swallow the body of the oesophagus becomes progressively more dilated (Fig. 1.1d) and tortuous, and food debris accumulates within its lumen.

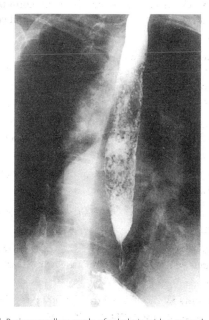

Fig 1.1d Barium swallow study of achalasia with a smooth narrowing of the lower oesophagus and food residue retained in the lower oesophagus.

Patients suspected of having motility disorders in the oesophagus are best investigated by oesophageal manometry. This is performed by passing a fine bore tube

- *Manometry*: the swallowing pressure peaks occur simultaneously throughout the oesophageal body and are uncoordinated.

- *Endoscopy*: the oesophagus is found dilated with food debris and secretions in the lower portion. The endoscope traverses the lower oesophageal sphincter without difficulty.

- *Treatment*:

  - *dilatation* is an effective non-surgical treatment for achalasia. This aims to produce mechanical disruption of the circular muscle fibres at the oesophagogastric junction. The effect of dilatation is usually short lasting and patients often require repeated dilatations.

  - *endoscopic injection* of *Clostridium botulinus* toxin into the muscle fibres of the oesophagogastric junction achieves similar results to dilatation.

  - *surgery* in the form of a cardiomyotomy remains the most effective treatment of achalasia. The operation divides the muscle fibres at the oesophagogastric junction and provides excellent results.

Diffuse oesophageal spasm

This condition occurs less commonly than achalasia.

- *Clinical features*: the hallmark of the disease is chest pain, which can often be intense. The pain may be cramp-like in character, felt in the substernal region, and radiating into the arms and neck like cardiac pain. The pain may occur on eating/drinking or spontaneously. The degree of dysphagia varies considerably and is often precipitated by cold or carbonated drinks. Regurgitation and weight loss are usually absent.

- *Radiology*: on barium swallow the oesophagus may be normal or may show features of tortuosity (so-called 'corkscrew oesophagus'). The range between these extremes can be encountered.

- *Endoscopy*: the oesophagus may be normal or may show evidence of mucosal inflammation or frank ulceration.

- *Manometry*: the oesophagus has not completely lost its peristaltic activity and lower oesophageal sphincter relaxation, but many swallows result in pressure peaks of abnormal amplitude and duration.

- *Treatment*: medical and surgical treatments of diffuse oesophageal spasm are often disappointing. Reassurance about the absence of serious disease (particularly cardiac disease) is essential. Symptomatic relief of pain is important.

Hypertensive peristaltic oesophagus (nutcracker oesophagus)

This is an uncommon condition affecting mainly young females.

- *Clinical features*: patients usually present with non-cardiac chest pain mimicking angina. The pain is usually spontaneous and often wakes the patient at night. Dysphagia is usually absent.

- *Manometry*: the contraction pressure peaks are found to be abnormally high.

- *Treatment*: reassurance about the benign nature of the disease is particularly important when the predominant symptom is angina-like chest pain. Symptomatic analgesia is essential for patients experiencing frequent symptoms. Spontaneous, long-term symptomatic improvements are seen in a number of patients.

Cancer of the oesophagus

Cancer of the oesophagus usually affects people after the sixth decade of life, and is more common in men. The incidence of adenocarcinoma of the lower third of the oesophagus has now overtaken squamous cancer. Squamous cancer is associated with tobacco and alcohol intake, adenocarcinoma with gastro-oesophageal reflux.

- *Cancer of the upper third (cervical) of the oesophagus*. This is usually squamous in type. Because the cervical

TABLE 1.1a	Comparison of oesophageal motility disorders		
	Achalasia	**Diffuse oesophageal spasm**	**Hypertensive peristaltic oesophagus**
Symptoms	Nocturnal vomiting	Cramping chest pain	'Angina-like' chest pain
Dysphagia	Variable dysphagia	Variable dysphagia precipitated by cold drinks	No dysphagia
Imaging	Dilated tortuous oesophagus	Normal to 'corkscrew' oesophagus	No abnormality
Manometry	Simultaneous peak pressures	High amplitude peak pressures	High contraction pressures
Treatment	Dilatation	Reassurance	Reassurance

region is rather limited in volume and connective tissue, the majority of patients with a malignant neoplasm of the oesophagus have locally advanced disease at the time of presentation. The management of these patients is by radiotherapy as their tumour is usually not amenable to surgical resection.

- *Cancer of the middle third of the oesophagus.* This may be squamous or adenocarcinoma; it is rarely resectable and may invade the trachea or bronchi to form a fistula. Surgery is possible in only one-third of patients. Treatment is by stent placement to maintain the lumen or laser to create a lumen, radiotherapy, chemotherapy, or chemoradiotherapy.

- *Cancer of the lower third of the oesophagus.* This is usually adenocarcinoma often associated with Barrett's metaplastic columnar epithelium, which becomes firstly dysplastic then an invasive adenocarcinoma. Treatment options are similar to that of carcinoma of the middle third of the oesophagus.

Diagnosis

Urgent upper gastrointestinal endoscopy and biopsy is indicated in all patients who present with dysphagia. If an ulcerated, polypoidal, or stenotic lesion is present, it must be biopsied to confirm the diagnosis. If endoscopy is not immediately available, then barium swallow (Fig. 1.1e) usually shows features suggestive of malignancy, a shouldered lesion, which must be confirmed by endoscopy and biopsy.

Management

1. *Resectional surgery* is the only chance of a 'cure' in early cancers, provided the tumour is removable, there is no metastatic disease, and the patient is fit and willing to undergo such major surgery. Giving chemotherapy preoperatively (neoadjuvant) may shrink the cancer and improve long-term survival.

   For assessment of operability and metastatic disease, the following must be undertaken:

   - physical examination to assess cervical lymphadenopathy, hepatomegaly, and general health

   - CT scan of chest and abdomen to assess locally advanced disease and metastatic spread to liver and lymph nodes. This may be combined with barium studies to assess the length of a tumour. Generally, tumours more than 5 cm are usually inoperable

   - for upper and middle thoracic oesophageal lesions, a bronchoscopy may determine tracheal involvement, if this is suspected from CT

   - pulmonary function tests, echocardiography, etc. to determine fitness of the patient to undergo the procedure, if there is doubt about these systems

   - endoscopic oesophageal ultrasound to assess tumour invasion and lymph nodes adjacent to the cancer and laparoscopy to look for peritoneal spread.

2. Radical radiotherapy or chemoradiotherapy can be considered if there is a contraindication to surgery. This can offer similar results to surgery in this group of patients.

3. *Palliative measures.* Stent placement, laser recanalization, radiotherapy, and chemoradiotherapy aim to palliate dysphagia. The method of choice should achieve palliation of dysphagia with least complications and minimum hospital stay and will vary from patient to patient.

4. *Stenting.* This involves placing a stent (metal wire or plastic tube) in the oesophagus at the site of the stenotic tumour. It maintains the patency of the oesophageal lumen and improves dysphagia. The stents can be placed endoscopically and in the majority of patients this can be done under sedation.

5. *Laser.* A laser can be used to vaporize a tumour occluding the lumen of the oesophagus. Several treatment episodes may be required to maximize the palliation.

6. *Palliative radiotherapy.* This can be used, targeting the cancer either alone or in combination with stenting or chemotherapy to provide longer lasting palliation.

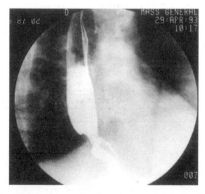

Fig 1.1e Barium swallow study of carcinoma of the oesophagus, showing characteristic 'shoulders' and irregular lumen.

Fast facts—Oesophageal cancer (malignant disease of the oesophagus)

Epidemiology

◆ M/F = 3:1, ↑ incidence with age

Aetiology

◆ Alcohol and cigarettes (squamous)

◆ Chronic oesophagitis and Barrett's oesophagus (adenocarcinoma)

Pathology

◆ Histologically

—40% squamous carcinoma (upper two-thirds)

—60% adenocarcinoma (lower third)

◆ Local, lymphatic and vascular spread

Clinical features

◆ Progressive dysphagia

◆ Weight loss

Investigations

◆ Oesophagoscopy to obtain histology

◆ CT scanning to assess the extent of the cancer and the degree of local spread

Management

◆ Curative resection (applicable in only one-third of patients)

◆ Palliation

—intubation or laser ablation of tumour to allow food to pass

—chemoradiation to slow the growth

Prognosis

◆ 5-year survival with resection 15%, 0% if only palliation possible

Conditions of stomach and duodenum

Scenario 1: acute upper abdominal pain

A 45-year-old man is brought into the A&E department after collapsing at work with sudden onset of severe upper abdominal pain.

ABC Because of the history of collapse remember the ABC—is the Airway patent, is he Breathing, and is the Circulation adequate (see Section 2 on ABC). Having established the airway is not blocked and putting on an oxygen mask to assist breathing (remember—ill patients need oxygen), it is essential that this patient's vital signs (pulse, BP, temperature, respiratory rate) are assessed quickly. Venous access must be established using a wide bore cannula and blood drawn for group and cross-match, baseline FBC, and biochemistry. IV fluid resuscitation should begin while a full assessment of the patient takes place.

On taking a history it is established that the onset of the pain was sudden, severe, and has not diminished since onset.

Key points in this history are the speed of onset of the pain, its severity, site, radiation, and any aggravating or relieving factors. Localized abdominal pain of sudden onset, which rapidly becomes generalized, is the hallmark of a perforated hollow viscus (i.e. oesophagus, stomach, small or large intestine) causing generalized peritonitis.

The pain becomes worse if he moves.

Aggravation of pain by movement is a key feature in patients with peritonitis. This is due to irritation of nerve endings of the parietal peritoneum by the contents of the gastrointestinal tract.

The pain was initially in the epigastrium, rapidly spread across the entire abdomen, and is now felt in both shoulder tips.

The spread of the pain reflects the spread of peritoneal contamination. The site of origin of the pain, in the epigastrium, makes perforation of a duodenal or gastric ulcer the most likely diagnosis. **Shoulder tip pain implies irritation of the peritoneal surface of the diaphragm** by peritoneal fluid and/or the contents of a ruptured viscus.

After the patient receives opiate analgesia a more detailed history is sought. He reports a history of indigestion over many years. These episodes come in 6- to 8-week bouts and then resolve for a time. He regularly takes over-the-counter antacids when he wakes at night with epigastric pain. He is a heavy drinker and smoker.

The major symptom of peptic ulceration is epigastric pain when the patient has not eaten for a while, hence waking at night. The disorder is episodic and is more common in males in their 30s and 40s with a history of heavy drinking and smoking.

> On physical examination the patient is sweating, tachycardic, and hypotensive.

The sweating and tachycardia are initially a result of pain and its autonomic (sympathetic system) sequelae. As the peritonitis develops, tissue fluid seeps into the peritoneal cavity and local tissues in response to the acute inflammation caused by the highly irritant gastrointestinal fluid—it is similar to acid burning a very large surface area in all parts of the abdominal cavity; this results in hypovolaemia and consequent hypotension.

> Examination of the abdomen reveals a rigid abdomen with absent bowel sounds.

Rigidity is caused by reflex tensing of the abdominal wall muscles in response to underlying peritonitis irritating the parietal peritoneum. Frequently there is right iliac fossa peritonism, as the leaked duodenal contents track down the right side of the abdomen.

The absence of bowel sounds is due to the autonomic response to pain leading to the bowel becoming immobile (paralytic ileus).

These features on examination support the diagnosis of a generalized peritonitis. **The key investigation is an erect CXR** (Fig. 1.1f). Look for subdiaphragmatic gas,

present in 70% of patients, which is the hallmark of a ruptured viscus. This is most easily seen under the right diaphragm above the liver on erect chest X-ray with gas. On the left-hand side, gas in the stomach can cause confusion.

> Gas is evident under both hemidiaphragms.

This confirms the suspected diagnosis. Remember it is important to ask for an **erect** CXR as this vital diagnostic sign of gas under the diaphragm may not be visible on a CXR if the patient is lying on his back. **If there is no gas under the diaphragms (30% of cases of perforated upper gastrointestinal tract) then the patient can be given dilute water soluble radiographic contrast.** This will pass out of any hole in the upper gastrointestinal tract into the peritoneal cavity and make the diagnosis.

After perforation of an ulcer is confirmed, the patient is prepared for a laparotomy, and the perforation is closed with a suture.

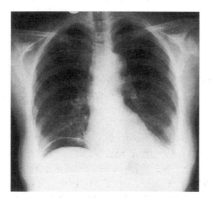

Fig 1.1f Erect chest X-ray showing gas under the right diaphragm (depending on the history and examination) usually associated with a perforated duodenal ulcer (or a normal early post-laparotomy appearance).

Clinical key points in perforated duodenal ulcer

- There is usually a history of sudden onset of localized upper abdominal pain

- Aggravation of pain by movement is a key feature in patients with peritonitis

- Shoulder tip pain implies irritation of the peritoneal surface of the diaphragm by peritoneal fluid

- There may be a history of indigestion or epigastric pain at night, suggesting chronic duodenal ulcer disease

- Examination will reveal upper abdominal peritonism or even rigidity (and frequently right iliac fossa peritonism, as the leaked duodenal contents track down the right side of the abdomen)

- The key initial investigation is an erect CXR, which will reveal subdiaphragmatic gas ('pneumoperitoneum') in 70% of patients. If pneumoperitoneum is not present and the diagnosis is not clear, then a CT scan with oral contrast is useful to confirm the diagnosis

- If the diagnosis is clear, with obvious peritonism, the patient usually proceeds straight to laparotomy

Scenario 2: vomiting and weight loss

> A 64-year-old man is admitted with a 6-month history of intermittent vomiting, and feeling full after small meals (early satiety). Over the past week he has been vomiting undigested food an hour after eating any meal. The vomit does not contain bile (i.e. not green-stained vomit). He has a decreased appetite. He smokes 40/day and has a long history of indigestion, for which he occasionally takes ranitidine (an H_2 antagonist).

This patient's history is quite long (6 months) and is suggestive of a long-standing subacute high intestinal obstruction. The long-standing complaint of **early satiety implies delay in gastric emptying**. This has now progressed to virtual complete gastric outlet obstruction.

Vomiting of undigested food usually means that the stomach is not emptying properly. The fact that there is no bile in the vomit suggests that there may be an obstruction to the outlet of the stomach (i.e. the pylorus), which is above where the bile comes into the duodenum (at the ampulla in the second part of the duodenum).

> On examination he is dehydrated and thin. He also has a succussion splash.

The patient is dehydrated due to his vomiting and he requires fluid resuscitation. U&Es should be checked, paying particular attention to possible low serum potassium (hypokalaemia). He is thin probably due to a degree of malnutrition.

An epigastric mass may be palpable in late presentation gastric cancer. **A succussion splash is elicited by shaking the abdomen and listening over the stomach**, when a splashing liquid noise is heard. This is caused by an accumulation of fluid sloshing around the stomach, which is failing to empty and is a classical sign of gastric outlet obstruction.

> He underwent a gastroscopy and biopsy.

Gastroscopy is the initial diagnostic investigation. This confirmed a large amount of fluid and undigested food debris within the stomach. The gastroscope could not enter the pylorus, which was replaced by a fungating, ulcerated mass. Biopsy confirmed the mass was an adenocarcinoma.

CT scan demonstrated a distal gastric cancer invading local structures, including the pancreas and was therefore unresectable. Other potential causes are pan-

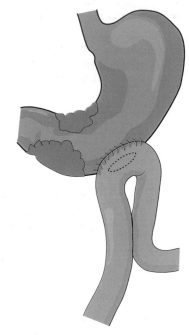

Fig 1.1g Diagram of gastroenterostomy showing a loop of small bowel anastomosed to the stomach to allow gastric contents to 'bypass' a pyloric stenosis).

Clinical key points in gastric outlet obstruction

- Ask about a history of vomiting of undigested food—this usually means that the stomach is not emptying properly—if the obstruction is in or above the first part of the duodenum, then the vomit is NOT bile stained

- The patient may have early satiety (easily feeling full after a meal)

- On examination the patient may be dehydrated due to repeated vomiting

- Examine for an epigastric mass, which may be palpable

- A succussion splash is elicited by shaking the abdomen and listening—there is a noise of fluid sloshing around in a distended stomach (like a hot water bottle)

- It is usually investigated by an upper gastro-intestinal endoscopy and a CT scan of the abdomen (with oral contrast)

creatic cancer or fibrosis secondary to chronic peptic ulceration

> He underwent a gastroenterostomy, with subsequent improvement in his symptoms.

The gastroenterostomy works by allowing the stomach to empty directly into the jejunum, effectively bypassing the obstruction at the pylorus (Fig. 1.1g).

Scenario 3: haematemesis

> A 50-year-old male presents with a history of massive haematemesis (vomiting blood). He collapsed, feeling faint.

Upper gastrointestinal bleeding can present with fresh blood or coffee-ground vomiting (blood that when mixed with the acid gastric contents looks like coffee grounds).

> While on the ward the patient passes a large amount of smelly black stool.

Blood has a marked purgative effect, causing it to pass through the gut rapidly remaining relatively unaltered. It appears as red–black tarry stools (melaena) with a characteristic never to be forgotten odour.

> The patient has chronic back pain and takes frequent regular non-steroidal anti-inflammatory drugs (NSAIDs). There is no past history of peptic ulceration. He is a non-smoker and only drinks at social occasions.

NSAIDs are the commonest cause of haematemesis, followed by chronic peptic ulceration. Smoking is a causative factor for peptic ulceration and alcohol for peptic ulceration and oesophageal varices.

> On examination his pulse is 120/min with a BP of 90/60. There is no lymphadenopathy, hepatomegaly, splenomegaly, or dilated abdominal wall veins.

For the patient to have a hypotension means the normal compensatory methods (vasoconstriction and tachycardia) have been overwhelmed by the amount of blood loss. The patient should be regarded as in established hypovolaemic shock.

If examination had revealed **hepatomegaly or lymphadenopathy then a gastric cancer would have been a distinct possibility**. The presence of **splenomegaly or dilated abdominal veins would have suggested portal hypertension and oesophageal varices**, as a potential cause of the haemorrhage.

ABC with active resuscitation. The patient requires immediate resuscitation with oxygen and IV fluids including blood replacement. Investigation would therefore include a FBC and **cross-matching of 4 units of blood.**

An upper gastrointestinal endoscopy is performed once the patient is stable. The underlying cause of the bleeding can range from:

♦ duodenal (Fig. 1.1h) or gastric ulcer

♦ gastritis, oesophagitis

♦ gastro-oesophageal varices or gastritis, and

♦ gastro-oesophageal cancer.

If a localized cause is identified, such as a bleeding vessel at the base of a duodenal ulcer, or a bleeding oesophageal varix, endoscopic treatment with adrenaline injection or banding, respectively, can be used to halt further blood loss.

Background: stomach and duodenum

The stomach is a muscular reservoir which functions to accommodate ingested food, commence the process of digestion, and deliver churned boluses of food to the duodenum. In addition, the stomach acts as an endocrine organ producing hormones which control the secretion of substances necessary for the digestive process and intrinsic factor for the absorption of vitamin B12 from the distal ileum:

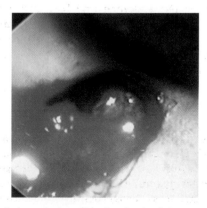

Fig 1.1h Endoscopic view of bleeding duodenal ulcer.

Clinical key points in upper gastrointestinal haemorrhage

- Upper gastrointestinal bleeding usually presents with fresh blood or coffee-ground vomiting. Red–black tarry smelly stools (melaena) are also a feature

- Ask the patient about drug history—e.g. aspirin, NSAIDs, warfarin. Ask about any history of previous indigestion or stomach problems. Check whether they smoke and how much alcohol they consume

- Check the ABCs and begin resuscitation

- Examine the patient for signs of portal hypertension (dilated abdominal wall veins, splenomegaly), in case the cause of the bleeding is oesophageal varices

- The patient requires immediate resuscitation with IV fluids, and blood as required

- Upper gastrointestinal endoscopy is performed once the patient is stable

- the stomach is an expansile reservoir, enabling a person to eat a complete meal without experiencing an uncomfortable sense of fullness

- the stomach mixes ingested food into a suspension, liquefying and mixing the contents with saliva, pepsin and hydrochloric acid

- the stomach and duodenum regulate the entry of nutrients into the upper small bowel and thus promote processing and absorption.

Conditions:

- peptic ulceration
  - duodenal ulceration
  - gastric ulceration
  - gastritis.
- gastric cancer.

Duodenal ulceration

The vast majority (80%) of duodenal ulcers occur in men. Duodenal ulcers are five times more common than gastric ulcers. Aetiological factors in the causation of duodenal ulcers include:

- *Helicobacter pylori* infection—the commonest cause of peptic ulceration.

- Use of NSAIDs, aspirin, and steroids: stopping the use of these agents usually results in healing of the ulcer. If these agents have to be used then the concurrent use of a mucosal protecting agent (such as misoprostil) reduces the incidence and improves the healing rate of NSAID peptic ulcers.

- Smoking.

- Alcohol.

- Zollinger–Ellison syndrome: a rare tumour of the pancreas, which produces a hormone resembling gastrin. This results in excessive secretion of acid, which gives rise to therapy resistant duodenal ulceration.

- Stress: trauma and burns patients develop stress ulcers. These patients are best given sucralfate suspension, as a prophylactic agent to form a barrier between the mucosa and gastric acid.

Helicobacter pylori

H. pylori is the commonest aetiological factor in peptic ulcers and present in 95% of patients with chronic duodenal ulcers. It inhabits the mucous layer which overlies the gastric epithelial cells. The organism is infective and is transmitted by the orofaecal route. It may also be responsible for many gastric ulcers, although the evidence for a causal association is less convincing than it is for duodenal ulcers. It may also be implicated in the pathogenesis of gastric cancer. Diagnosis of *H. pylori* infection is by the following methods:

- *Urease production.* In this test, commonly known the CLO (Campylobacter Like Organism) test, an endoscopic gastric biopsy is placed in a substrate that contains urea with a pH indicator. In the presence of *H. pylori*, ammonia is released, the pH rises and the indicator changes colour from yellow to red. An alternative non-invasive technique uses carbon-labelled urea. This solution is taken by mouth and expired air is collected. *H. pylori*, in the stomach, degrade the urea and labelled carbon dioxide is detected in the breath, hence its name the 'urea breath test'.

- *Serological tests.* *H. pylori* is very antigenic and ELISA (enzyme-linked immunosorbent assay) methods can reliably detect serum antibodies to *H. pylori* with a high degree of accuracy.

In duodenal and gastric ulcers, if *H. pylori* is eradicated, ulcer relapse is unlikely. *H. pylori* eradication regimen is called 'triple therapy', as it uses three drugs: for example omeprazole (a proton pump inhibitor that inhibits acid production), and two antibiotics, usually amoxycillin or clarithromycin with metronidazole, taken for a

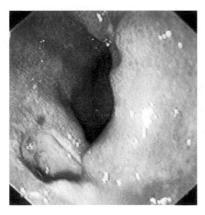

Fig 1.1i Endoscopic view of gastric ulcer (only biopsy will indicate whether it is malignant or not).

week. If the organism is completely eradicated, reinfection rate is very low. The majority of relapses are due to incomplete eradication.

Gastric ulceration

Gastric ulcers can be divided into ulceration of the body of the stomach and ulceration of the antrum (Fig. 1.1i). Antral ulcers behave similarly to duodenal ulcers, and are treated in the same fashion. The aetiological factors for ulceration in the body of the stomach are less clear: a proportion of gastric ulcers is attributable to infection with *H. pylori*, but other aetiological factors, such as mucosal ischaemia and duodenogastric bile reflux, have been implicated.

The complications of gastric ulceration are the same as those for duodenal ulcers: perforation, haemorrhage, and scarring. The other important consideration in the stomach is that chronic inflammation leads to a change in the differentiated state of the cells, leading to intestinal metaplasia, predisposing to dysplasia and subsequent carcinoma.

Complications of peptic ulceration

1. *Ulcer perforation* results in the release of gastroduodenal contents into the peritoneal cavity, leading to peritonitis. Gas may escape through the perforation and accumulate under the diaphragm and can be seen on a CXR taken in the erect posture (see Scenario 1) in about 70% of patients. Management of peptic ulcer perforation is by surgery to suture the perforated ulcer and wash out of the peritoneal cavity. A few patients are not fit to have surgical treatment and may be managed by nasogastric intubation (used to keep the stomach empty), IV fluids,

and antibiotics until the ulcer is healed. If this conservative approach is taken the patient may still need an operation if he deteriorates.

2. *Haemorrhage*. Bleeding gastric and duodenal ulcers are the commonest cause of upper gastrointestinal haemorrhage with a mortality rate of about 10%. Posterior duodenal ulcers and lesser curve gastric ulcers in the body of the stomach can erode into large vessels (such as the gastroduodenal artery behind the duodenum) and result in major, even fatal, haemorrhage. Patients can present with haematemesis (vomiting blood), melaena (dark tarry stool with a characteristic sickly sweet smell), or both. Bleeding does not usually occur at the same time as perforation. Management of these patients consists of the following:

   ◆ ABC *Resuscitation*. In addition to oxygen, restoring the circulating blood volume, should be achieved without delay. The amount of blood loss can be estimated from the patient's history and from continuing losses. More accurately, a central venous catheter and monitoring urine output provides an assessment of blood loss and adequacy of its replacement.

   ◆ *Diagnosis*. Upper gastrointestinal endoscopy is the preferred way of diagnosing the source of upper gastrointestinal haemorrhage. Endoscopy should be carried out at the earliest opportunity, after resuscitation, to identify the site of the bleed.

   ◆ *Haemostasis*. A number of drugs can be used in the acute management of bleeding peptic ulcer.

   ◆ *Acid inhibiting drugs*. H_2 antagonists (e.g. ranitidine) and proton pump inhibitors (e.g. omeprazole).

   There is sufficient evidence that therapeutic endoscopy is associated with significant reduction in further bleeding, requirement for surgery, and death. A number of therapeutic measures can be used, including injection of adrenaline (1:10 000) around the bleeding point. Surgery remains the only option for the patient with continued, life-threatening bleeding which cannot be controlled by endoscopic methods. Surgery should aim at dealing with the eroded vessel in the base of the ulcer by undersewing the vessel.

3. *Stenosis*. This is fibrosis due to chronic ulceration, resulting in narrowing (stenosis) of the affected part. This usually occurs in the pylorus, producing pyloric stenosis. Patients present with recurrent vomiting, which may be projectile. They may have weight loss

Fast facts—Peptic ulcer (break in the epithelial surface of upper gastrointestinal tract caused by gastric secretions)

Epidemiology

- M/F = 4:1, 25–50 years

Aetiology

- *Helicobacter*, alcohol, cigarettes, and NSAIDs

Clinical features (duodenal ulcer/pyloric/antral)

- Epigastric pain
  - —hunger pain, relieved by food
  - —episodic
- Haematemesis
- Vomiting if develops pyloric scarring and stenosis

Clinical features (gastric body)

- Epigastric pain
- Vomiting
- Weight loss

Investigations

- FBC
- Faecal occult blood
- Endoscopy

Management

- Avoid smoking
- Antacids
- Medical
  - —H$_2$ blockers
  - —proton pump inhibitors
  - —triple therapy (for *Helicobacter*)
- Surgery for complications
  - —haematemesis (endoscopic control)
  - —perforation (oversew)
  - —outlet obstruction (gastroenterostomy)

and usually have a succussion splash (due to the stomach being full of fluid, as it fails to empty). They usually have electrolyte abnormalities (metabolic alkalosis and low serum potassium, due to the vomiting of H$^+$/K$^+$) and may be in renal failure due to the recurrent vomiting and dehydration. Pyloric stenosis is treated surgically by pyloroplasty (operating up the pyloric) or bypassed by a gastroenterostomy.

Gastritis

An inflammatory response of the gastric mucosa to injury is very common. The definition and classification is confused mainly because the endoscopic appearances correlate poorly with the histopathological findings. Ideally, the diagnosis and classification of gastritis should be based on histology. Based on histopathology two basic morphologies of gastritis are recognized.

1. *Acute gastritis*. Several conditions may lead to acute damage of the gastric mucosa. These include the following:

   - *stress-related acute gastritis*: this is usually in association with serious injury, sepsis, and hypovolaemic shock. Prophylaxis with acid suppression and/or a mucosal protective agent is indicated.

   - *drug-induced acute gastritis*: aspirin and NSAIDs can cause acute mucosal injury and inflammation. Treatment with acid suppression and/or mucosal protective agents is necessary for some patients.

2. *Chronic gastritis*. This condition is usually progressive until eventually mucosal atrophy develops. Chronic gastritis carries a three- to fourfold increase in the risk of gastric cancer. There are two types:

   - *microbial chronic gastritis*: this is the common variety and is caused by infection with *H. pylori*. Whenever the organism is found in the gastric mucosa, histological gastritis is present. Peptic ulcer disease is also increased 10-fold in the presence of *H. pylori* chronic gastritis.

   - *autoimmune chronic gastritis*: an uncommon form of chronic gastritis and effects up to 10% of individuals. Circulating antibodies to gastric intrinsic factor, and to parietal cells are found in patients with pernicious anaemia. There is a three- to fourfold increase in the risk of gastric cancer in pernicious anaemia.

Gastric cancer

Over the last 100 years gastric cancer has shown a dramatic decrease in incidence probably due to the use of refrigeration rather than pickling or nitrates for food

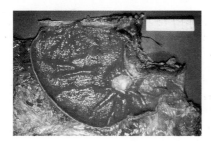

Fig 1.1j Pathological specimen of gastric cancer showing rolled edges and an irregular base.

preservation. There is also evidence that *H. pylori* plays a part in gastric carcinogenesis. Patients with a number of conditions are known to have a higher than average risk of gastric cancer:

◆ *chronic gastritis*: continuing inflammatory damage to the mucosa leads to chronic atrophic gastritis

◆ *gastric polyps (adenomas)*: these occur predominantly in the antrum with a risk of malignant transformation in up to 40% of those adenomas greater than 2 cm in diameter.

Pathology

◆ *Adenocarcinomas*. Approximately 90% of all malignant tumours of the stomach are adenocarcinoma (Fig. 1.1j) . It mainly presents late in its natural history and is the sixth commonest cause of cancer death in the UK.

◆ The majority of the remaining tumours are either malignant lymphomas or stromal tumours.

Management of gastric cancer

Following the endoscopic diagnosis and biopsy of gastric cancer, accurate staging of the disease requires CT and laparoscopy for peritoneal disease.

The best results are obtained by gastric resection. The extent of resection is dictated by the site of the tumour. Proximal tumours are best managed by a total gastrectomy with resection of adjacent lymph nodes. Patients with early adenocarcinoma in which the tumour is limited to the mucosa or submucosa, with no lymph node metastases, have an excellent prognosis with a 95% 5-year survival; however, the overall 5-year survival is 15% due to late presentation.

Two-thirds of gastric cancers are irresectable and are treated by palliation, either by chemotherapy to reduce the disease burden, or surgical bypass (gastroenterostomy) if the cancer is causing gastric outlet obstruction.

Gastrointestinal stromal tumours (GIST). These used to be called leiomyomas and leiomyosarcomas. They are now considered to be derived from undifferentiated stromal fibroblasts and hence have been referred to as stromal tumours. These tumours tend to ulcerate and present with upper gastrointestinal haemorrhage.

Lymphomas. The stomach is the most common site for gastrointestinal lymphomas. The commonest type of lymphoma in the stomach is the B-cell lymphoma of the

Fast facts—Gastric cancer

Epidemiology

◆ M/F = 2:1, ↑ incidence with age

Aetiology

◆ Diet (nitrosamines)

◆ Atrophic gastritis

◆ Previous partial gastrectomy

◆ *Helicobacter* infection

Pathology

◆ Adenocarcinoma

◆ Locally, lymphatic spread

◆ Peritoneal spread

Clinical features

◆ Pain, vomiting

◆ Weight loss

◆ Anaemia

◆ Malignant disease of the stomach

Investigations

◆ FBC

◆ Endoscopy and biopsy

◆ Staging CT scan of abdomen and chest

Management

◆ Curative resection

◆ Palliation by gastroenterostomy, chemotherapy

Prognosis

◆ Overall 5-year survival 15%

Mucosa Associated Lymphoid Tissue (MALTOMA). Up to 90% are associated with *H. pylori* infection. Treatment is by eradication of *H. pylori*, resection, and adjuvant chemotherapy. Generally they have excellent survival rates with 90% 5-year survival rates.

Small bowel

Chapter contents

Scenario 1: acute right lower abdominal pain *17*

Scenario 2: vomiting and abdominal distension *18*

Scenario 3: recurrent abdominal pain *19*

Scenario 4: abdominal pain and weight loss *20*

Background: small bowel *21*

Scenario 1: acute right lower abdominal pain

> A 19-year-old woman is admitted with abdominal pain, which began in the centre of the abdomen but has localized to the right iliac fossa. She has felt unwell with nausea and vomiting for the last 24 hours. Her GP is concerned she might have appendicitis.

This is one of the most frequent indications for urgent admission to a surgical unit. Most patients with appendicitis present like this with a history of periumbilical pain with nausea and vomiting, with the pain shifting to the right iliac fossa.

> Three weeks ago she had an upper respiratory tract infection with a sore throat, there are no gynaecological symptoms, she is sexually active, and her last period 2 weeks ago was normal.

There are numerous causes of abdominal pain, especially in young women, that may cause confusion with appendicitis. A careful history and physical examination are vital. **For women of child-bearing age, pregnancy (excluded by a pregnancy test), and gynaecological conditions need to be considered.**

> She was flushed, had low-grade fever (37.5°C), no tachycardia. Abdominal examination reveals a vague central abdominal tenderness with no other features. Rectal examination is normal, urinary beta-HCG (pregnancy) test is negative, and there is no evidence of a urinary tract infection. A white cell count is normal.

Flushing with a low-grade pyrexia are fairly non-specific. Although she may have an early appendicitis, mesenteric adenitis (inflamed mesenteric lymph nodes) is also a possibility following her recent upper respiratory tract infection. The decision is taken to keep her under observation, regularly recording her vital signs, and a plan made to re-examine her 4 hours later.

> Four hours later she remains febrile but has developed a tachycardia (pulse 110/min) and she says her pain is worse especially when she moves. A repeat abdominal examination shows she is now tender with guarding in the right iliac fossa. She also experiences pain localized to the right iliac fossa with coughing and on gentle percussion.

Clearly the clinical signs have changed. **Tenderness with guarding in the right iliac fossa associated with localized peritonitis (as demonstrated by pain**

Clinical key points in appendicitis

- Most patients with appendicitis present with periumbilical pain with nausea and vomiting, with shifting of the pain to the right iliac fossa

- For women of child-bearing age pregnancy (excluded by a pregnancy test) and gynaecological conditions need to be considered

- On examination the patient may have a flushed appearance, a tachycardia, and a slight pyrexia

- On examination tenderness with guarding in the right iliac fossa associated with localized peritonism (as demonstrated by pain on coughing and percussion) is highly suggestive of appendicitis

- Repeated examination is important to assess deterioration (or improvement) of symptoms and signs

- Plain abdominal X-ray is usually unhelpful

- In females, there may be causes of right iliac fossa pain other than appendicitis (e.g. ruptured or twisted ovarian cyst, ectopic pregnancy, retrograde menstruation, urinary tract infection) — ALL females of child-bearing age should have a pregnancy test (beta-HCG) performed

- Treatment of appendicitis is appendicectomy—all females of child-bearing age should have a laparoscopy initially to rule out other causes of right iliac fossa peritonism

with coughing and on percussion) suggests, but is not diagnostic of, appendicitis. Non-invasive tests, such as ultrasound, or plain abdominal radiology often add little to the diagnosis of abdominal pain in younger patients.

A decision is taken to perform a diagnostic laparoscopy. During laparoscopy the contents of the peritoneal cavity including the gynaecological organs can be inspected. In this case, the examination confirms an acute appendicitis and an appendicectomy is performed. She makes an uneventful recovery.

Scenario 2: vomiting and abdominal distension

> An 82-year-old lady presented with a 2-day history of abdominal pain and distension, brown foul smelling vomiting, and confusion. On examination the abdomen was tympanitic and auscultation revealed high pitched bowel sounds.

Abdominal colic, distension, and vomiting are hallmarks of intestinal obstruction. If the bowel becomes obstructed for whatever reason, then the proximal bowel dilates with gas and intestinal contents, which normally pass through the bowel. This leads to a distended and tympanitic abdomen. High pitched (or obstructive) bowel sounds are caused by active peristalsis in the dilated proximal bowel. **Stagnant, partially digested gut contents result in a brown discoloration and foul-smelling (so-called faeculent) vomiting.**

> Further examination revealed a 3-cm tender swelling in the right groin with surrounding erythema. The swelling was below and lateral to the pubic tubercle.

ALWAYS check for groin hernia or abdominal scars (previous surgery) in patients with small bowel obstruction, as hernia and adhesions are the commonest causes of small bowel obstruction. The pubic tubercle is an important landmark in the identification of groin hernia. If the hernia is below and lateral to the pubic tubercle, then it is a femoral hernia. An inguinal hernia would come out above and medial to the pubic tubercle (Fig. 1.2a). The fact that the hernia is tender and red implies that the small bowel within the hernia is ischaemic.

The patient is given oxygen and a nasogastric tube is passed to decompress the stomach and to avoid further vomiting and potential aspiration of vomit. An IV drip is started as the patient will be dehydrated, due to the

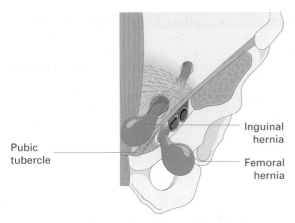

Fig 1.2a Diagram of the anatomy of the inguinal canal and femoral/inguinal hernias.

Pubic tubercle

Inguinal hernia

Femoral hernia

fluid and electrolytes lost within the small bowel and vomiting.

A urinary catheter and central venous line may be required to titrate fluid resuscitation.

A plain abdominal X-ray confirmed small bowel obstruction (Fig. 1.2b).

The key initial investigation in small bowel obstruction is a plain abdominal X-ray (which will reveal dilated loops of small bowel) and an erect CXR (to exclude pneumoperitoneum).

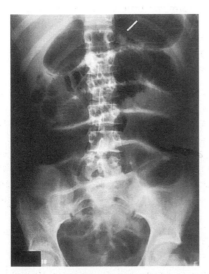

Fig 1.2b Plain abdominal X-ray showing multiple loops of dilated small bowel indicating small bowel obstruction.

Initial treatment was by the insertion of a nasogastric tube and an IV drip, followed by emergency surgery.

As soon as possible after rehydration, the patient is taken to theatre as the potential of ischaemic bowel is a surgical emergency. If the bowel within the hernial sac is ischaemic then that portion of the bowel needs to be resected, and the hernial defect closed. An obstructed femoral hernia is an important cause of small bowel obstruction in the thin elderly female patient.

Clinical key points in small bowel obstruction

- There is usually a history of abdominal colic, abdominal distension, and vomiting. These are hallmarks of intestinal obstruction
- Brown, faeculent vomit is a sign of obstructed, stagnant bowel content
- On examination ALWAYS check for groin hernia or abdominal scars (from previous surgery), as these are the commonest causes of small bowel obstruction
- Erythema around the hernia suggests ischaemia of the underlying bowel in the hernia, and is an indication for urgent surgery
- The key initial investigation in small bowel obstruction is a plain abdominal X-ray (which will reveal dilated loops of small bowel) and an erect CXR (to exclude pneumoperitoneum)

Scenario 3: recurrent abdominal pain

A 38-year-old man presents with an 18-month history of intermittent abdominal pain. He thinks he has lost at least 1 stone in weight and complains that he always feels tired. The pain is mainly in the lower abdomen and colicky in nature. Episodes last 2–3 weeks and are associated with loose stools with excessive mucus and occasionally some red blood. There is a past history of perianal diseases.

Abdominal pain and weight loss point towards a digestive disorder. A full gastrointestinal and dietary history should be obtained.

On examination the patient appears thin, pale, and on abdominal examination there is an ill-defined mass palpable in the right iliac fossa.

Weight loss, long-standing abdominal pain and a mass in the right iliac fossa in a young patient point to Crohn's disease. The history is too long and does not fit with appendicitis. In **an older patient with similar findings a diagnosis of caecal cancer would need to be considered.**

Some patients who develop small intestinal Crohn's disease begin with symptoms of perianal Crohn's disease (recurrent perianal sepsis) earlier in life. In this patient the previous history of perianal sepsis is therefore also of significance. Similarly, **Crohn's disease can rarely present with extraintestinal features (eyes, joints, skin, liver problems).**

His FBC, serum inflammatory markers, and nutritional indices must also be checked. A **barium follow-through X-ray would be the investigation of choice** to examine the distal small bowel (Fig. 1.2c).

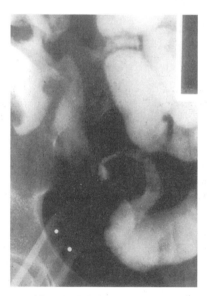

Fig 1.2c Barium follow through showing 'string' sign of Kantor.

The patient is anaemic (Hb 10.8 g/dl) and his C-reactive protein elevated at 85 u/l. The serum albumin is 28 g/dl (normal range 35–48 g/dl). The barium study shows a 10-cm stricture in the terminal ileum associated with ulcers and fissures. The proximal small intestine appears dilated.

The anaemia is due to blood loss from inflamed bowel. The C-reactive protein is an acute phase protein, which is elevated when there is an inflammatory process. These findings are in keeping with active Crohn's disease in the terminal ileum, which is the most frequent site of the disease.

Clinical key points in Crohn's disease

- Weight loss, long-standing abdominal pain, and a mass in the right iliac fossa in a young patient point to Crohn's disease

- It may present acutely with a right iliac fossa inflammatory mass, or with general ill health, anaemia, abdominal pain, and diarrhoea

- It can occasionally present initially with severe perianal disease (perianal sepsis, or anal fistula)

- It can rarely present with extraintestinal features (eyes, joints, skin, liver problems)

- A small bowel barium follow through is the key investigation

- If the patient was elderly, then a caecal cancer is a possibility and a barium enema would be more appropriate

This patient's symptoms initially respond to treatment with high-dose steroids but his symptoms could not be controlled on a maintenance dose. He eventually required a limited right hemicolectomy, including the terminal ileum, to resect the diseased segment of intestine.

Scenario 4: abdominal pain and weight loss

A 72-year-old female smoker with peripheral arterial disease presents with an 8-month history of periumbilical pain after eating and weight loss of 2 stones.

Always think about mesenteric ischaemia in a patient with other manifestations of occlusive arterial disease (e.g. intermittent claudication) with abdominal pain. In mesenteric ischaemia the blood supply to the small intestine is impaired. After eating, the bowel needs more blood to digest the food; however, as the vessels are narrowed the bowel does not get sufficient blood and becomes ischaemic leading to pain—so-called abdominal angina.

On examination the patient is thin, but there is no abdominal tenderness. An abdominal bruit is heard over the umbilicus.

The patient has been having symptoms for 8 months and in that time the food in the bowel has not been properly absorbed due to the ischaemia, with resultant weight loss. **The abdominal bruit is caused by the irregular flow of the blood through a narrowed vessel.**

The patient undergoes a mesenteric angiogram.

The appropriate investigation would be a mesenteric angiogram. Using a fine bore catheter inserted into the femoral artery and positioned at the origin of the coeliac, superior and inferior mesenteric arteries, a mesenteric angiogram injects dye into the blood vessels of the gut. In this patient the superior and inferior mesenteric arteries are blocked ('occluded'). As the blood supply of the gut is normally very good, it usually requires two of the three arteries to be blocked before symptoms arise, as collateral vessels usually open up to help the blood flow to the gut. A single stenosis may be suitable for dilation via the angiogram catheter.

The patient is nutritionally fed by a central line and then undergoes a laparotomy.

The patient's condition is optimized by feeding her via a central vein for a while to improve her nutritional status. At operation the small bowel is noted to be slightly purple rather than the normal pink but viable. The patient undergoes a 'bypass' of the blocked superior mesenteric artery, and at the end of the operation, the bowel is noted to be pink. No bowel required resection as the bowel was viable. She was put on warfarin anticoagulation after the operation, so that the 'bypass' does not occlude.

An arterial embolus can also lodge in the visceral arteries causing sudden bowel ischaemia. This is usually severe and is often diagnosed too late to save the patient. Any patient with an irregular pulse and abdominal pain (classically described as out of proportion to the physical findings) should raise the possibility of gut infarction secondary to a mesenteric embolus. A high white cell count (>15) and high amylase (>300) and acidosis support the clinical diagnosis of acute intestinal ischaemia.

Background: small bowel

The small bowel lies between the stomach/duodenum and the colon. Its purpose is to digest and absorb the majority of the nutrients within food. To enable this to occur, pancreatic enzymes and bile salts are added to the small bowel from the pancreas and liver.

Conditions:

- appendicitis (dealt with here, although comes off the caecum!)
- small bowel obstruction
- Crohn's disease
- mesenteric ischaemia
- malabsorption.

Appendicitis

Acute appendicitis is one of the most common surgical emergencies. Appendicitis is rare in infants but becomes increasingly frequent in childhood and reaches a peak incidence in young adults declining through the older age groups. The appendix is a diverticulum that arises from the caecum close to the ileocaecal valve. Usually the appendix lies alongside the caecum but it can also hang down into the pelvis, or lie behind the caecum or between the loops of small intestine. It is these anatomical variations that are responsible for some of the unusual clinical presentations of acute appendicitis, which can lead to a delay in diagnosis.

Pathophysiology

Most episodes of acute appendicitis are caused by obstruction of the appendix lumen either by faecoliths, intestinal worms or parasites, or by lymphoid hyperplasia in the wall of the appendix. Secretions build up behind the obstruction, become infected, and the appendix swells as the inflammation spreads from the mucosa, through the muscular wall of the appendix to the serosa.

Untreated, the appendix will become gangrenous as the venous drainage then arterial blood supply are cut off in turn by the swollen appendix. Eventually a gangrenous appendix will burst releasing pus and bacteria into the peritoneal cavity causing peritonitis.

Clinical features

The earliest symptoms and signs of acute appendicitis are often quite variable and vague. Patients may complain of any combination of nausea, vomiting, loss of appetite, or central abdominal discomfort. As the inflammatory process progresses and the inflamed serosa of the appendix irritates the overlying parietal peritoneum,

---

Clinical key points in mesenteric ischaemia

- Always think of mesenteric ischaemia in patients with peripheral vascular disease, postprandial pain, and weight loss
- Examine the patient for signs of weight loss; examine for all the peripheral pulses and listen to the abdomen for an abdominal bruit
- A mesenteric angiogram is the key diagnostic investigation

the pain moves (localizes) to the right iliac fossa. By this stage many patients complain that the pain is aggravated by movement (walking, or coughing) and physical examination will reveal maximal tenderness in the right iliac fossa and percussive (rather than rebound) tenderness, which is **best elicited by gentle percussion**.

Some patients will show non-specific signs of sepsis—flushing, low-grade fever (less than 38°C), or a tachycardia.

Three of four patients with acute appendicitis will fit this clinical picture. However, it is important to realize that the absence of these symptoms and signs does not rule out the diagnosis of acute appendicitis:

- if the appendix is retrocaecal, the caecum will cushion the appendix from the examiner's hand and will reduce abdominal tenderness

- when the appendix lies in the pelvis there may be no abdominal tenderness and the diagnosis will only be suspected after a rectal examination elicits tenderness

- in those patients with an anatomically 'high' caecum, tenderness may be maximal in the loin and the diagnosis will be confused with a pyelonephritis.

The diagnosis is especially difficult in four groups of patients:

1. in young women where acute gynaecological pathology is mistaken for acute appendicitis

2. the very young, who cannot give a history

3. the elderly, in whom other pathologies may be more likely

4. during pregnancy where the enlarging uterus may confuse the diagnosis.

If the initial symptoms are overlooked, patients can present with signs of generalized peritonitis after the appendix has ruptured, or with a mass in the right iliac fossa, caused by the adjacent intestines and omentum wrapping around the appendix and walling off the inflammatory process from the rest of the peritoneal cavity—called an appendix mass.

The key on examining the patient is to decide whether there is peritonism or not—this is best done by asking the patient to cough (which irritates the inflamed peritoneum in the right iliac fossa), and by gentle percussion over the right iliac fossa. If both of these tests reveal pain in the right iliac fossa, then the patient probably has peritonism and usually requires an operation.

Laboratory tests and investigations have little role to play in making the diagnosis. Many patients will have a raised white cell count (leucocytosis), but a normal white cell count does not rule out appendicitis. In addition a plain abdominal X-ray or ultrasound is generally unhelpful.

Treatment

The treatment of acute appendicitis is surgical removal of the appendix (appendicectomy) either through an open wound in the right iliac fossa (grid-iron incision) or by laparoscopic 'keyhole' surgical techniques.

Fast facts—Acute appendicitis (acute inflammation of the vermiform appendix)

Epidemiology

- Commonest surgical emergency, usually in second and third decades; rare under 2 years

Pathology

- Luminal obstruction with super-added infection

Clinical features

- Initially periumbilical pain
- Shifts and localizes to right iliac fossa
- Right iliac fossa peritonism
- Possible appendix mass

Investigations

- WCC
- Laparoscopy (in females of child-bearing age)

Differential diagnosis

- Mesenteric lymphadenitis
- Gynaecological conditions
- Urinary tract infection
- Non-specific abdominal pain

Management

- Appendicectomy
- If appendix mass, IV fluids/antibiotics

  —if settles, delayed appendicectomy (after 6–8 weeks)

  —if not appendicectomy

When there is doubt about the diagnosis after a period of observation, many surgeons will undertake a diagnostic laparoscopy as a first step, proceeding to appendicectomy if the diagnosis is confirmed. A preliminary laparoscopy is especially helpful in young women who may have acute gynaecological pathology, such as a ruptured ovarian cyst or inflammation of the fallopian tube (salpingitis), and reduces the number of times that a normal appendix is removed.

Outcome

Wound infection is the most frequent specific complication following appendicectomy. Mortality rates are low (less than 1 in 1000), but deaths still occur usually in patients at the extremes of life because the diagnosis has been delayed and the appendix perforates.

> All women of child-bearing age with right iliac fossa peritonism should have a diagnostic laparoscopy carried out to check for a gynaecological cause for their symptoms, as well as to check the appendix.

Small bowel obstruction

A simple mechanical obstruction of the small intestine causes progressive distension of the bowel above the point of obstruction, as a result of accumulation of gastrointestinal secretions, swallowed air, food, and fluids. This distension leads to fluid build-up and subsequent vomiting. Loss of electrolyte-rich fluids in the vomit causes dehydration and electrolyte imbalance. As the small intestine is about 12 feet long, the clinical picture in patients with small bowel obstruction will vary depending on the distance of the obstruction from the duodeno-jejunal flexure.

The most common causes of small bowel obstruction are:

* adhesions (postoperative or congenital)
* irreducible hernias, e.g. femoral, inguinal (Fig. 1.2d) or incisional hernia

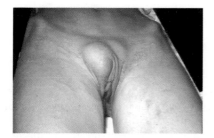

Fig 1.2d Clinical photograph of an irreducible inguinal hernia.

* a carcinoma of the caecum that obstructs the ileo-caecal valve.

Clinical features

Repeated episodes of small intestinal colic (a central abdominal pain that builds up to a crescendo and then subsides) are the hallmark of small bowel obstruction. Other clinical features will vary depending on the level of the obstruction:

* A proximal small bowel obstruction is characterized by profuse vomiting caused by obstruction to the flow of saliva, gastric, pancreatic, and biliary secretions. These patients rapidly become dehydrated and lose large amounts of sodium, chloride, and potassium in the vomit. Often, such patients are remarkably pain free.

* A distal small bowel obstruction is characterized by abdominal distension (caused by large amounts of swallowed air and gastrointestinal secretions trapped in the obstructed intestine), severe colicky abdominal pain, and vomiting. Electrolyte disturbances and vomiting are less marked compared with proximal small bowel obstruction.

Unlike large bowel obstruction, constipation is not a feature of small bowel obstruction. Most patients will show signs of dehydration (reduced skin turgor, dry tongue, etc.). The abdomen may be distended and tympanitic with tinkling (obstructed) bowel sounds on auscultation. In a proximal obstruction, the distension will be less and sometimes the bowel sounds will be normal. It is important to search for clues as to the cause of the obstruction.

In a patient with small bowel obstruction, it is important to look for abdominal scars (pointing to adhesions as a potential cause) and inspect the groins for either an inguinal or femoral hernia as a cause of the obstruction.

Strangulation is a life-threatening complication of small bowel obstruction and is caused by interruption of the blood supply to the obstructed intestine. It is more common in:

* *an irreducible groin hernia*: where the tight neck of the hernia obstructs the blood flow to the trapped intestine
* *a closed loop obstruction*: where a single loop of bowel becomes obstructed between two fixed points and rapidly distends

It is vital to detect signs of strangulation as these patients require urgent surgery. Strangulation should be suspected in any obstructed patient with:

* fever, tachycardia, leucocytosis

◆ localized abdominal tenderness

◆ colicky abdominal pain, which becomes constant.

Management

Baseline blood tests are important. A leucocytosis raises suspicion of strangulation and the blood urea, creatinine, and electrolytes on admission are a guide to the fluid resuscitation that is required. A plain abdominal X-ray will usually clinch the diagnosis (Fig. 1.2b). Centrally placed loops of distended small intestine are characteristic, with the mucosal folds extending right across the bowel (called the plicae circulares or valvulae coniventes), showing the typical 'step ladder' or 'stacked coin' appearance. All patients require rehydration and correction of any electrolyte imbalance as the first step. Thereafter, the management depends upon the cause of the obstruction:

◆ urgent surgery after resuscitation is indicated in patients with suspected strangulation or obstructed hernia

◆ if adhesive obstruction is the most likely diagnosis then a period of conservative management is appropriate, as approximately one-half of all episodes of adhesive obstruction will resolve without operation.

The key steps of conservation management are:

◆ stop all oral intake

◆ insert a nasogastric tube and apply nasogastric suction, to deflate the distended bowel

◆ give IV fluids

◆ correct any fluid or electrolyte imbalance.

Any small bowel obstruction that persists after 24–48 hours conservative management usually requires surgery.

Operative treatment will vary depending upon the cause of the small bowel obstruction. Adhesive bands can be simply divided (called division of adhesions or adhesiolysis); bowel trapped in a hernia can be freed and the hernia repaired; a caecal cancer causing a small bowel obstruction can be resected (a right hemicolectomy). If the bowel is strangulated relieving the obstruction, if carried out in time, may restore the blood supply to the intestine. In neglected cases, where the bowel has infarcted and died, it is necessary to resect the strangulated segment of intestine.

Outcome

Outcome is excellent after surgery for simple mechanical small bowel obstruction. If strangulation develops 1 in 10 patients will die as a result.

Fast facts—Small bowel obstruction (blockage of the small bowel)

Causes

◆ Adhesions from previous surgery

◆ Hernias (inguinal, femoral, umbilical, incisional most common)

◆ Caecal cancer obstructing the bowel

Clinical features

◆ Vomiting with abdominal distension and constipation

Examination

◆ Distended, tympanitic abdomen with high pitched bowel sounds

◆ Check for abdominal scars, groin hernias

◆ Look for evidence of bowel strangulation (erythema around hernia, severe constant pain)

Investigations

◆ Check urea and electrolytes (? dehydration)

◆ Check FBC (if WCC↑, ? bowel strangulated)

◆ Plain abdominal X-ray/erect CXR

Management

◆ IV fluids ('drip')

◆ Nasogastric tube ('suck'—to decompress the bowel)

◆ Treat conservatively (i.e. 'drip & suck') for 24–48 hours if adhesions likely and no signs of strangulation

◆ Laparotomy for possible strangulated bowel, and repair of irreducible obstructed hernias

◆ Excision of non-viable bowel (infarcted) if present

◆ Excision of right colon (right hemicolectomy) if caused by caecal cancer

---

Crohn's disease

Crohn's disease is a chronic inflammatory disease that can affect anywhere along the gastrointestinal tract from the mouth to the anus. It is most common in patients aged 20–50 years. The small intestine is affected in over one-half of all patients with Crohn's disease and the terminal ileum is the most frequently affected segment of small intestine. Other common sites are the perineum where Crohn's disease may present with perianal abscesses, fissures, and fistulae, and the large intestine. Perianal and large intestine Crohn's often coexist with small bowel Crohn's disease. The cause of Crohn's disease remains unknown.

The key pathological and histological features of Crohn's disease are:

- inflammatory changes involving the full thickness of the bowel wall—in contrast to ulcerative colitis, which is characterized by inflammatory changes only in the mucosa and submucosa

- deep fissures that spread from the mucosa and penetrate the bowel wall—these arise as a result of the full thickness inflammation

- non-caseating granulomas in the bowel wall or adjacent lymph nodes.

Affected loops of small bowel are rigid and thick walled. The attached mesentery appears to extend over the serosal surface of the intestine (fat encroachment). Repeated bouts of inflammation lead to scarring and healing by fibrosis, which can narrow (stricture) the lumen of the small bowel and cause obstructive symptoms. **Fistulae (an abnormal communication between two epithelial surfaces, e.g. small bowel to skin (entero-cutaneous), colon to bladder (colo-vesical))** between adjacent bowel loops or interloop abscesses are caused by fissures that extend through the full thickness of the bowel wall.

If the lining of the intestine is examined it has a 'cobblestone' appearance caused by multiple fissures and aphthous ulcers separated by oedematous folds of normal mucosa. 'Skip' lesions—diseased segments of intestine, separated by apparently normal small intestine—are another characteristic of Crohn's disease. All of these pathological changes interfere with the function of the small intestine causing failure of the absorptive function and/or chronic mechanical obstruction.

Clinical features

Crohn's disease should be suspected in any patient with a history of **recurrent colicky abdominal pains and diarrhoea**. Vomiting is uncommon. The abdominal pain is caused by exaggerated peristalsis as a result of chronic obstruction of the diseased intestine.

Diarrhoea in Crohn's disease is principally the result of failure of the absorptive function of the small intestine. Anaemia and weight loss caused by malnutrition will develop if the disease continues untreated.

Occasionally, small bowel Crohn's disease will present acutely and mimics acute appendicitis.

Early on in the disease abdominal examination can be normal. The perineum should always be inspected as evidence of perianal disease might be the first clue to the diagnosis. As the disease progresses, thickened, tender loops of intestine can be felt in the right iliac fossa or a Crohn's mass may be evident in patients who develop a fistula or abscess between adjacent loops of bowel.

Diagnosis

A **barium follow through is the key diagnostic test** in small bowel Crohn's disease. The distinctive features are segments of thickened bowel wall with a luminal stricture ('string' sign of Kantor) (Fig. 1.2c), and 'rose thorn' fissures. These patients are usually anaemic and have elevated inflammatory markers (C-reactive protein, plasma viscosity). Patients with colonic Crohn's may be investigated with either **barium enema or colonoscopy** with biopsies.

Complications

The main complications of Crohn's disease are:

- stricture formation, leading to intestinal obstruction and fistula formation

- fistula formation: fistulae commonly occur between bowel loops, between bowel and bladder or vagina, and between bowel and the anterior abdominal wall

- toxic dilatation of the colon, similar to ulcerative colitis (see large bowel conditions)

- bleeding, caused by a large raw inflamed area of bowel

- malignant change in the colon

- extraintestinal manifestations: such as erythema nodosum, ankylosing spondylitis, sclerosing cholangitis.

(Table outlining the key elements of Crohn's disease and ulcerative colitis can be found at the end of sections on p. 26 and p. 41.)

Treatment

The natural history of Crohn's disease is of spontaneous relapses and remissions (getting worse and better by itself). This makes evaluation of any therapy difficult. Usually, the first line treatment is medical with surgery kept in reserve for the management of complications.

1. *Medical therapy.* Steroids and/or immunosuppressive drugs form the backbone of medical treatment. Nutritional support will also be necessary in some

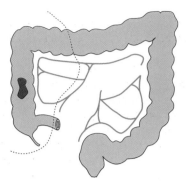

Fig 1.2e Diagram of a right hemicolectomy.

malnourished patients but is unlikely to influence the course of the disease.

♦ **Prednisolone is the most commonly used steroid drug**. Intermittent courses of high doses (usually 40 mg/day) are used alone or in combination with other medications. Newer preparations of oral steroids are being developed to limit systemic absorption of the drug and thus prevent unwanted steroid side-effects such as osteoporosis and weight gain. Avoiding these side-effects is especially important in patients with Crohn's disease because they may require long-term treatment. Azathioprine and cyclosporin (immunosuppressant drugs) are sometimes used alongside steroids to help suppress the chronic inflammatory reaction associated with Crohn's disease. Other drugs such as metronidazole (an antibiotic) or the sulphasalazines are less effective in small bowel Crohn's disease and are used mainly in perianal or colonic Crohn's disease.

2. *Surgery*. **Obstruction, perforation, abscess, and fistula** are the main indications for surgery in Crohn's disease and are often difficult operations. Usually the terminal ileum/caecum are affected and a conservative resection of these areas (a limited right hemicolectomy (Fig. 1.2e)) is required.

Outcome

Three of four patients with small bowel Crohn's disease will need surgery at some point during their lives. Many require two to three operations over a lifetime with the disease. Patients with Crohn's disease are twice as likely to die prematurely, compared with an age-matched population because of the disease.

Fast facts—Crohn's disease (a transmural inflammation of the gut)

Epidemiology

♦ M/F 1:6, young adults

Pathology

♦ Can affect anywhere from mouth to anus, but most commonly terminal ileum and anus
♦ Inflammatory changes involving the full thickness of the bowel
♦ Non-caseating granulomas in the bowel wall or adjacent lymph nodes
♦ Deep fissures that spread from the mucosa and penetrate the bowel wall

Clinical features

♦ Recurrent abdominal colic and diarrhoea
♦ Anaemia/weight loss
♦ Perianal sepsis

Investigations

♦ FBC/C-reactive protein/albumin
♦ Plain abdominal X-ray/?obstruction
♦ Barium follow through
♦ CT for intra-abdominal abscesses

Management

♦ Oral steroids
♦ 5-amino salicylic acid, e.g. mesalazine
♦ Metronidazole—for small bowel Crohn's and perianal sepsis
♦ Azathioprine—an anti-inflammatory drug
♦ Surgery for the complications of Crohn's—most common is resection of terminal ileum and caecum (right hemicolectomy)

Complications

♦ Malnutrition
♦ Obstruction
♦ Abscess and fistula
♦ Colonic cancer

Mesenteric ischaemia

Mesenteric ischaemia or infarction develops when the blood supply to the small or large intestine (or rarely, the stomach) is interrupted.

The initial damage is seen in the submucosa and mucosa where a haemorrhagic infarction occurs leading to sloughing of the intestinal mucosa and bleeding into the intestinal lumen. At this stage the damage is reversible and the mucosa will regenerate if the blood supply is restored. If ischaemia persists, the full thickness of the bowel wall becomes ischaemic and perforation will eventually occur causing a potentially fatal peritonitis.

The main sources of blood to the stomach and intestines are the **coeliac artery** (the artery to the foregut supplying the stomach, duodenum, pancreas, and liver), the **superior mesenteric artery** (the artery to the midgut supplying the small intestine, appendix, and large intestine as far as the transverse colon), and the **inferior mesenteric artery** (the artery to the hind gut, supplying blood to the remaining colon and upper rectum) (Fig. 1.2f). An extensive network of collateral blood vessels link these three major arteries and blood flow through them will almost always sustain the intestine when there is a gradual occlusion of one or two of the major vessels.

The severity of the vascular insult to the intestine depends on the site and extent of the vascular occlusion and its speed of onset. Atheromatous narrowing of one or more vessels may go unrecognized because of the collateral circulation until a critical point is reached or thrombosis develops within the atheromatous vessel. In contrast, a mesenteric embolus is usually a catastrophic event that precipitates a surgical emergency because there is no time for a collateral circulation to develop.

Ischaemia implies a reversible vascular injury, but once infarction develops, the damage is permanent. Although all three major arteries to the gut can be affected most surgical emergencies arise as a result of an acute vascular event affecting the superior mesenteric artery.

Clinical features

Mesenteric ischaemia is one of many causes of an acute abdomen. A superior mesenteric artery embolus is characterized by a sudden onset of severe abdominal pain, vomiting, diarrhoea, and cardiovascular collapse. Almost always the patient is an arteriopath with evidence of cardiac or peripheral vascular disease. They may have a source of an embolus—e.g. atrial fibrillation, when a mural thrombus may form in the left ventricle. Often these patients are so ill that the diagnosis is only made at laparotomy, which is undertaken after a period of vigorous fluid resuscitation.

A mesenteric thrombosis is often preceded by weight loss (through failure of the intestine to absorb nutrients). Patients often complain of severe postprandial pain (called abdominal angina). This is caused by failure of the intestinal blood supply to meet demand during digestion. Eventually, these patients present with increasingly severe abdominal pain, vomiting, and bloody diarrhoea. They may also have an abdominal bruit (caused by irregular flow of blood through the narrowed vessel).

Investigation

When the diagnosis is suspected a **mesenteric angiogram is the key diagnostic test** (Fig. 1.2g) and will demonstrate occlusion or narrowing of one or more of the major mesenteric vessels.

Treatment

The goals of treatment are to restore the blood supply to the intestine and to excise surgically (resect) any

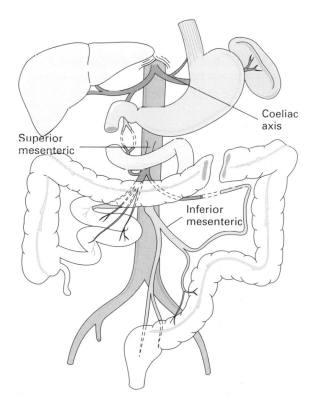

Fig 1.2f Diagram of blood supply to gut.

Coeliac axis

Superior mesenteric

Inferior mesenteric

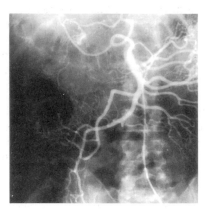

Fig 1.2g A mesenteric angiogram of the superior mesenteric artery with its cascades of vessels supplying the small and proximal large bowel.

infarcted (gangrenous) intestine. Sometimes removal of an occluding arterial embolus (embolectomy) is possible. In other patients with arterial thrombosis, blood may have to be routed from the aorta to a point beyond the thrombosed segment of the vessel using a vascular graft (aortomesenteric bypass).

Infarcted segments of intestine have to be excised, but sometimes, after restoring the blood supply to a segment of ischaemic intestine it can be difficult to decide if the bowel will remain viable. In these patients a 'second look' laparotomy is performed 24 hours later to check whether or not a further segment of intestine needs to be resected.

Prognosis

Despite the treatment options, the outlook is extremely poor for these patients and only one in four will survive. Frequently, by the time these patients undergo surgery there is massive small intestinal infarction stretching from the duodenal flexure to the caecum and little can be done.

The best results are obtained in patients who present with abdominal angina and weight loss who undergo mesenteric bypass surgery before they develop a small bowel infarction.

Malabsorption

Proteins, fats, and complex carbohydrates are broken down into absorbable units mainly in the small intestine. The overall digestive process begins in the stomach and duodenum and depends on gastric, biliary, and pancreatic secretions being delivered in the appropri-

---

Fast facts—Mesenteric ischaemia (poor blood supply to the gut)

Anatomy: 3 Arteries

- Foregut—coeliac artery (stomach to duodenum)
- Midgut—superior mesenteric artery: duodenum to transverse colon
- Hindgut—inferior mesenteric artery: transverse colon to rectum

Causes of ischaemia

- Thrombus gradually occluding the vessel— usually need occlusion of two main arteries before develop symptoms of ischaemia
- Embolus (usually to superior mesenteric artery) —of sudden onset and catastrophic
- Ischaemia can be reversible, but if irreversible leads to bowel infarction

Clinical features

- Thrombus—history of abdominal colic after food, and weight loss; may have abdominal bruit; usually have peripheral vascular disease as well
- Embolus—sudden onset of severe abdominal pain; may have atrial fibrillation (leading to left ventricular thrombus)

Investigation

- Mesenteric angiogram

Management

- Oxygen
- Fluid resuscitation
- Laparotomy—either bypass of occluded mesenteric vessel or embolectomy. Excision of non-viable bowel
- Occasionally small bowel non-viable from duodenum to colon and the patient is dying— keep comfortable

Prognosis

- Poor

ate amount and in the correct sequence to the intestinal tract. In the intact gastrointestinal tract, a variety of neural and endocrine pathways control this activity.

Malabsorption, failure of this absorptive pathway, can be caused by disease or as a result of a surgical operation, which interferes with this digestive process.

Stomach

Most malabsorptive syndromes related to the stomach are the result of gastric surgery either for malignancy or less often for ulcer disease. Generally, symptoms are worse following total gastrectomy than after a partial gastrectomy and depend on the technique used to restore gastrointestinal continuity after all or part of the stomach is removed.

Often there is a lack of storage capacity for ingested food and inadequate mixing of food and enzymes in the stomach remnant. In all these patients gastric emptying is no longer regulated by neural and hormonal pathways and food is dumped into the proximal small intestine or duodenum out of sequence with biliary and pancreatic secretion. As a result, patients may become malnourished because of inadequate carbohydrate, fat, and protein absorption. Iron and B12 absorption will also be affected because of the loss of gastric acid and intrinsic factor production resulting in anaemia.

Although surgery for peptic ulcer disease has been supplanted by H_2 antagonist drugs and proton pump inhibitors there are still many patients who have undergone truncal vagotomy plus a gastric drainage procedure as primary treatment for this condition. The vagus nerve in addition to stimulating gastric acid production has a regulatory function in small bowel motility. Some of these patients will develop severe diarrhoea, caused by rapid small bowel transit, which with the unregulated gastric emptying will contribute to malabsorption.

Hepatobiliary system

Bile emulsifies fat, an essential step in its absorption. Failure to produce bile (as a consequence of hepatocellular disease) or failure to deliver bile to the small intestine (e.g. by mechanical obstruction of the common bile duct causing obstructive jaundice) will reduce absorption of fat and the fat soluble vitamins A, D, E, K, and calcium. Many of these patients will be jaundiced and the failure of fat absorption will cause steatorrhoea.

Pancreas

Pancreatic insufficiency is usually an end result of chronic pancreatitis or major surgical resection of the pancreas gland for cancer. The exocrine function of the pancreas is to secrete digestive enzymes (trypsin and chymotrypsin, amylase and lipase), which play a major role in protein, carbohydrate, and fat digestion. These patients usually present with severe weight loss and steatorrhoea caused by failure of fat absorption.

Small intestine

Absorption of the products of nutrition occurs mainly in the small intestine. Small bowel Crohn's disease, or surgical resection of the small intestine, are the main causes of absorptive failure.

Up to 50% of the small intestine can be removed before malabsorption becomes a problem. With adequate nutritional support some patients with as little as 40 cm of small intestine will survive. Patients with less small intestine than this will require long-term home parenteral nutrition in order to survive.

The most critical segment of the small intestine is the terminal ileum, which is the site of vitamin B12 and bile salt absorption. This section of the intestine along with the ileocaecal valve may be removed in patients with Crohn's disease. These patients will become B12 deficient causing a megaloblastic anaemia. A few will develop steatorrhoea because of depletion of the bile salt pool affecting fat absorption especially in those patients with Crohn's disease who have had large segments of terminal ileum resected.

Large intestine

In health, the colon absorbs water. Removal of the entire large intestine in patients with inflammatory bowel disease is well tolerated with adaptive changes in the small intestine to compensate for the change in water balance.

Patients with acute inflammatory bowel disease affecting the entire colon may lose large amounts of water, electrolytes, and nutrients from the inflamed colon and if the disease continues untreated, they become dehydrated and malnourished.

Clinical features

Taking a careful case history is essential. Diarrhoea, steatorrhoea, weight loss, and symptoms of anaemia are the most common features of malabsorption. These may be superimposed on the background symptoms of the disease responsible for the malabsorption, for example Crohn's or pancreatic disease or there may be a history of previous gastric, intestinal, or pancreatic surgery.

A baseline nutritional assessment of the patient should include anthropomorphic measurements (weight, height, fat, and muscle indices) along with haematological tests (FBC, serum B12, folate levels, and serum ferritin), and liver function tests.

Treatment

The management of these patients can be complex and is best achieved with a multidisciplinary nutrition team with input from surgeons, physicians, and nutritionists. The treatment for most of these patients is based on adequate nutritional support either by dietary modification, or oral nutrition supplements to maintain an adequate caloric and nitrogen intake. Vitamin and calcium supplements are given as required. Whenever possible the enteral route is used either by direct oral supplementation or by overnight nasogastric feeding regimens. In patients with pancreatic disease oral pancreatic enzyme supplements will improve absorption.

If these methods fail then parenteral nutrition is used. This requires central venous access. This technique, called total parenteral nutrition (TPN), can be used to deliver all a patient's nutritional requirements. Once patients are trained to care for these catheters themselves nutritional support can be continued at home.

The role of surgery is to treat any underlying disease process, for example resection of Crohn's disease or relief of an obstructive jaundice. Occasionally, complex revisional surgery will be required for some of the malabsorptive syndromes caused by previous gastric surgery.

Fast facts—Malabsorption (failure to absorb nutrients form gut)

Stomach

- Postsurgery
  - —dumping/inadequate mixing
  - —bypassing biliary and pancreatic secretions
- Lack of intrinsic factor (B12 anaemia)

Hepatobiliary

- Posthepatic disease and biliary obstruction
  - —lack of fat emulsification
  - —reduced fat absorption
  - —reduced fat soluble vitamin (A, D, E, K) uptake
- Steatorrhoea

Pancreatic

- Postchronic pancreatitis
  - —reduced digestive enzymes
  - —reduced carbohydrate, fat, and protein digestion
- Severe weight loss and steatorrhoea

Small bowel

- Postextensive small bowel resection
  - —lack of absorptive area
  - —reduced B12 absorption (B12 anaemia)
- Severe weight loss

Large bowel

- Post-total colectomy—slight disturbance in fluid absorption
- Rapid adaptation

Colorectal and perianal disorders

Chapter contents

Colorectal conditions *31*

Scenario 1: blood per anum *31*

Scenario 2: recurrent diarrhoea and cramping abdominal pain *32*

Scenario 3: severe left lower abdominal pain *33*

Scenario 4: abdominal pain and constipation *34*

Background: colon and rectum *36*

Perianal conditions *46*

Scenario 1: bleeding on painful defecation *46*

Scenario 2: painless bleeding on defecation *47*

Scenario 3: perianal pain and swelling *47*

Background: perianal disorders *48*

Colorectal conditions

Scenario 1: blood per anum

> A 55-year-old male notices dark blood streaked on his faeces.

Bleeding per anum is an important symptom and should always be taken seriously. Blood *on* the stool rather than separate from it, suggests a lesion in the colon or rectum, which bleeds when stool passes. The fact that the blood is dark also means that the blood is not fresh and coming from the colon. Bleeding from piles is usually bright red (fresh) and noticed separate from the stool.

> He also has lower abdominal pain associated with intermittent constipation and diarrhoea.

Change of bowel habit is an equally important symptom. It may be caused by a partially obstructing colonic lesion. When it is due to a colonic cancer it usually indicates a tumour in the left side of the colon where stools are more solid (as water has been reabsorbed from the large bowel contents as they pass the length of the colon).

If a tumour arises in the rectum then occasional fresh rectal bleeding and mucus discharge are possible. **There may also be a feeling of incomplete evacuation with defecation (tenesmus).**

Tumours of the left colon spread in the bowel via the bowel wall lymphatics, which encircle the bowel pro-

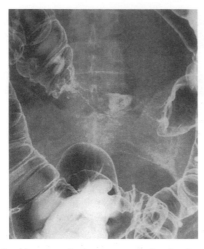

Fig 1.3a Double contrast barium enema of a long 'apple-core' malignant stricture of the transverse colon.

ducing a circular (annular) lesion. This produces the classical 'apple-core' lesion seen on barium enemas (Fig. 1.3a).

> His father had a colostomy and he has two aunts who have had bowel operations.

The family history is suggestive of a familial predisposition to colorectal carcinoma. If all the relatives have indeed had the disease, this patient will be at significantly increased risk.

> He has lost 1 stone in weight over a period of 3 months.

Weight loss is a worrying feature and indicates that if the underlying diagnosis is a tumour, it may be locally advanced or that there are distant metastases.

This patient has the typical presenting features of colonic cancer, and will need careful investigation of rectum and colon.

A digital rectal examination must be performed with a barium enema and sigmoidoscopy. If this does not reveal a lesion, then colonoscopy is indicated. As chronic blood loss is common the patient may also be anaemic.

Cancer of the right colon, where the faeces are relatively liquid, allows the faeces to pass without restriction. The tumour can still bleed but as it takes time to get from the right colon frank blood is not apparent. Patients with right colonic tumours therefore tend not to see blood on the stool but can present with anaemia due to chronic occult blood loss.

Clinical key points in colorectal cancer

- Any patient with altered bowel habit or bleeding per rectum should be investigated

- A patient with symptoms and a strong family history should be investigated

- Weight loss is a worrying feature and indicates that if the underlying diagnosis is a tumour, it may be locally advanced or that there are distant metastases

- Ask about alteration in bowel habit, per rectum bleeding or mucus, tenesmus (a feeling of incomplete evacuation), abdominal pain, and anorexia and weight loss

- All patients should be examined for an abdominal mass, hepatomegaly, and most IMPORTANTLY have a rectal examination

- The minimum investigation should be a flexible sigmoidoscopy and barium enema

---

Scenario 2: recurrent diarrhoea and cramping abdominal pain

> A 35-year-old female has a 3-month history of blood-stained diarrhoea with the passage of mucus (slime) and cramping lower abdominal pain. She opens her bowels between six and 20 times per day.

In this case, the **patient's age (20–40 years old) and the diarrhoea associated with the bleeding suggest inflammatory bowel disease. The large bowel is inflamed, exuding mucus, and as it represents an ulcerated raw area it can also bleed.**

> She has lost a stone in weight over this time period.

The relatively long history makes an infective cause unlikely, and the weight loss is also in keeping with ulcerative colitis or colonic Crohn's disease (inflammatory bowel disease).

> She also complains of sore joints. Baseline investigations reveal anaemia and a raised C-reactive protein.

The basis of ulcerative colitis is an autoimmune disease and it is associated with inflammation in other structures such as joints (25% of patients) and eyes (10% of patients). As there is chronic blood loss the patients are often anaemic (iron deficient). In acute ulcerative colitis, C-reactive protein, an acute phase protein and marker of inflammation, is raised. **Stool cultures should also be sent, however, as infective colitis cannot otherwise be ruled out.**

The most appropriate investigation here is colonoscopy and biopsy of the colonic mucosa.

Clinical key points in ulcerative colitis

- Usually presents in patients aged 20–40

- A history of diarrhoea, associated with bleeding, is suggestive of either infective colitis or inflammatory bowel disease

- The patient can also occasionally present with extra-intestinal symptoms (eyes, joints, skin, liver problems)

- Stool cultures should also be sent, however, as infective colitis cannot otherwise be ruled out

- Flexible endoscopy (either sigmoidoscopy or colonoscopy) is the most appropriate investigation as the mucosa should be biopsied for diagnostic purposes

---

Scenario 3: severe left lower abdominal pain

An 83-year-old female presents with severe left iliac fossa pain. She has a history of similar but less severe episodes.

Pain localizing to the left iliac fossa usually indicates a problem in that area. It may indicate irritation of the underlying peritoneum and implies an inflammatory or infective process. In the left iliac fossa the most likely diagnosis is acute diverticulitis of **the sigmoid colon (the commonest site for diverticular disease).**

Diverticulitis is inflammation of out-pouchings from the distal large bowel, usually the sigmoid colon. **It is due to chronic constipation, caused by a low-fibre diet.** As the large bowel has to work hard to move constipated faeces this causes a significant rise in intraluminal pressure. This in turn causes the inner lining of the bowel (mucosa) to herniate through the muscle layers of the bowel wall. These mucosal projections are called diverticulae.

As this is a chronic condition there may be a prolonged intermittent history of intermittent left iliac fossa pain and altered bowel habit.

These episodes are accompanied by either constipation or alternating constipation and diarrhoea.

As the diverticulae become swollen by inflammation the bowel can become less active and narrowed and hence constipation can result.

There is no history of bleeding per rectum.

A diverticulum can be the underlying cause of bleeding (occasionally torrential). It is thought to be due to erosion of the small artery that is at the neck of the diverticulum. However, just because someone has diverticular disease does not mean that the cause of the bleeding is diverticular. Other causes must be actively ruled out, i.e.:

- haemorrhoids
- colonic cancer
- angiodysplasia
- duodenal ulcer
- vascular malformation
- aortoenteric fistula.

On examination the patient is unwell with pyrexia. The abdomen is distended. She is tender in the left iliac fossa with a palpable mass.

The diverticulitis can become an inflammatory mass of tissue, which may be palpated as a mass in the left iliac fossa. The abdomen is distended as the inflammatory mass has occluded the large bowel. Repeated attacks of diverticulitis may result in scarring of the bowel with a fibrous stricture of the bowel causing recurrent subacute obstruction.

The acute inflammation may progress to perforation of the diverticulum that gives rise to a sealed-off abscess. The abscess in turn can adhere to adjacent structures (bladder, vagina, small bowel) and in turn develop into a faecal fistula. The perforation may also allow faeces into the abdominal cavity, giving rise to faecal peritonitis.

There are no signs of generalized peritonitis.

Without generalized peritonitis, the patient may be treated conservatively without an operation. In these circumstances **the symptoms must be investigated** by barium enema and flexible sigmoidoscopy to rule out other potential diagnoses.

However, if the patient's condition deteriorates then a laparotomy may be indicated. If an operation is required then the affected segment of bowel is excised and usually a proximal colostomy performed with closure of the rectum (Hartmann's procedure—Fig. 1.3b). The bowel can be joined together again about 6 months later.

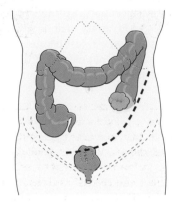

Fig 1.3b Diagram of Hartmann's procedure, the sigmoid colon excised, the rectal stump closed and the proximal bowel (descending colon in this example) brought out as a stoma.

Clinical key points in diverticular disease

- Low-fibre diet is the underlying cause

- Diverticular disease affects the sigmoid colon predominantly

- Ask about abdominal pain—a history of intermittent left iliac fossa pain and altered bowel habit may be caused by diverticular disease. They present acutely with left iliac fossa pain and pyrexia as diverticulitis

- Can be a cause of per rectum bleeding (occasionally torrential)

- On examination, there may be a mass in the left iliac fossa, due to inflammation around the sigmoid colon

- There may be fistulae to surrounding structures (most commonly to the bladder)

- Barium enema and flexible sigmoidoscopy are the two most pertinent investigations

Scenario 4: abdominal pain and constipation

> A 67-year-old man presents with a 3-week history of colicky lower abdominal pain. He has not moved his bowels for 5 days. He feels bloated and has been vomiting for 48 hours.

Constipation, vomiting, abdominal distension, and colic are the hallmark of an intestinal obstruction. On taking a detailed history some of the features of the previous colorectal cancer (Scenario 1) may be present.

> The patient looks grossly dehydrated with reduced skin turgor and a dry mouth and furred tongue.

In bowel obstruction dehydration is due to fluid entering the lumen of the bowel (and so is no longer available to the cardiovascular system) and also fluid being lost from the body by vomiting.

> His abdomen is distended and tympanitic but does not appear tender. The bowel sounds are frequent, tinkling, and high pitched. The rectum is empty.

The abdomen is distended due to fluid and gas within the bowel. The gas comes from swallowed air and gas produced within the bowel. This produces a tympanitic (drum-like) quality on percussion. Tinkling bowel sounds are caused by the air/fluid interface in the lumen of the bowel moved sloshed around by the active peristalsis. The rectum is empty simply because nothing gets there.

> There are no obvious hernias or surgical scars.

It is important to rule out trapped bowel within a hernia (particularly inguinal, femoral, and incisional) as the cause of a small bowel obstruction. Such trapped bowel may become ischaemic (due to strangulation), possibly leading to infarction, necrosis, and perforation of the bowel.

The above features would be in keeping with a distal small bowel or a large bowel obstruction.

The initial management steps comprise ABC oxygen (as usual for ill patients), IV fluid resuscitation, restriction of oral intake, and gastrointestinal decompression using a nasogastric tube, which allows fluid or swallowed air to be emptied.

Blood should be drawn for baseline haematology and biochemistry and a plain abdominal X-ray obtained to determine the type of obstruction (always remember to get an erect CXR as well, to look for free air under the diaphragms, a sign of bowel perforation).

The FBC may show a microcytic anaemia (chronic blood loss from a carcinoma); a raised white cell count raises the possibility of bowel infarction; biochemistry may show a raised urea or creatinine, due to dehydration.

> The plain X-ray confirms large bowel obstruction (Fig. 1.3c).

A plain abdominal film in large bowel obstruction shows:

◆ Grossly distended loops of colon, which are characterized by a 'picture frame' distribution around the perimeter of the abdominal cavity. (The picture frame distribution relates to gas within the large bowel which 'frames' the abdomen.)

◆ Mucosal folds (haustra), which do not cross the lumen of the distended intestine. (Loops of centrally placed smaller diameter intestine where the mucosal folds cross the lumen of the intestine.)

It is important to look at the outline of the caecum in any patient with a large bowel obstruction. As it is thin walled, it is the most common site of perforation in neglected large bowel obstruction.

If the diameter of the caecum is greater than 10 cm, then the patient should be considered for urgent surgery, before the caecum ruptures.

> After 24 hours fluid resuscitation and intestinal decompression (nasogastric tube) the patient's condition is much improved.

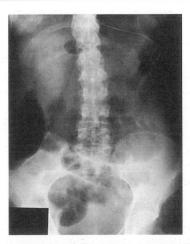

Fig 1.3c Plain radiograph in a patient with a three-day history of constipation showing distension of both small and large bowel.

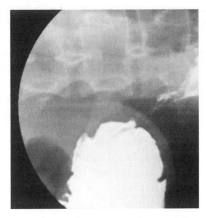

Fig 1.3d Single contrast barium enema with tumour (supplied X-ray).

Careful resuscitation is important and unless there is imminent danger of caecal rupture, time can be taken. **Replacement of fluid lost to the gut and with vomiting optimizes the patient for probable surgery. Decompression allows the patient to feel more comfortable, reduces the risk of aspiration, and stops splinting of the diaphragms** in which the distended abdomen pushes the diaphragms upward reducing ventilation of the bases of the lungs.

> A single contrast enema performed with water soluble contrast shows a shouldered stricture in the sigmoid colon (Fig. 1.3d).

One of the causes of large bowel obstruction is pseudo-obstruction, in which no mechanical obstruction is present (see p. 44). A single contrast barium enema can rule out this diagnosis.

> The following day, having excluded pseudo-obstruction, he is taken to theatre and undergoes a resection of an obstructing cancer in the sigmoid colon and a colostomy (Hartmann's procedure).

There is no single opinion as to the optimum treatment for an obstructing cancer in the sigmoid colon. In this case the surgeon felt the safest option was to resect the sigmoid colon containing the tumour closing off the remaining rectal stump and exteriorizing the proximal end of the colon to create an end colostomy (called a Hartmann's procedure). This still leaves an option to restore continuity of the intestine later, when the patient is better, at a second operation.

> ### Clinical key points in large bowel obstruction
>
> ◆ The history is usually that of abdominal pain (colic) associated with constipation, vomiting, and abdominal distension. There may be a preceding history of alteration in bowel habit
>
> ◆ Examine for evidence of dehydration (poor urine output, dry mouth)
>
> ◆ On abdominal examination, look for a distended, tympanitic abdomen. Examine for an abdominal mass, hepatomegaly, and DO a rectal examination
>
> ◆ The cause of a large bowel obstruction is usually either a colorectal cancer or pseudo-obstruction.
>
> ◆ A single contrast enema is the key investigation to identify the site of the obstruction and to exclude pseudo-obstruction (see section on intestinal obstruction, p. 44)

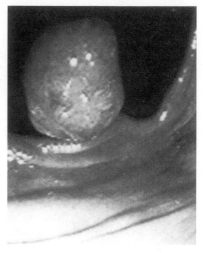

Fig 1.3e Colonoscopic view of a peduculated colonic polyp.

Background: colon and rectum

The colon, or large intestine, is the portion of the bowel from the terminal ileum to the rectum. It consists of the caecum, ascending colon, transverse colon, descending colon, and sigmoid colon. The rectum is below the peritoneal cavity (extra-peritoneal) within the pelvis. Its purpose is to act as a reservoir for the stool and to absorb fluid from the stool. Disorders of the colon arise from its mucosa (polyps, cancer, inflammatory bowel disease), its wall (diverticular disease), and twisting of its mesentery (volvulus)

Conditions:

◆ colonic polyps

◆ colorectal tumours

◆ ulcerative colitis

◆ diverticular disease

◆ angiodysplasia

◆ colonic volvulus

◆ intestinal obstruction.

Colonic polyps

Polyps can occur anywhere in the gastrointestinal tract.

1. *Juvenile polyps.* These occur in infants and young children. They are mainly found in the rectum and distal colon; they may be single or multiple. There is a family predisposition and they occur mostly in boys. They have little malignant potential but should be removed endoscopically when identified.

2. *Adenomatous polyps.* These are pedunculated (i.e. on a stalk), varying in size from a few millimetres to centimetres. They occur mainly in the rectum and colon. They are usually asymptomatic but can produce anaemia from chronic occult blood loss. Adenomatous polyps have a malignant potential and should be removed when identified (Fig. 1.3e).

3. *Villous polyps.* Villous polyps are sessile and spread around the circumference of the bowel, secreting large amounts of mucus. As such, they can produce spurious diarrhoea. They have a significant malignant potential and should be excised when identified.

4. *Familial polyposis.* This is an autosomal dominant condition and can be identified by genetic typing. It is characterized by hundreds of adenomatous polyps throughout the colon in the patient's second decade. With so many polyps, bleeding and abdominal pain are possible symptoms. The malignant potential is 100% within 15 years. The entire colon should be removed with formation of an ileal-pouch anal anastomosis.

Colorectal tumours

There are two main types of colorectal tumour—adenomatous polyps and adenocarcinoma, and it is believed that **most, if not all, carcinomas arise from pre-existing polyps.** Colorectal cancer is the second most common cause of cancer death in the UK after lung cancer, with some 28 000 new cases arising each year. The sex incidence is almost equal, although rectal cancer is slightly more common in men, and colonic cancer in women. The rectum, followed by the sigmoid colon, is the commonest site for both polyps and cancers and 5% of tumours are multiple.

Aetiology

The aetiology is unknown, although a strong family history is important and a diet rich in animal fat is associated with developing the disease. Risk factors include:

- ulcerative colitis
- pre-existing polyps
- familial adenomatous polyposis
- strong family history.

Familial adenomatous polyposis is a dominantly inherited condition, characterized by the appearance of multiple colorectal adenomatous polyps, usually at about the age of 20, which inevitably progresses to malignancy. It is treated by total colectomy soon after the polyps appear.

Spread of colorectal cancer

- *Lymphatic*: to regional lymph nodes lying alongside the blood vessels that supply and drain the colon and rectum.
- *Local*: through the bowel wall and into adjacent structures, such as abdominal wall, small bowel, bladder, vagina, stomach, or ureter.
- *Blood*: the commonest sites for blood-borne metastases are the liver, lungs, and pleura. Spread also occurs to the bones and brain.
- *Transcoelomic*: throughout the peritoneal cavity, producing multiple nodules of tumour.

Clinical features

The presentation of colorectal cancer depends largely on its site.

- *caecum and right colon*: anaemia (caused by blood loss from an ulcerating tumour), abdominal mass or small bowel obstruction. Caecal tumours tend to be quite large on presentation because the faecal material is still liquid on the right side of the colon, and obstruction of the bowel occurs at a late stage.
- *left colon*: abdominal pain, change of bowel habit and bleeding.

- *rectum*: bleeding (again from an ulcerated tumour), pain, and a feeling of incomplete evacuation (called tenesmus). Tenesmus occurs because the tumour fills the lumen of the rectum, leading to a full rectum sensation, and a feeling that the rectum has not completely emptied following evacuation of the bowels.

Patients may also present with the symptoms of advanced disease—weight loss, jaundice, due to liver metastases, abdominal distension due to ascites, or breathlessness owing to pulmonary or pleural metastases.

Currently, 20% of patients with colorectal cancer present as emergencies, most commonly with intestinal obstruction.

When examining a patient with suspected colorectal cancer, the following should be sought specifically:

- clinical evidence of weight loss, jaundice, or anaemia
- abdominal mass
- hepatomegaly
- abdominal swelling due to intestinal obstruction or ascites
- mass palpable on rectal examination.

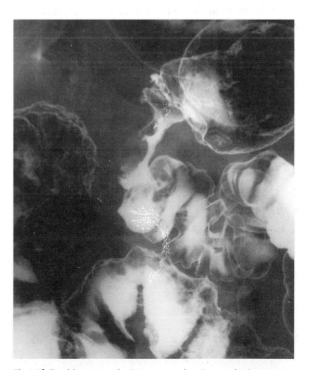

Fig 1.3f Double contrast barium enema showing a colonic tumour filling the lumen of the bowel.

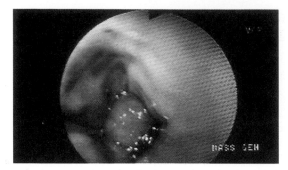

Fig 1.3g Colonoscopic view of a carcinoma of the colon, seen as an irregular mass filling the colonic lumen.

Investigation

When colorectal cancer is suspected, the patient should have complete colorectal visualization with a sigmoidoscopy, and a barium enema (Fig. 1.3f). If there is any doubt about the quality of the barium enema or if the patient has continuing symptoms, a colonoscopy should be carried out, which can examine the sigmoid colon in more detail (Fig. 1.3g).

FBC will indicate whether the patient is anaemic. Liver ultrasound or CT of the abdomen and pelvis (for rectal cancer) should be performed preoperatively to stage the disease.

Faecal occult blood testing can be used for screening asymptomatic populations, but it is not useful in making a diagnosis in a symptomatic patient.

Carcinoembryonic antigen is a tumour marker expressed in the blood in about 60% of patients with colorectal cancer. However, it is also found in other types of cancer, and while it is useful in monitoring the results of treatment when it is raised, it is of little diagnostic value.

TABLE 1.3a	Stages of colorectal cancer	
Duke's classification/staging		**5-year survival**
A Tumour has not invaded all the way through the muscle layer of the bowel wall		80%
B Tumour has invaded through the muscle layer but the local lymph nodes do not contain tumour		60%
C Tumour has spread to the regional lymph nodes		30%
D Distant metastases present		<5%

Fast facts—Colorectal cancer (malignant disease of the colon and rectum)

Epidemiology

- M/F = 1.3:1, ↑ incidence with age

Aetiology

- ↓ fibre diet, ↑ animal fat
- Adenomatous polyps
- Ulcerative colitis
- Familial polyposis coli

Pathology

- 75% of tumours are adenocarcinoma
- Within 60 cm of anal margin
- 5% have a second tumour (synchronous), 3% will get a second tumour (metachronous)
- Spread—direct local invasion, via lymphatics, and via portal vein to the liver
- Duke's staging

Clinical features

- Alteration in bowel habit
- Blood per rectum
- Tenesmus
- Anaemia

Investigations

- Digital rectal examination
- FBC
- Flexible sigmoidoscopy **and** double contrast barium enema, **or** colonoscopy
- Carcinoembryonic antigen (↑ in advanced disease)
- CT of abdomen (and pelvis for rectal cancer) for staging

Management

- Resection
- Adjuvant chemotherapy
- Resection of liver metastases

Prognosis

- 5-year survival depends on staging, 37% overall

Management

The main principle of management is surgical excision of the primary tumour.

If the tumour is stage C, there is evidence that a course of chemotherapy containing 5-fluorouracil can improve survival. This is known as **adjuvant chemotherapy**.

In rectal cancer, preoperative radiotherapy can reduce the rate of local recurrence and may improve survival.

In metastatic disease, chemotherapy is usually the only option, although partial liver resection may be useful in some cases, when there are metastases confined to the liver only. Patients with inoperable rectal cancer may benefit from radiotherapy.

Outcome

Overall, the 5-year survival in colorectal cancer is 37%, but this is highly dependent on the stage at presentation. The stage of colorectal cancer is most commonly described by Duke's classification (Table 1.3a).

Anal carcinoma

Unlike true colorectal carcinoma, anal cancer is usually squamous in origin (as opposed to adenocarcinoma of the colon or rectum). **Spread is usually to the inguinal lymph nodes**, although distant metastases can occur. The mainstay of treatment is a combination of radiotherapy and chemotherapy. Only if this fails is excision of the anal canal and rectum required, termed abdominoperineal resection as a combined operation is required from the abdomen and perineum.

Ulcerative colitis

Ulcerative colitis is an inflammatory condition, which in the intestine **only affects the colon and rectum**. It affects the rectum and distal colon predominantly, although the whole of the large bowel can be involved.

Histologically, the inflammatory exudate forms crypt abscesses coalescing to form shallow ulcers that destroy the mucosa and penetrate as far as the muscularis mucosa. The intervening mucosa becomes oedematous and swollen, and can form inflammatory pseudo-polyps. **The inflammatory process does not penetrate the whole thickness of the bowel wall**, but in chronic cases fibrosis supervenes and the colon can become thickened and rigid, losing its haustrations.

During a severe acute attack, however, due to destruction of the myenteric plexuses, with subsequent loss of the bowel muscle tone, the bowel wall can become very thin and grossly dilated (toxic dilatation). **Toxic dilatation is an indication for emergency surgery**, as the dilated bowel may perforate.

Complications

The main complications of ulcerative colitis are:

* bleeding

* stricture

* toxic dilatation leading to perforation

* malignant change

* extraintestinal manifestations.

Malignant change tends to occur in long-standing active colitis, which affects the whole of the large bowel, especially if it started at an early age. The precise risk is difficult to estimate, but it is reckoned that 10% of patients with disease of 10 years' duration and 20% of patients with disease of 20 years' duration will develop carcinoma. The average age of developing colonic malignancy is 43 years among colitis patients compared with 63 years in the general population.

The extraintestinal manifestations of ulcerative colitis include:

* skin (erythema nodosum, pyoderma gangrenosum)

* eyes (iritis)

* liver (hepatitis, sclerosing cholangitis), and

* musculoskeletal system (arthritis and ankylosing spondylitis).

If permanent changes have not occurred, these conditions resolve with removal of the diseased colon.

Presentation

Generally, ulcerative colitis presents with attacks of blood-stained diarrhoea, sometimes with mucus or pus, with or without abdominal pain. Most attacks are mild, but in severe disease, diarrhoea can occur 10–15 times per day. In severe attacks, urgency to defecate and weight loss are prominent symptoms.

On abdominal examination, there may be little to find in mild disease, but when severe there can be marked tenderness. A tachycardia and pyrexia are also indicative of severe disease. Rectal examination may reveal a thickened 'velvety' mucosa, and there may be blood and/or mucopus on the finger. Other systemic manifestations (listed above) may also be present.

Diagnosis and investigation

1. *Endoscopy*. The diagnosis is best made at colonoscopy where the mucosa will be seen to be granular, friable, and ulcerated, and biopsies can be taken to confirm the diagnosis. However, this is not advisable during an acute attack if there is any suggestion of toxic dilatation with its attendant risk of perfora-

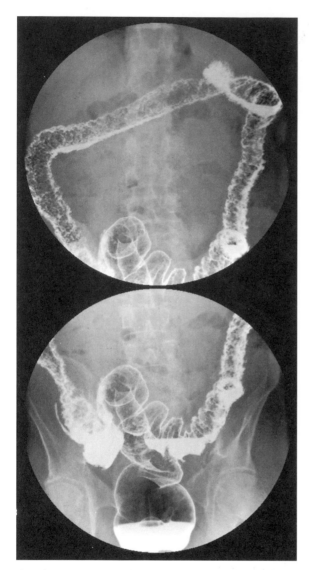

Fig 1.3h Barium enema study showing ulcerative colitis with diffuse ulceration shown as an irregular bowel wall.

tion, and here a limited sigmoidoscopy with rectal biopsies will suffice.

2. *Barium studies.* A barium enema will demonstrate ulceration in the acute phase (Fig. 1.3h), and in chronic disease, a featureless 'drainpipe' colon lacking haustrations will be seen. Biopsies are still required to establish the diagnosis.

3. *Plain radiography.* A plain abdominal X-ray is useful in the acute phase of severe disease in order to establish whether or not toxic dilatation is occurring (Fig. 1.3i). An erect CXR should also be performed to look for air under the diaphragm indicating perforation.

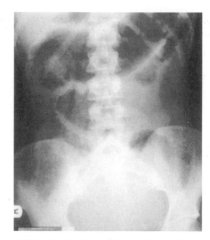

Fig 1.3i Plain abdominal radiograph in a patient with severe ulcerative colitis showing dilatation of the transverse colon and mucosal islands.

4. *Stool microscopy and culture.* These should be performed to exclude infective causes of colitis.

5. *Blood tests.* A FBC should be carried out to check for anaemia and leucocytosis. U&Es are important when there has been severe diarrhoea, and C-reactive protein will be raised in active disease.

Management

The management of ulcerative colitis is **medical in the first instance**, with non-steroidal anti-inflammatory drugs for mild cases and steroids for more advanced cases.

The mainstay of the treatment of mild disease is 5-amino salicylic acid in the form of mesalazine. This can be given orally, or, in the case of localized distal disease, as an enema, so that the treatment is given directly to the inflamed area. Mesalazine is also used to maintain remission if the colitis tends to relapse.

More severe disease requires steroid therapy, and the standard dose is 40 mg prednisolone orally per day, in divided doses, for about 4 weeks and then tailing off the dose. In very severe disease requiring hospital admission, high doses of IV steroids may be required.

The **surgical treatment of ulcerative colitis consists of either subtotal colectomy leaving a rectal stump or panproctocolectomy, with ileostomy or ileoanal pouch** (see Section 2). This is indicated for the following situations:

◆ complications of ulcerative colitis (see above)
◆ severe acute disease not responding to medical treatment
◆ severe chronic disease not responding to medical treatment

Fast facts—Ulcerative colitis (chronic inflammatory disease of the colon)

Epidemiology

◆ M/F = 1:16, age 30–50

Aetiology

◆ Genetic (10% incidence in relatives)

◆ ? autoimmune disease

Pathology

◆ Rectum (always involves the rectum) and colon

◆ Mucosal ulceration only

◆ Crypt abscesses, inflammatory polyps, granulation tissue

Clinical features

◆ Diarrhoea, passage of mucus (slime) and blood per rectum

◆ Abdominal pain, weight loss

◆ Anaemia

◆ Extraintestinal manifestation—arthritis (10%), uveitis (10%)

◆ Severe disease

—6–20 bloody stools/day

—fever, dehydration

—colonic dilatation/perforation

Investigations

◆ FBC

◆ Flexible sigmoidoscopy/biopsy

◆ Barium enema

◆ Plain abdominal film—colonic dilatation/gas under the diaphragm

Management

◆ Medical

—high-fibre diet

—anti-inflammatory drugs (salazopyrine, steroids)

—immunosuppressive agents

◆ Surgical (failure of medical management/complications/cancer risk)—panproctocolectomy with ileostomy/ileal pouch

Prognosis

◆ Incidence of colonic cancer

◆ long-standing disease with dysplasia to prevent malignancy from developing.

Diverticular disease

Diverticular disease is a common condition of the Western world, thought to be **secondary to a low-fibre diet**. The primary pathology seems to be hypertrophy of the colonic muscular wall, **particularly in the sigmoid colon**. This generates high intraluminal pressures, which in turn lead to outpouchings, or diverticulae of the colonic mucosa, at sites of weakness in the muscular wall where it is penetrated by blood vessels. The condition is uncommon before the age of 40, but is present in **at least 40% of the elderly population**.

Complications

The complications of diverticular disease are mostly related to inflammation of one or more of the diverticulae:

◆ inflammation of the diverticulae—called diverticulitis

◆ bleeding

◆ paracolic abscess

◆ faecal peritonitis

◆ fistula

◆ diverticular stricture.

Bleeding occurs as a result of erosion of a colonic wall vessel at the point where the diverticulum penetrates the muscle wall, and can be profuse, although often self-limiting.

Diverticulitis may progress to perforation of a diverticulum, which in turn may lead to the formation of a paracolic abscess or, if not localized, to life-threatening faecal peritonitis. If diverticulitis erodes into an adjacent hollow organ (bladder, small bowel, or vagina) a fistula will result. Recurrent attacks of inflammation cause fibrosis and subsequent stricturing, usually in the sigmoid colon.

Presentation

A patient with uncomplicated diverticular disease is usually constipated, but whether this is caused by the condition or vice versa is not clear. **Diverticulitis and paracolic abscess present with left iliac fossa pain and tenderness, and a mass may be felt.** Systemic upset (pyrexia and other signs of sepsis) is often present. Both a paracolic abscess and a fibrous diverticular stricture may give rise to change in bowel habit progressing to large bowel obstruction.

When massive bleeding occurs, the patient will present with copious rectal bleeding, usually red with clots, sometimes accompanied by signs of hypovolaemia.

Presentation of a fistula will depend on its anatomy. A vesicocolic fistula will cause recurrent urinary tract infections, or rarely bubbles of air in the urine (pneumaturia). A fistula between the small bowel and the sigmoid colon may lead to diarrhoea, and a patient with a colovaginal fistula leaks faeculent discharge from the vagina.

Diagnosis and investigation

FBC may show a raised white cell count (and accompanying raised C-reactive protein) in diverticulitis, paracolic abscess, or faecal peritonitis.

1. *Barium studies.* Most cases of diverticular disease are diagnosed on barium enema, which demonstrates the characteristic diverticulae well (Fig. 1.3j). Barium enema also outlines diverticular strictures and will often demonstrate fistulae

2. *Endoscopy.* Colonoscopy or flexible sigmoidoscopy will show the mouths of the diverticulae (Fig. 1.3k), and endoscopy with biopsy is essential in cases of sig-

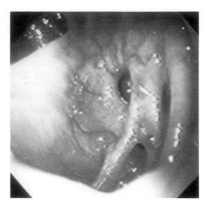

Fig 1.3k Colonoscopic view of diverticulosis with a small entrance to the diverticulum.

moid stricture where it is impossible to distinguish between a diverticular and a malignant aetiology.

3. *CT.* This investigation is useful when a paracolic abscess is suspected.

Management

The patient with uncomplicated diverticular disease requires no specific treatment, but the accompanying constipation will usually respond to a high-fibre diet.

The majority of patients with diverticulitis or even paracolic abscess can be treated conservatively with IV fluids and antibiotics (usually a cephalosporin and metronidazole), but **if the symptoms and signs do not settle on this regimen, a CT scan may demonstrate ongoing inflammation, abscess formation, or perforation then an operation is sometimes necessary.** In this case, it is preferable to resect the diseased segment of sigmoid colon, close off the rectum, and bring the distal colon out as an end colostomy (Hartmann's procedure).

Faecal peritonitis is a surgical emergency, requiring ABC fluid resuscitation, IV antibiotics, and early surgery. At operation, the affected colon (usually sigmoid) is resected and the peritoneal cavity thoroughly washed and the patient given a colostomy. Symptomatic strictures and fistulae also require sigmoid resection, but unless there is severe inflammation or contamination, it is often possible to achieve a primary anastomosis.

Angiodysplasia

Angiodysplasia is a rare condition that refers to vascular malformations in the submucosa, which have a tendency to bleed. They are most commonly found in the right colon, but they may occur anywhere in the intestine. The aetiology is unclear, but they generally occur

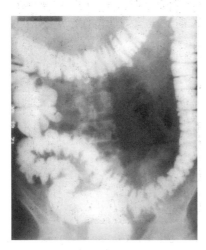

Fig 1.3j Barium enema study of diverticulosis with multiple small pockets of contrast lying alongside the bowel.

Fast facts—Diverticular disease (constipation—a cause or a result)

Epidemiology

♦ M/F = 1:1.5, ↑ incidence with age

Aetiology

♦ ↓ fibre diet, with ↑ intracolonic pressure

Pathology

♦ Diverticulae are most common in the sigmoid colon

♦ Wall of diverticulum is mucosa (i.e. no muscle layers)

Clinical features

♦ Mostly asymptomatic

♦ Left iliac fossa pain

♦ Acute diverticulitis

—malaise, fever

—left iliac fossa tenderness ± left iliac fossa mass

♦ Perforation—abscess/peritonitis

♦ Mucosal herniation of the left colon

♦ Large bowel obstruction

♦ Fistula (to bladder, vagina, small bowel)

Investigations

♦ FBC

♦ Flexible sigmoidoscopy

♦ Barium enema

♦ Erect CXR for perforation (free gas)

♦ CT scan abdomen

Management

♦ Medical—high-fibre diet

♦ Surgical (failed medical management/complications)—resection ± primary anastomosis/defunctioning colostomy

Prognosis

♦ Significant mortality and morbidity from complications

in elderly individuals, and are thought to represent degenerative change.

Presentation

These lesions present with rectal bleeding, which may be massive and/or recurrent.

Diagnosis

The diagnosis can be made at colonoscopy, or during active bleeding, by emergency mesenteric angiography, when contrast is injected through a catheter threaded via the femoral artery to see if there is a 'leak' of the contrast at the bleeding site. Sometimes it is possible to embolize the bleeding point at the time of the angiogram.

Management

ABC Bleeding may cease spontaneously. With ongoing bleeding, embolization or resection may have to be carried out. In the 'cold' case, colonoscopic electrocoagulation may be effective in preventing recurrent bleeding.

Volvulus of the colon

Caecal volvulus

If the caecum is poorly fixed to the posterior abdominal wall and is on a long mesentery a clock-wise torsion is possible. This produces obstruction, gangrene of the caecum, and perforation. Treatment is by surgical excision of the caecal volvulus (right hemicolectomy).

Sigmoid volvulus

Volvulus of the sigmoid colon is most commonly seen in elderly institutionalized patients. A redundant loop of

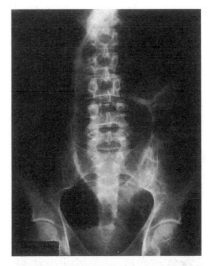

Fig 1.3l A plain abdominal film showing a sigmoid volvulus with massively dilated loop of gas-filled large bowel.

sigmoid with a narrow mesentery may twist on its mesentery to a greater or lesser extent producing a spectrum of results from subacute obstruction to infarction.

The abdomen is usually grossly distended, readily seen on a plain abdominal film (Fig. 1.3l). It may be decompressed with a sigmoidoscope or flatus tube. It usually requires elective resection, as with caecal volvulus.

Intestinal obstruction

Intestinal obstruction can be mechanical or due to paralytic ileus in which there is cessation of peristalsis. The latter may be secondary to intra-abdominal sepsis, surgery, trauma, or drugs, or it may be idiopathic. A particular form of paralytic ileus, colonic pseudo-obstruction, can mimic a distal mechanical large bowel obstruction. Pseudo-obstruction can be caused by chest infection and low serum potassium (hypokalcaemia)

Distinction between colonic pseudo-obstruction and colonic mechanical obstruction must be made prior to treatment, usually by a single contrast enema. In pseudo-obstruction, this shows dilatation of the whole bowel down to the rectum, with no obstructing lesion and does not usually need an operation; mechanical obstruction requires a laparotomy. The rest of this section will concentrate on mechanical obstruction.

Aetiology

Mechanical intestinal obstruction can be thought of as affecting the large bowel or small bowel and as originally extramural (outside the wall), intramural (in the wall), or intraluminal (in the lumen) (Table 1.3b).

Pathophysiology

When the bowel is obstructed, the proximal segment becomes dilated with gas (swallowed and from bacterial fermentation) and with fluid (produced by net secretion of extracellular fluid from the gastrointestinal tract).

Increased peristaltic activity in an attempt to overcome the obstruction leads to waves of intestinal colic. Owing to distension of the bowel, its blood supply becomes impaired, and this can lead to ischaemia, infarction, and perforation.

The blood supply can also be cut off by strangulation of the mesenteric vessels by an adhesive band or a tight hernial orifice and lead to gangrene and perforation of the ischaemic bowel. When bowel becomes ischaemic, it is unable to contain bacteria and their toxins, so that ischaemic bowel within the peritoneal cavity can lead to infected peritonitis before perforation occurs.

The main hazards of intestinal obstruction are:

1. Dehydration owing to loss of fluid and electrolytes into the bowel lumen and from vomiting.

2. Toxaemia and septicaemia owing to migration of toxins and bacteria through ischaemic bowel wall or via a perforation.

Presentation

The symptoms of intestinal obstruction are:

- pain
- vomiting
- abdominal distension
- absolute constipation (absence of faeces *and* flatus).

It is important to realize, however, that the symptoms reflect the *site* of the obstructing lesion, and that all four are not always present.

1. *Pain.* This is colicky in nature, i.e. waves of gripping pain lasting a few minutes at a time. It is most marked in small bowel obstruction.

2. *Vomiting.* Vomit may be pale and opaque (from gastric secretions) in gastric outlet obstruction, green or brown (bile stained) when from upper small bowel and dark brown and smelly (faeculant) in the late stages of intestinal obstruction as more distal small bowel content is vomited. (*This is to be distinguished from true faecal vomiting, which can only result from a gastrocolic fistula.*) Vomiting occurs earlier the more proximal the obstruction.

3. *Distension.* This is marked in distal large bowel obstruction, but not obvious in a proximal small bowel obstruction.

4. *Absolute constipation.* An early feature of distal large bowel obstruction, this may take several days to develop in a more proximal obstruction.

Examination

On examination, the abdomen is usually distended and tympanitic, unless the obstruction is very proximal. **An abdominal scar will suggest an adhesive cause for**

| TABLE 1.3b | Aetiology of intestinal obstruction |

Extramural	Intramural	Intraluminal
Hernia	Tumours (malignant or benign)	Faecal impaction
Adhesions	Diverticular disease	Food bolus
Peritoneal tumour	Crohn's disease	Foreign body
Volvulus	Hirschsprung's disease	Gallstone ileus
Intussusception	Congenital atresia	

the obstruction, and a careful examination of the groin is important, to exclude an obstructed hernia.

Tenderness, with or without guarding, suggests strangulation. A raised temperature and rapid pulse rate will tend to reinforce this suspicion.

In mechanical obstruction, the bowel sounds tend to be prominent and high pitched or tinkling as waves of peristalsis try to overcome the obstruction. Rectal examination is vital, as it may reveal an obstructing rectal cancer, faecal impaction, or a mass in the pouch of Douglas, suggesting pelvic tumour.

Diagnosis and investigation

The most important diagnostic procedure in suspected intestinal obstruction is the **plain abdominal X-ray**. The supine film is particularly useful for determining the gas pattern, and small and large bowel distension can be distinguished in the following ways:

♦ *small bowel*: central distribution, with ladder pattern indicating the valvulae conniventes (circular mucosal folds).

♦ *large bowel*: peripheral distribution, with haustrations, not extending across the whole width of the bowel (Fig. 1.3c). Note: a caecum that is distended to 10 cm or more is in danger of perforation, as this indicates a closed loop obstruction (i.e. colon obstruction with a competent ileocaecal valve—if the valve is competent, then gas cannot flow back into the small bowel and therefore the caecum expands rapidly).

Erect X-ray films will show fluid levels, confirming the diagnosis of obstruction but add little to a standard film. Occasionally, when there is a lot of fluid in the obstructed bowel, the characteristic gas patterns are not seen on the supine film, and only the erect film will give the diagnosis.

In the case of large bowel obstruction, it is important to arrange a contrast enema to exclude pseudo-obstruction (Fig. 1.3m), or to identify the site of a true obstruction (e.g. in the transverse colon or sigmoid colon—Fig. 1.3d) as this may influence the operation performed.

In the case of small bowel obstruction, it is important to examine the abdomen for scars (as adhesions from previous surgery may cause the obstruction) and to check for irreducible hernias, which may cause the obstruction, particularly in the groin where they may be hidden by abdominal skin fat folds.

In all cases, it is necessary to send blood for FBC and U&Es to check for anaemia (from the obstructing lesion), leucocytosis (due to strangulation), electrolyte imbalance, and extracellular fluid deficit secondary to intraluminal fluid loss and vomiting.

Management

1. *Initial management.* ABC Oxygen, pain relief, and IV replacement of fluids and electrolytes (normal saline with added potassium where appropriate) should be started as soon as possible. This must be accompanied by gastric aspiration by nasogastric tube suction to decompress the bowel and to reduce the risk of aspiration of gastric contents. Pain relief must not be forgotten.

2. *Conservative management.* If there are no symptoms or signs suggesting strangulation or perforation, and if the likely cause is adhesions (e.g. the patient has a previous abdominal surgical scar), a trial of conservative management as above is reasonable, as on many occasions the condition will resolve.

3. *Operative management.* Surgery for intestinal obstruction is indicated when:

   ♦ there are signs of strangulation or perforation

   ♦ there is an obstructed hernia

   ♦ contrast enema confirms large bowel obstruction

   ♦ conservative measures (IV fluids, nasogastric tube suction, analgesics) fail.

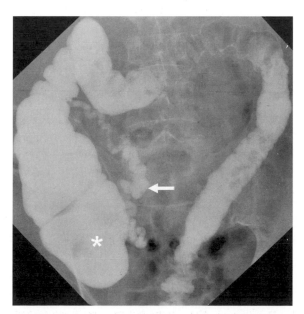

Fig 1.3m A single contrast barium enema which has passed into the small bowel through an incompetent ileocaecal valve—no lesion.

Fast facts—Large bowel obstruction (complete or incomplete obstruction of the large bowel lumen)

Causes

- Intramural—tumours, diverticular disease
- Intraluminal—faecal impaction, foreign bodies
- Motility disorder (pseudo-obstruction)

Pathophysiology

- Bowel proximal to obstruction dilates and becomes oedematous
- Bowel distal to the obstruction collapses
- As bowel wall distends the wall's blood supply is compromised—leading to infarction, perforation

Clinical features

- Colicky abdominal pain, vomiting, absolute constipation (no flatus, no faeces)
- Abdominal distension
- Dehydration (if severe ↓ BP)
- Empty rectum

Investigations

- FBC (Hb/WCC)
- U&Es
- Abdominal X-ray
- Contrast study to define site and cause of obstruction

Management

- Oxygen and analgesia
- Decompression of the gut (nasogastric tube)
- IV fluids to replace losses
- Operation to relieve the obstruction
  - if a failure of conservative management of adhesion obstruction
  - if signs of peritonitis or strangulation of bowel
  - if cause requires surgical treatment (cancer, hernia)

Prognosis

- Significant mortality and morbidity, particularly if serious underlying cause (e.g. cancer)

At operation, the procedure carried out will depend on the site of the obstruction, its cause and the state of the obstructed bowel. With adhesions or a hernia (where it is usually the small bowel that is affected) it may be sufficient to relieve the obstruction by dividing the adhesions or reducing the hernia. If a segment of the bowel is non-viable, however, it must be resected. Signs of non-viability are as follows:

- black or green colour
- lack of mesenteric arterial pulsation
- loss of sheen
- loss of peristalsis.

If there is doubt, the bowel can be observed for about 10 minutes after release to see if it recovers.

When small bowel has been resected, it is nearly always safe to perform a primary anastomosis. With large bowel, however, where a resection for an obstructing lesion (e.g. a carcinoma) has been performed, this is not always the case. With a right-sided lesion, a right hemicolectomy with primary ileocolic anastomosis is usually safe, but with a left-sided lesion, a Hartmann's procedure (closure of the rectal stump with proximal end colostomy—see section on gastrointestinal operations) may be necessary. This is because the blood supply of the colon is not as rich as that of the small bowel, and in the presence of an unprepared bowel full of faeces, a colonic anastomosis is likely to leak. Primary anastomosis can be carried out in selected patients after intraoperative bowel cleansing, but this requires a high level of expertise.

Perianal conditions

Scenario 1: bleeding on painful defecation

A 25-year-old female has noticed bright red rectal bleeding on defecation. At the same time she experiences severe, sharp, anal pain like passing broken glass. Following defecation there is severe, persistent anal discomfort.

Painful defecation is typical of an anal fissure. The tear or ulcer in the mucosa of the anal canal gives rise to both the pain and the fresh bleeding, but only when the bowels are opened. The persistent discomfort is due to anal sphincter spasm

She explains that there have been other similar episodes. On examination there is a perianal skin tag and a longitudinal fissure (Fig. 1.3n).

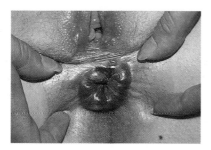

Fig 1.3n Clinical photograph showing perianal fissure (at 12 o'clock) and blue-red haemorrhoids.

The diagnosis can be confirmed by inspection of the anal canal alone—digital rectal examination in this patient is likely to be very painful. The skin tag ('*sentinel pile*') is due to previous episodes and is positioned at the outside end of the fissure.

She is treated by the use of locally applied muscle relaxant cream (nitrates). If this fails the internal sphincter is cut (lateral sphincterotomy) to reduce the anal tone.

Scenario 2: painless bleeding on defecation

A 50-year-old male has large amounts of fresh bleeding immediately after opening his bowels. The blood tends to drip into the toilet bowel afterwards. There is no pain. There are no other symptoms.

Again, these are symptoms of anal canal bleeding; the blood is fresh, and there is no history of change in bowel habit. The pattern of bleeding experienced by this patient is entirely typical of haemorrhoidal bleeding, triggered by the passage of faeces past the engorged vascular anal cushions.

Blood on the toilet paper is a very common symptom with haemorrhoids. It is experienced by about 80% of the population from time to time. It is usually due to internal haemorrhoids in most instances. In a young patient with no other symptoms, a normal rectal examination should be sufficient to provide reassurance, but further investigations must be carried out if the bleeding is persistent. **In older patients this could represent a worrying symptom until proved to be perianal in origin.**

Digital rectal examination is unremarkable. Proctoscopy reveals three purple vascular cushions (Fig. 1.3o).

Rectal examination is important, but may not provide the diagnosis of haemorrhoids. Proctoscopy will give

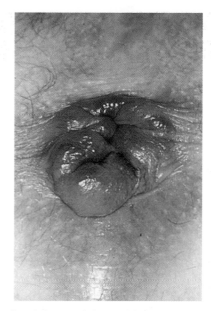

Fig 1.3o Clinical photograph showing haemorrhoids.

the diagnosis, but in view of the patient's age, fuller investigation of the large bowel (e.g. sigmoidoscopy) would be appropriate.

Treatment is by high fibre laxatives, injection sclerotherapy, or 'banding'. Banding uses elastic loops to pinch off the haemorrhoid. Rarely is formal excision of the haemorrhoids (haemorrhoidectomy) required.

Scenario 3: perianal pain and swelling

A 42-year-old man notices a painful swelling in the perianal region. He feels shivery and unwell.

A painful perianal swelling is in keeping with a perianal abscess (Fig. 1.3p).

This discharges pus, and the pain settles. Subsequently, however, he has a persistent blood-stained discharge from a small perianal lump associated with pruritus.

The abscess discharged spontaneously and with the consequent development of a fistula-in-ano. The pruritus is due to the chronic discharge from the fistula track. Recurrent perianal abscesses are usually due to a persistent fistula-in-ano. Further **evaluation requires transanal examination and ultrasound under anaesthesia.**

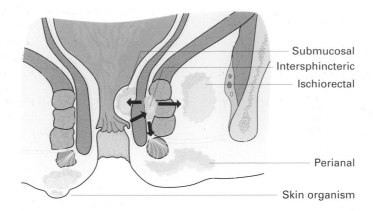

Fig 1.3p Diagram of the anatomy and naming of perianal abscesses.

Submucosal
Intersphincteric
Ischiorectal
Perianal
Skin organism

Clinical key points in perianal condition

- Ask about pain on defecation—this is usually due to a perianal fissure

- Ask about rectal bleeding—this is a worrying symptom until proved to be perianal (e.g. by flexible sigmoidoscopy)

- Tender perianal swelling with possible fever and rigors usually indicates perianal sepsis. The two most important investigations are transanal ultrasound and examination under anaesthesia

Background: perianal disorders

Conditions:

- haemorrhoids
- perianal abscess and fistula-in-ano
- pilonidal sinus
- anal fissure
- perianal haematoma
- rectal prolapse.

Haemorrhoids

Haemorrhoids are congested vascular cushions in the anal canal, which prolapse to a varying degree. There are usually three main haemorrhoidal masses, situated at 3, 7, and 11 o'clock (12 o'clock being anterior) around the anal canal. They are classified as follows:

- *first degree*: confined to the anal canal; they do not prolapse, but can bleed

- *second degree*: prolapse on defecation, but reduce spontaneously

- *third degree*: prolapse spontaneously, but can be reduced

- *fourth degree*: prolapsed, irreducible.

They are usually idiopathic but haemorrhoids may be precipitated by factors which cause congestion of the superior rectal veins, such as pregnancy or a pelvic tumour.

The symptoms of haemorrhoids are bright red bleeding and discomfort produced by prolapse. Prolapsing haemorrhoids can also give rise to mucus discharge and pruritus.

Diagnosis is made by inspection of the anal canal and if the haemorrhoids have not already prolapsed, proctoscopy. Haemorrhoids may be complicated by anaemia when bleeding is severe and by thrombosis when the anal sphincter grips large prolapsed haemorrhoids. The latter condition is very painful.

Management

Symptomatic haemorrhoids can be treated as follows:

- first and second degree—diet, injection of sclerosant, or banding

- third and fourth degree—haemorrhoidectomy (see section on gastrointestinal operations).

Thrombosed haemorrhoids are usually treated by analgesia, bed rest, and cold compresses. However, immediate haemorrhoidectomy may be indicated.

Perianal abscess and fistula-in-ano

1. *Perianal abscess*. A perianal abscess arises as a result of infection of an anal gland. These glands are situated between the internal and external sphincters, and empty into the anal canal at the level of the dentate line (Fig. 1.3q).

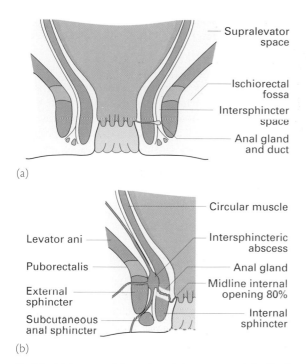

(a)

(b)

Fig 1.3q (a) Anatomy of the anal canal showing an anal gland in the intersphincteric space, with the glandular duct opening in the anal canal at the dentate line: (b) coronal section of an anal canal, showing the relationship between the anal gland, an intersphincteric abscess, and the possible paths fistula tracts can take within the sphincter complex.

The infection usually tracks down between the sphincters to present at the anal verge (intersphincteric or perianal abscess), but it may track across the external sphincter into the ischiorectal fossa (ischiorectal abscess). Occasionally, the infection may pass upwards to form a pelvic abscess, but this is very unusual; a pelvic abscess generally arises from infection in pelvic organs (e.g. diverticular abscess).

2. *Fistula-in-ano.* When a perianal abscess discharges through the skin or is surgically drained, it usually heals by secondary intention, but occasionally the connection between the anorectal mucosa and the perianal skin persists as a fistula-in-ano. Conventionally, these fistulae are classified as low if they do not traverse the external sphincter and high if they do. Alternative terms are intersphincteric, transsphincteric, and suprasphincteric.

Presentation

The patient with a perianal or ischiorectal abscess presents with a throbbing pain in the perianal region, and there will usually be a tender, red, fluctuant mass. With a deep-seated ischiorectal abscess or abscess between the sphincter muscles; however, there may be little to find on examination other than tenderness on palpation.

In a patient with a fistula-in-ano there is usually, but not always, a clear history of a previous abscess that has discharged or been drained. This is followed by the development of a small, intermittently discharging lump in the perianal region, which is usually painless but can be uncomfortable. The discharge may lead to perianal itching (pruritus ani).

Management

A perianal or ischiorectal abscess is treated by surgical drainage and antiseptic dressing until healing is achieved. If a fistula develops or is diagnosed primarily, the treatment will depend on whether it is low or high. A low fistula is cut open to heal by secondary intention, and as the external sphincter is not involved this carries very little risk.

Laying open of a high fistula, however, may lead to faecal incontinence, owing to division of part or all of the external sphincter. Management of high fistulae is complex and involves establishing good control of sepsis by means of a seton (a suture passing along the fistula tract, which is left in place to establish drainage of the sepsis).

Pilonidal sinus and abscess

'Pilonidal' means 'nest of hairs', and a pilonidal sinus is an acquired condition, usually in men with hairy but-

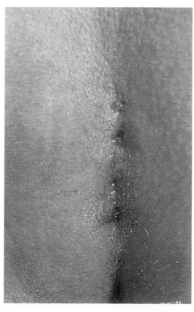

Fig 1.3r Clinical photograph showing pilonidal sinuses in the upper natal cleft.

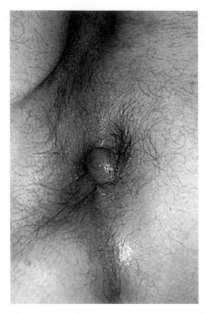

Fig 1.3s Clinical photograph showing perianal haematoma which appears as a small polypoid lesion, the base of which is from the perianal skin rather than the anal canal.

tocks, in which a sinus or series of sinuses of varying complexity form in the natal cleft (Fig. 1.3r). These sinuses are lined by granulation tissue, contain loose hair, and are prone to becoming infected and forming abscesses. The precise aetiology of this condition is unknown, but it is probably caused by hairs being driven into the skin by the movement of the skin in this area.

Presentation

A pilonidal sinus is frequently asymptomatic, and only found as a series of pits in the natal cleft. When infect-

ed, however, it will present either as an abscess (red, hot tender swelling) or as chronic discharge from the sinus.

Management

A pilonidal abscess is drained, deroofing the cavity and cleaning out the hairs and granulation tissue. With a quiescent sinus that has been symptomatic, the whole area is excised, and if possible, sutured primarily. Sometimes primary closure is impossible, and the skin defect has to be left open to heal by a secondary intention, a process that can take many weeks. Unfortunately, recurrence is not uncommon even after radical treatment. For this reason, the asymptomatic or minimally symptomatic sinus is best left alone.

Anal fissure

An anal fissure is a linear ulcer in the anal canal (90% posterior, 10% anterior). It is thought to be caused by ischaemia secondary to a high internal sphincter pressure compressing the blood supply to the anal canal.

There is usually a history of constipation and straining to pass stool. Defecation should be a product of muscle relaxation not effort (straining).

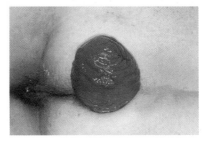

Fig 1.3t Clinical photograph of a rectal prolapse showing the rectal mucosa.

Fig 1.3u Diagram showing a rectal intussusception (a) passing into the anal canal (arrow) to become a full thickness rectal prolapse (b) arrow.

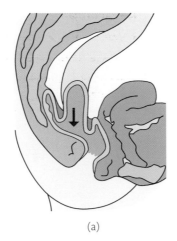

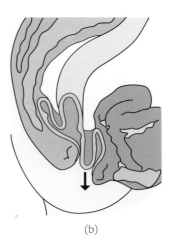

(a)   (b)

Patients usually present with painful rectal bleeding and diagnosis is made by inspection of the anal canal.

Management is by high-fibre diet and 0.2% GTN cream to relax the internal sphincter. If this fails, a lateral sphincterotomy (in which the internal sphincter is divided) is recommended to reduce the internal sphincter tone. A side-effect of this, however, can be either flatus incontinence or minor faecal incontinence.

Perianal haematoma

This is the result of a small bleed into the perianal skin. It produces an exquisitely tender small blue lump at the anal margin (Fig. 1.3s).

It usually resolves spontaneously but if the patient is very distressed the blood clot can be evacuated through a small incision done under local anaesthetic. This produces immediate relief from a very grateful patient.

Rectal prolapse

Rectal prolapse can be partial or complete. In partial prolapse only the mucosa is involved and protrudes only a centimetre or two from the anal verge. Complete prolapse, on the other hand, involves all layers of the rectal wall, and this may protrude many centimetres (Fig. 1.3t, 1.3u). It is uncomfortable, and, by stretching the anal sphincter, it may lead to faecal incontinence. It is largely confined to elderly females.

Management

Management is surgical. Partial prolapse can be treated by means of excising the mucosa. Full thickness prolapse, however, is best dealt with by means of a resection rectopexy, which involves mobilizing the rectum, removing a length of colon, and rejoining the two ends.

Fast facts—Benign perianal conditions (problems around the anus)

Haemorrhoids

◆ Submucosal vascular plexus
  —painless bleeding with defecation
  —may prolapse with defecation

Perianal abscess

◆ Painful tender perianal swelling
  —originates in anal glands
  —may give rise to fistula-in-ano

Fistula-in-ano

◆ Abnormal communication between perianal skin and anal canal
  —chronic discharge
  —recurrent perianal abscesses

Pilonidal sinus

◆ A blind ending tract form a 'nest' of hairs in the natal cleft—may give rise to pilonidal abscess

Anal fissure

◆ Anal tear causing exquisite pain with defecation—initially treated by GTN cream

Perianal haematoma

◆ Very painful subcutaneous blood clot in rescued region—immediate relief if incised and evacuated

Rectal prolapse

◆ Protrusion of rectal mucosa from the anus
  —usually due to poor anal sphincter tone
  —produces mucus discharge, bleeding per rectum

Disorders of the pancreas, biliary tree, liver, and jaundice

Chapter contents

Pancreatic disorders 53

Scenario 1: severe upper central abdominal pain 53

Background: pancreas 55

Disorders of the biliary system 61

Scenario 1: repeated right upper abdominal pain 61

Scenario 2: upper abdominal pain and vomiting 61

Background: biliary tract 63

Jaundice 61

Scenario: abdominal pain and jaundice 64

Background: jaundice 66

Background: liver 68

Pancreatic disorders

Scenario 1: severe upper central abdominal pain

> A 63-year-old man presents to an A&E department with a short history of upper abdominal pain of increasing severity. The pain is epigastric and radiates through to the back. It is not made worse by movement but he does seem more comfortable leaning forward. This patient tells you he has been admitted twice in the last 12 months with similar symptoms and that he drinks on average half a bottle of whisky each night.

Pancreatitis usually presents with sudden onset of upper abdominal pain radiating through to the back and associated with nausea and vomiting.

The history of recurrent hospital admissions coupled with a heavy alcohol intake should make you think of acute pancreatitis **as a possible diagnosis. All patients presenting with upper abdominal pain should have their serum amylase checked to exclude acute pancreatitis**.

Having established that the airway is not blocked and putting an oxygen mask on the patient to assist breathing (remember ill patients need oxygen), venous access is established using a wide bore cannula and blood drawn for baseline FBC and biochemistry. IV fluid resuscitation should begin while a full assessment of the patient takes place.

On examination he is clearly in severe pain. He looks flushed, he is tachycardic with an increased respiratory rate but a BP of 140/80 mmHg. His abdomen is generally tender particularly in the epigastrium. Bowel sounds are present. On examination of the chest it is dull to percussion at both bases with absent breath sounds and coarse crackles above this.

Epigastric tenderness, a tachycardia, and fever indicates an inflammatory or infective process within the area of the upper abdomen. Owing to intraperitoneal inflammation by pancreatic enzymes, the chest can also be affected with a sympathetic pleural effusion and lung changes.

The serum amylase level is greater than 2000 IU/dl (normal range 50–250 IU/dl).

TABLE 1.4a Investigation in patients with pancreatitis

Arterial blood gases	Examines respiratory function through the effect on oxygen content due to increased oxygen usage and pulmonary damage causing blood to pass through the lungs without being oxygenated (right-to-left shunt)
CXR	Examines cardiovascular system through evidence of heart failure due to toxins depressing myocardial function, pleural effusion secondary to cardiac and pulmonary damage
Blood glucose	Examines pancreatic function through insulin secreting islet cell dysfunction due to local oedema and toxic damage
Serum calcium	Reduced serum calcium as it is bound to fat released from damaged fat cells following autolysis by pancreatic enzymes released into the tissues
Serum creatinine	Renal tubular necrosis through fluid loss (as oedema) and the release of cellular toxins
LFTs (alanine transaminase, bilirubin, alkaline phosphatase)	Damage to the liver as toxins released from damaged cells cause hepatocellular dysfunction
White cell count	Haematological system through a white cell response to systemic inflammatory response syndrome (SIRS)
C-reactive protein	As a measure of inflammatory response

A serum amylase of greater than three times the upper limit of normal is diagnostic of acute pancreatitis.

Once confirmed a range of **tests is undertaken to establish the severity of the attack on the cardiovascular, respiratory, and renal systems (Table 1.4a).**

His arterial pO_2 is 7.6 kPa (normal range 9–13 kPa). All other blood tests are within normal limits. Within 1 hour of admission his systolic BP drops from 140 to 110 mmHg. His fluid balance chart shows that he has not passed urine.

Treatment is supportive and this patient will require supplemental oxygen therapy and careful monitoring of his blood gases. Almost all attacks of acute pancreatitis are associated with large fluid losses into the retroperitoneal space from the inflamed pancreas. The effect is likened to a large internal burn. Untreated this will lead to dehydration, cardiovascular collapse, renal failure, and death.

Fluid balance is of critical importance in patients with acute pancreatitis. This patient will need to be catheterized (a catheter placed in the bladder to monitor the urine output) and careful fluid replacement given to maintain an adequate urine output (at least 30 ml per hour). A central venous line to measure central venous pressure may be required to ensure sufficient fluid is given to maintain the central venous pressure at 3–8 cm water. This helps more accurate monitoring of the patient's response to IV fluid.

After 72 hours careful fluid resuscitation and supplemental oxygen therapy this patient's condition steadily improves. An ultrasound of the biliary system showed no evidence of gallstones and a non-dilated common bile duct.

Most patients with acute pancreatitis make a recovery without further intervention. However, occasionally the acute pancreatitis will be severe with failure of one or more of the following organ systems: respiratory, cardiac, renal. These patients require a high level of supportive care (intensive care); in severe cases, multiorgan failure may occur leading to death. In these circumstances **a CT scan is required to assess the state of the pancreas as there is likely to be pancreatitic necrosis with or without super-added infection.**

Clinical key points in acute pancreatitis

- Ask about abdominal pain—pancreatitis usually presents with sudden onset of upper abdominal pain radiating through to the back and associated with nausea and vomiting

- Ask about alcohol intake

- Examination usually shows epigastric tenderness and a tachycardia. There may be an associated fever

- Usually diagnosed by a rise in the serum amylase —ALL patients with upper abdominal pain should have their serum amylase checked

- The patient should have a plain abdominal X-ray and an erect CXR initially to exclude a perforated duodenal ulcer as the cause of the symptoms

- The severity of the attack can be gauged by the results of a number of tests assessing the cardiac, respiratory, and renal systems

- Pancreatitis is usually caused by gallstones or alcohol—the best initial investigation is an abdominal ultrasound to check for gallstones

- Patients will require a CT scan of the abdomen if the pancreatitis is predicted to be severe

Most attacks of pancreatitis are caused by either gallstones or alcohol. This patient's ultrasound showed no evidence of gallstones and therefore it was likely that his pancreatitis was related to his alcohol intake. He was advised to abstain from alcohol, to prevent further recurrences of his pancreatitis.

Background: pancreas

The pancreas is situated in the upper abdomen, below and behind the stomach. It is divided into head, body, and tail. The head is 'framed' by the duodenum and the tail by the spleen. It is both an exocrine gland (secreting digestive enzymes into the bowel) and an endocrine gland (secreting insulin into the circulation).

Conditions:

- acute pancreatitis

- chronic pancreatitis

- cancer of the pancreas.

Acute pancreatitis

Acute pancreatitis is an acute inflammation of the pancreas characterized by upper abdominal pain with raised concentration of pancreatic enzymes in the blood and urine. Severe acute pancreatitis carries a significant mortality rate at about 10%.

Causes

Most attacks (about 75%) of acute pancreatitis are caused by either gallstones or alcohol. Gallstones cause pancreatitis by passing from the gall bladder via the cystic duct and into the common bile duct (Fig. 1.4a), where they can get stuck at the ampulla of Vater. Here they can either block off the common bile duct leading to obstructive jaundice or block off the pancreatic duct, causing pancreatitis.

Alcohol leads to pancreatitis as a toxic effect. Persistent alcohol drinking leads to recurrent attacks of pancreatitis, resulting in chronic pancreatitis.

Occasionally, pancreatitis may be caused by endoscopic retrograde cholangiopancreatography (ERCP, see below). Other, rarer, causes of pancreatitis include viruses (e.g. mumps), direct trauma to the abdomen overlying the pancreas with the pancreas squashed up against the thoracic vertebra, drugs (e.g. azothioprine), and metabolic causes, like a raised serum calcium (hypercalcaemia) or raised serum lipids.

Causes of acute pancreatitis

- Gallstones

- Alcohol

- ERCP

History and examination

The diagnosis of acute pancreatitis should be considered in all patients who present with a history of upper abdominal pain. Usually the pain radiates to the back (as the pancreas is a retroperitoneal organ) and is associated with nausea and vomiting.

Examination reveals epigastric tenderness (due to the inflamed pancreas) and occasionally the patient may be shocked (due to the oedema and fluid loss around the pancreas). These features may occur in several other acute abdominal diseases, and a diagnosis of acute pancreatitis is often unreliable if made on the clinical findings alone.

Diagnosis

In the majority of cases the diagnosis of acute pancreatitis is made by a serum amylase activity three to four

Fig 1.4a Anatomical diagram of gall bladder/bile duct anatomy in relationship to the duodenum and pancreas.

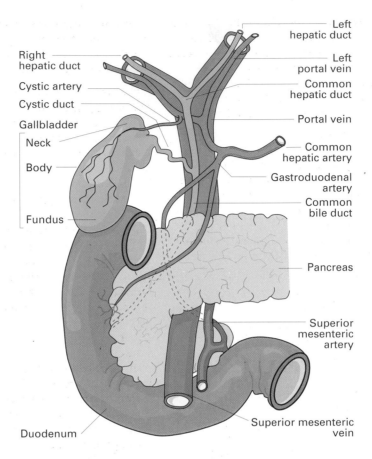

Right hepatic duct

Cystic artery

Cystic duct

Gallbladder

Neck

Body

Fundus

Duodenum

Left hepatic duct

Left portal vein

Common hepatic duct

Portal vein

Common hepatic artery

Gastroduodenal artery

Common bile duct

Pancreas

Superior mesenteric artery

Superior mesenteric vein

times above normal. A raised serum amylase together with upper abdominal pain, however, can occur in other serious conditions such as mesenteric ischaemia, duodenal perforation, acute cholecystitis, and leaking abdominal aortic aneurysm. Other radiological tests should therefore be carried out routinely to exclude other pathology and to provide a baseline picture.

◆ *Plain chest and abdominal X-rays*:

- a *CXR* may show a pleural effusion, particularly on the left, which is a reaction to the inflamed pancreas just below the diaphragm (Fig. 1.4b). In severe cases, diffuse alveolar interstitial shadowing may suggest acute respiratory distress syndrome (ARDS).

Fig 1.4b CT scan of the lower chest/upper abdomen showing pleural effusion (arrowed) associated with pancreatitis.

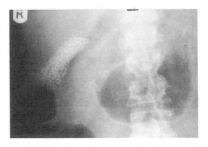

Fig 1.4c Plain abdominal film showing radio-opaque gallstones.

- *abdominal X-rays* may show dilated local loops of small bowel, due to the bowel being paralysed by the inflammation (called localized paralytic ileus). Ten per cent of gallstones are radio-opaque and may be seen on an abdominal X-ray (Fig. 1.4c). Rarely, in chronic pancreatitis the pancreas may be calcified, due to repeated attacks of inflammation.

- *Ultrasonography*: ultrasound examination of the abdomen may be helpful in confirming the diagnosis, as a swollen pancreas may be detected. However, it is most useful in detecting gallstones in the gall bladder, and to measure the diameter of the common bile duct, which may be dilated if there is a stone blocking the distal end of the common bile duct. **ALL patients with pancreatitis should have an ultrasound to exclude gallstones as the cause**.

- *CT scanning*: A CT scan is indicated for diagnostic purposes if the clinical and biochemical findings are inconclusive. It is also required in patients with severe pancreatitis, to look for pancreatic necrosis or complications such as pseudocyst formation (see below)

Assessment of severity

An attack of pancreatitis can be divided into mild or severe, depending on several parameters—this has important implications in the management and prognosis of the patient.

A variety of biochemical and objective criteria have been described to stratify patients into mild and severe groups. The Glasgow scoring system discriminates between mild and severe pancreatitis—three or more positive criteria based on initial admission score and subsequent repeat tests over 48 hours, constitute severe disease (see Table 1.4b).

Another simple way to predict severe pancreatitis is to measure the C-reactive protein—this usually rises 2–3 days after the onset of the pancreatitis, but if it rises to >150 mg/l, predicts a severe pancreatitis.

Management of pancreatitis

Mild acute pancreatitis usually runs an uneventful self-limiting course. These patients can be managed by basic monitoring (of pulse, temperature, BP, and urine output), stopping oral intake, and giving IV fluid therapy until the attack subsides, which usually takes 48–72 hours.

If the arterial oxygen saturation (SaO_2) is decreased the arterial blood gasses should be checked (see Section 2).

Severe acute pancreatitis patients should be managed in a High Dependency Unit (HDU) or Intensive Care Unit (ICU). The initial management involves full resuscitation and monitoring of organ function. Occasionally, the inflammation of the pancreas is so great that portions of the pancreas may become ischaemic and necrose (called pancreatic necrosis). A collection of fluid may gather behind the stomach in the lesser sac (pseudocyst).

Secondary infection of areas of fluid collection and pancreatic necrosis leads to abscess formation, and these patients are usually desperately ill. CT scanning should be obtained in patients with severe pancreatitis within 5–10 days following the onset of the attack, to detect pancreatic necrosis. If detected, infected pancreatic necrosis should be managed aggressively with a broad-spectrum antibiotic, draining any abscesses by surgical exploration of the pancreas, and removing the dead bits of pancreas (called necrosectomy).

Failing organs (such as the kidneys and lungs) should be supported artificially (by dialysis or ventilation) until resolution of the pancreatitis. Nutrition should be supplemented during a protracted period of fasting—this should be preferably by nasojejunal feeding (a fine tube is passed via the nose to the first part of the jejunum) to maintain gut mucosal integrity, or by venous catheter.

Further management of the cause of the pancreatitis is then considered. If gallstones are responsible, bile duct clearance and cholecystectomy is indicated (see Biliary section).

Chronic pancreatitis

A continuing inflammatory disease of the pancreas, characterized by repeated attacks of pancreatitis, eventually leading to loss of normal pancreatic function. This is a relatively uncommon condition occurring more often in men. **It is usually caused by alcohol,**

TABLE 1.4b Criteria in the Glasgow scoring system for the initial prediction of severity in acute pancreatitis (more than three criteria constitute severe disease)

Age	>55 years
White blood cell count	>15 × 10⁹/l
Glucose	>10 mmol/l
Urea	>16 mmol/l
PaO₂	<8 kPa (60 mmHg)
Calcium	<2 mmol/l
Albumin	<32 g/l
Lactate dehydrogenase	>600 units/l

Fast facts—Acute pancreatitis (inflammation of the exocrine pancreas)

Aetiology

- Gallstone and alcohol abuse (80%)
- Post-ERCP
- Idiopathic

Pathophysiology

- Digestive enzymes released by injured pancreas
- Release of digestive pancreatic enzymes leads to local inflammation and systemic effects
- Secondary effects:
  - —kidneys: acute tubular necrosis
  - —lungs: $\downarrow pO_2$; right to left shunt
  - —metabolic: $\downarrow$ calcium; $\downarrow$ glucose; $\downarrow$ pH
  - —myocardial depression

Clinical features

- Mild/moderate pancreatitis
  - —upper abdominal/back pain
  - —nausea, vomiting, pyrexia
- Severe pancreatitis
  - —severe pain, hypovolaemia
  - —respiratory, renal, and cardiovascular impairment

Investigations

- Amylase (for diagnosis)
- Severity scoring—C-reactive protein, LFTs, glucose, white cell count, and arterial blood gas (for severity)

Management

- Oxygen
- IV fluids
- Nasogastric tube if vomiting
- Monitor SaO_2 and glucose
- HDU/ITU if severe pancreatitis
- ?ERCP/cholecystectomy if caused by gallstones
- ?Laparotomy and debridement of pancreas if necrotic tissue

Complications

- Renal failure
- Respiratory failure
- Pseudocyst
- Pancreatitic abscess
- Pancreatitic haemorrhage
- Chronic pancreatitis

Prognosis

- 10% mortality with severe pancreatitis

---

although rarer causes include congenital abnormalities, such as annular pancreas.

Clinical features

Pain is the most prominent symptom in the majority of patients. It is usually experienced in the epigastrium and radiates to the back (as it is a retroperitoneal organ). After many years, the pain may burn out when the gland atrophies. Continued alcohol use contributes to the persistence of pain.

Another feature is steatorrhoea (fatty, loose, smelly stool, which is difficult to flush), present in about 50% of patients with chronic pancreatitis. Patients tend to undergo progressive loss of exocrine function (secretion of pancreatic enzymes), leading to fat malabsorption. **Diabetes can occur in about 30% of the patients**, due to loss of endocrine function of the pancreas.

Fibrosis around the chronically inflamed pancreas can thrombose the peripancreatic vessels, including the splenic, superior mesenteric, and portal veins. These veins thrombose leading to an increase in pressure in the portal venous system (**portal hypertension**).

Investigations

- Contrast enhanced CT and ultrasonography provide imaging of the pancreas and the pancreatic duct.
- ERCP outlines the pancreatic duct and its branches showing strictures, dilatation, stone formation, or abnormal anatomy. This investigation may cause an episode of acute pancreatitis.

Management

The main symptom of chronic pancreatitis is pain. Avoidance of alcohol may prevent exacerbations and will reduce the severity of the pain.

Oral pancreatic enzyme supplements have a role in controlling pain in some patients by decreasing pancreatic secretion and reducing pressure in the pancreatic ducts.

Coeliac plexus block (ablation of the splanchnic nerves with alcohol) and splanchicectomy (surgical division of the splanchnic nerves) can provide analgesia of several months' duration.

Pancreatectomy may be used as a last resort in some patients, but results in a difficult to control (brittle) diabetes.

Malabsorption is best managed by calorie supplementation, in addition to calcium and vitamin supplements. Fat and protein malabsorption can be improved by the addition of oral pancreatic enzyme supplements, e.g. creon. These are sprinkled on food prior to eating.

The management of diabetes in chronic pancreatitis is the same as diabetes from other causes. However, carbohydrate restriction is undesirable in view of the malnutrition that is often present.

Carcinoma of the pancreas and ampulla of Vater

Cancer of the pancreas is an aggressive tumour with a poor prognosis. **More than 90% of patients die within one year of diagnosis**. Adjacent tumours, originating from the lower bile duct or from the ampulla, appear to have a better prognosis.

Risk factors

Cigarette smoking is associated with pancreatic carcinoma. Other factors such as diet, coffee, and alcohol consumption are less convincingly linked to pancreatic carcinoma.

Clinical features

Carcinoma of the pancreas can develop in the head, body, or tail. To some extent, the site of origin alters the mode of presentation, though the cardinal features of pain, weight loss, and jaundice are similar.

Pain is the presenting feature in some patients and is commonly dull, boring, and occurs in the epigastric region or back. Patients may also have prominent weight loss. It is generally rapid and progressive and is thought to be due to anorexia.

Jaundice is the presenting feature in up to 65% of patients and occurs at some stage in 90% of patients with carcinoma of the pancreas. Classically, the jaundice is described as painless, in fact is often accompanied by pain in the back. Jaundice is usually progressive until relieved by surgery, stenting, or drainage of the common bile duct. Pruritis often accompanies the jaundice and is caused by the deposition of bile salts under the skin. Jaundice most often occurs with tumours of the head of the pancreas and ampulla, but can be found in patients with tumours of the body and tail due to

hepatic metastases or obstruction of the bile duct by enlarged nodes in the porta hepatis.

Examination

Examination of the patient may reveal jaundice, caused by obstruction of the common bile duct by the tumour. The liver may be enlarged by metastases to the liver. A palpable gall bladder (**Courvoisier's sign**: a palpable gall bladder in the presence of jaundice) is often found, and is caused by the obstruction of the biliary tree and dilation of the gall bladder by obstructed bile.

Tumours of the body and tail of the pancreas often present with signs of distant spread such as hepatic metastases or ascites.

Investigation

In pancreatic cancer, investigation has three roles:

- to establish a definite diagnosis of pancreatic malignancy

- to determine whether resectional surgery is possible

- to select the best palliative therapy.

The following investigations should be undertaken:

- *CT scanning*. This gives information about the size and site of the primary tumour, the biliary and pancreatic ductal diameters, the presence or absence of lymph node or hepatic metastatic disease and the proximity of the disease to major vessels (such as the portal vein) (Fig. 1.4d). The CT scan should also include the chest to look for pulmonary metastases.

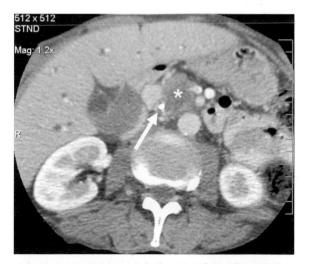

Fig 1.4d CT scan of the pancreas showing a pancreatic cancer adjacent to superior messenteric vessels (asterix) and the presence of a common bile duct stent (arrowed) placed to allow bile drainage and the relief of jaundice.

◆ *ERCP or percutaneous transhepatic cholangiography* (placing a needle into a dilated bile duct percutaneously via the liver) outlines the common bile duct and pancreatic duct directly. These investigations confirm the level of obstruction and exclude coincidental pathology and multiple obstructions.

Treatment

Surgery remains the only prospect of cure in this disease. However, this treatment is undertaken at the expense of considerable morbidity and some mortality, and careful preoperative assessment is required.

Curative surgery should be undertaken in patients less than 70 years old, with small tumours (less than 3 cm in diameter), with no evidence of local spread, vascular invasion, or metastatic disease.

A diagnostic laparoscopy (inserting a telescope into the abdomen via the umbilicus under a general anaesthetic) is usually performed initially to exclude small liver or peritoneal metastases not seen on CT scan. If this is clear then pancreaticoduodenectomy (Whipple's operation) with lymph node clearance should be undertaken for tumours of the head of the pancreas and ampullary tumours. Distal pancreatectomy is uncommonly performed for body and tail of pancreas cancers, as these are usually advanced tumours at presentation.

Palliation of symptoms should be considered for all patients unfit for surgery and those with advanced unresectable cancer. Obstructive jaundice can be relieved either by placing a stent (a plastic or metal tube) into the common bile duct to drain the bile into the duodenum—this is done by ERCP (Fig. 1.4e) or percutaneous transhepatic cholangiography.

If that fails then the common bile duct can be drained surgically. This is done by anastomosing a loop of jejunum to the dilated gall bladder (cholecysto-jejunostomy) or common bile duct (choledochojejunostomy). Obstruction of the duodenum by invading pancreatic cancer can be relieved by a gastroenterostomy (anastomosing a loop of jejunum to the stomach, bypassing the obstructed duodenum).

Prognosis

The prognosis of pancreatic cancer is poor with an 8% 5-year survival of patients treated by curative surgery and an average survival of 6 months in patients with cancer managed by palliation. The prognosis of cancer of the ampulla of Vater is significantly better with a 5-year survival of 35%.

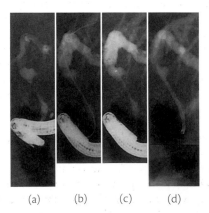

Fig 1.4e Intubation of a biliary stricture: (a) cholangiogram showing the obstruction; (b) cannula below the stricture and the guidewire across the stricture; (c) cannula and guidewire both across the stricture; and (d) stent 'railroaded' into place.

Fast facts—Pancreatic cancer (malignant disease of the pancreas)

Epidemiology

◆ M/F 2:1, age 50–70
◆ Risk factors
◆ Smoking/?alcohol

Pathology

◆ Adenocarcinoma—60% head, 25% body, 15% tail

Clinical features—can present with:

◆ Abnormal weight loss or back pain
◆ Jaundice
◆ Duodenal obstruction
◆ Malignant ascites

Investigations

◆ CT scan abdomen and chest—to assess for local spread by tumour and pulmonary metastases
◆ ERCP—for cytology and biliary stenting
◆ Laparoscopy—to assess for peritoneal seedlings

Management

◆ Stenting of obstructed duct
◆ Gastrojejunostomy for duodenal obstruction
◆ Pancreatectomy for localized tumours

Prognosis

◆ 90% mortality within 1 year (if not resected)

Disorders of the biliary system

Scenario 1: repeated right upper abdominal pain

A 53-year-old woman reports to her GP with repeated episodes of upper abdominal pain. These have affected her for the past 6 months and often come on in the evening after a meal. Further enquiry determines that the pain is principally in the epigastrium and beneath the right subcostal margin.

This patient appears to be describing repeated episodes of biliary colic caused by gallstones, which block off the cystic duct where it drains the gall bladder, leading to pain. **This classically is described as intermittent episodes of biliary colic and presents as epigastric/right upper quadrant pain, which comes on 2–3 hours after a meal and lasts for up to 6–8 hours.**

The pain is colicky, with each episode of colic lasting for about 30 minutes and the episodes of colic last for about 6–8 hours. The pain radiates between the shoulder blades. Nausea and belching without sickness accompany each episode.

Biliary colic differs from small bowel colic in that the waves of colic last for longer (many minutes) than small bowel colic (a few seconds).

She has not noticed any jaundice or change in colour of her stools or urine.

There are no features in the history to suggest episodes of obstructive jaundice caused by common bile duct stones.

She is overweight. No abnormalities are evident on abdominal examination, and she is apyrexial.

Between episodes of pain, physical examination in patients with symptomatic gallstones is usually normal. Gallstones (cholelithiasis) are associated with overweight females.

An ultrasound scan showed multiple gallstones with no gall bladder wall thickening. The intra- and extrahepatic biliary tree was not dilated and her LFTs were normal.

The most important diagnostic tests are an ultrasound examination of the liver, pancreas, and biliary tree together with LFTs.

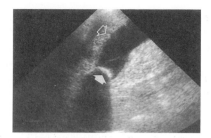

Fig 1.4f1 An acutely inflamed thick walled gallbladder (open arrow) with a large stone (closed arrow) impacted in Hartmann's pouch.

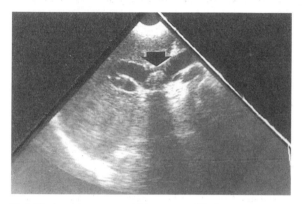

Fig 1.4f2 A very large stone within common bile duct.

An ultrasound scan is the key investigation (Fig. 1.4f1, 1.4f2). In this case the findings confirm the diagnosis of gallstones. Thickening of the gall bladder wall suggests episodes of inflammation (cholecystitis), which was not evident with this patient. In addition, patients with cholecystitis usually have a low-grade pyrexia, as opposed to biliary colic when there is no inflammation in the gall bladder.

As the LFTs are normal, the biliary tree is not dilated, and she has no history of pancreatitis, it is unlikely that she has associated common bile duct stones. The history and ultrasound findings suggest biliary colic, which is best treated by removal of the gall bladder (cholecystectomy). This patient's symptoms were completely resolved following an elective laparoscopic cholecystectomy.

Scenario 2: upper abdominal pain and vomiting

A 50-year-old woman is referred by her GP to the surgical admissions unit in the early hours of the morning with a history of upper abdominal pain and vomiting. This was the second time within a week that he had been called to see this patient with the same symptoms.

Abdominal pain and vomiting are common presenting problems. Although a careful history and examination will point towards the most likely diagnosis all these patients should undergo a screen of basic diagnostic tests at the time of admission to ensure that an important differential diagnosis is not overlooked.

> The patient describes the pain as abrupt in onset, mainly in the right upper quadrant with radiation around her costal margin and to her shoulder blade. It is worse if she tries to take a deep breath. The pain has usually lasted several hours in the past before it subsides. This episode has been more severe; she has been sick several times and feels hot.

Constant right upper quadrant pain radiating to the shoulder blade with pyrexia points to a diagnosis of acute cholecystitis. The cause of acute cholecystitis is usually gallstones. The stones impact in the neck of the gall bladder. This causes smooth muscle spasm, acute chemical inflammation of the gall bladder and bacterial infection of the obstructed gall bladder may follow.

Gram-negative bacteria such as *Escherichia coli* are the most common infecting organism in acute cholecystitis. The inflammatory process with or without infection makes the patient feel unwell with loss of appetite.

> The patient looks flushed and has a pulse rate of 120/min. Her temperature is 38.5°C. On examination she is generally tender in her upper abdomen especially in the right upper quadrant. On inspiration with the hand trying to palpate the liver edge she gasps.

Tenderness below the right ribs is a consistent finding in cholecystitis. When the inflammation extends to the outer covering of the gall bladder, localized peritonism develops affecting the abdominal peritoneum resulting in guarding, rigidity, and rebound tenderness.

Murphy's sign (suddenly catching her breath during inspiration with right upper quadrant palpation) is not diagnostic but reflects localized peritonism and may be the result of other conditions (such as a perforated duodenal ulcer). With the development of localized peritonitis the patient may complain of shoulder tip pain, due to referred pain from irritation of the diaphragm.

> The patient's temperature climbs to 39.5°C and she vomits several times.

After taking blood cultures this patient should be started on broad-spectrum IV antibiotics, which is effective against coliform organisms. Often patients with acute cholecystitis are more comfortable if oral intake is withheld, resting the gastrointestinal tract. IV fluid replacement will need to take into account any extra fluid losses caused by fever and vomiting.

> The diagnosis is confirmed the following day by an ultrasound of the abdomen. Multiple gallstones are identified in a swollen gall bladder with a thickened wall. The common bile duct is not dilated. 24 hours later the patient undergoes a laparoscopic cholecystectomy and makes an uneventful recovery.

Biliary colic should not be confused with acute cholecystitis. If the stone remains impacted, acute cholecystitis may follow. The severe pain starts abruptly, often after a fatty meal. It lasts for several hours often radiating through to the back, with sweating and vomiting. There is usually no pyrexia with biliary colic. With cholecystitis the gall bladder wall is usually thickened by repeated attacks of infection. With biliary colic the gall bladder wall is generally not thickened. Antibiotics are not required for biliary colic.

Despite the clinical picture there are other important diseases that may be mistaken for an acute cholecystitis. Most can be eliminated by some simple tests:

Clinical key points in gallstone disease

- Ask about abdominal pain—biliary colic presents as epigastric/right upper quadrant pain, which comes on 2–3 hours after a meal and lasts for up to 6–8 hours

- Infection in the gall bladder (cholecystitis) presents with pyrexia and right upper quadrant pain

- Ask the patient about previous episodes and whether they have ever been jaundiced (caused by a gallstone getting stuck in the common bile duct) or had episodes of fevers or rigors

- Examine the patient for signs of jaundice, check the temperature and pulse. Examine the abdomen for right upper quadrant tenderness or possibly a mass in the right upper quadrant

- A biliary ultrasound is the key investigation—this looks for gallstones in the gall bladder, thickening of the wall of the gall bladder (suggesting inflammation), and the diameter of the common bile duct

♦ *erect CXR*—this will detect a right basal pneumonia, or subdiaphragmatic gas from a perforated viscus

♦ *serum amylase*—this will diagnose pancreatitis. Remember gallstones cause one-third of all attacks of pancreatitis so this is an important test

♦ *ECG*—sometimes a myocardial infarction will present with upper abdominal pain.

Background: biliary tract

The biliary tract is a tree-like structure that transports bile from the liver to the duodenum. Bile is stored and released on demand in the gall bladder. Bile assists in the digestion of fats and the absorption of fats and fat soluble vitamins.

Conditions:

♦ asymptomatic gallstones

♦ symptomatic gallstones

♦ complications of gallstones.

Gallstone disease

Gallstones, or cholelithiasis, is an extremely common problem—**up to 30% of people over the age of 70 have gallstones**. The most common type of gallstone is composed of cholesterol. However, in some disease processes, pigment or mixed gallstones can be formed. Cholesterol gallstones are primarily caused by abnormally high secretion rates of cholesterol into bile relative to phospholipids and bile salts, producing supersaturation of bile with cholesterol. **Obesity, female gender, pregnancy, and ageing** are recognized risk factors for cholesterol gallstone formation.

Cholelithiasis may be divided into three clinical groups: asymptomatic, symptomatic, and complicated.

Asymptomatic cholelithiasis

This is very common. **Eighty per cent of subjects with gallstones remain asymptomatic**. As a result, no rationale exists for treating asymptomatic cholelithiasis in order to prevent complications. Watchful waiting is a safe strategy in this group.

Symptomatic cholelithiasis

The typical symptom of symptomatic cholelithiasis is biliary colic. This is a pain, which increases in intensity over 20–30 minutes, then subsides to a dull, less severe pain. The pain is typically in the right upper quadrant radiating round the chest wall to the back and right shoulder. The mechanism of the pain is that a gallstone is trapped in the neck of the gall bladder. Severe muscular contractions of the gall bladder wall try to move the stone. These muscular contractions cause severe pain described as colic.

Biliary colic is best treated by laparoscopic cholecystectomy to remove the gall bladder—the patient should be warned at the time of consent that there is a 5% chance of needing to convert from laparoscopic to open surgery, due to unforeseen circumstances, such as difficult anatomy.

Complications of cholelithiasis

Most patients with complications of gallstones (cholecystitis, empyema, or mucocoele of the gall bladder) require a cholecystectomy:

1. *Acute cholecystitis.* Cystic duct obstruction by an impacted gallstone initiates the process. Bacteria may be subsequently involved in maintaining the inflammatory process. The usual organisms involved are Gram-negative bacilli, typically *E. coli* or *Klebsiella*. The condition usually presents with constant right upper quadrant pain with a fever and leucocytosis.

   Diagnosis is confirmed at abdominal ultrasound by finding gallstones in a thick-walled gall bladder with tenderness over the gall bladder under the examining ultrasound probe.

   Management of these patients consists of antibiotics usually directed against Gram-negative bacilli (e.g. amoxicillin + clavulanic acid) and cholecystectomy at the earliest opportunity.

2. *Mucocoele of the gall bladder.* Cystic duct obstruction with inflammation in the gall bladder wall induces the gall bladder mucous membrane to secrete mucous. This accumulates in the obstructed gall bladder causing severe constant pain with local peritonism. Systemically, the patient may have a fever and leucocytosis. The distended gall bladder is viewed ultrasonographically and found to contain echogenic gallstones. Treatment is again by antibiotics and early cholecystectomy.

3. *Empyema of gall bladder.* When the obstructed gall bladder, filled with mucus, is secondarily infected and the mucous becomes pyogenic. The patient usually has systemic signs of sepsis, which may include rigors, or even septic shock. The management consists of resuscitation of the usually seriously ill patient with IV fluids and antibiotics.

   Urgent ultrasonography is required, followed by cholecystectomy, to remove the source of sepsis. Occasionally, the patient requires a cholecystectomy but is not fit—in this situation, the gall bladder is drained by inserting a tube into the gall bladder (either radiologically or surgically under local anaesthetic)—called a cholecystostomy. This drains the pus in the gall bladder.

4. *Choledocholithiasis* (stones in the common bile duct) (see also Jaundice section). When the cystic duct is wide or the stones very small, the gallstones within the gall bladder can slip into the common bile duct. Most small stones pass from the common bile duct through the ampulla of Vater and into the duodenum undetected. Larger stones may impact in the ampulla of Vater or cause oedema as they pass through and hence block the pancreatic duct causing acute pancreatitis.

The stones may also block the common bile duct, leading to obstructive jaundice (see Liver section). Bile within the obstructed bile duct may become secondarily infected causing cholangitis (inflammation of the bile duct). Patients with cholangitis have three signs (Charcot's triad):

  ◆ jaundice

  ◆ right upper quadrant pain

  ◆ rigors.

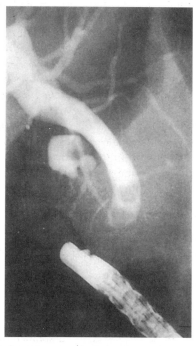

Fig 1.4g Endoscopic retrograde cholangiogram showing stones in the common bile duct. This patient has had a previous polya partial gastrectomy so that the endoscope approaches the ampulla backwards from the duodenojejunal flexure along the third part of the duodenum.

Patients with cholangitis (inflammation of the common bile duct) generally have jaundice, right upper quadrant pain, and rigors. These patients are ill and require careful fluid resuscitation, IV antibiotics, urgent removal of the stones from the common bile duct, and drainage of the biliary tree, usually by ERCP.

Drainage by ERCP and sphincterotomy (dividing the sphincter of Oddi at the ampulla, to allow gallstones to pass into the duodenum). Elective cholecystectomy can then be carried out to remove the source of the gallstones, unless surgery is contraindicated by other comorbid risks.

If ERCP is unsuccessful, then the patient requires a cholecystectomy and exploration of the common bile duct. At this operation, gallstones are removed from the bile duct surgically, and a T-tube left in the common bile duct, in addition to removal of the gall bladder. The T-tube allows for an X-ray to be done postoperatively (called a T-tube cholangiogram) to check that the gallstones have been cleared from the duct.

ERCP (Fig. 1.4g) is a useful therapeutic investigation and the common bile duct may be cleared by removal of common bile duct stones, or drained by placing a stent into the duct. However, it can cause pancreatitis, which can be severe and hence ERCP should be reserved for therapeutic interventions, rather than as a diagnostic tool, when MRI scanning of the common bile ducts (magnetic resonance cholangiopancreatography) should be used (see Jaundice section, pp. 64–72).

5. *Gallstone ileus.* Rarely, a large gallstone can erode through the wall of the gall bladder into the duodenum (causing a fistula to the duodenum). This large gallstone can migrate down the small bowel, but get stuck at the small diameter of the distal ileum, causing a small bowel obstruction, which is called (wrongly) gallstone ileus. A plain abdominal film will show dilated small bowel loops and may also show gas in the biliary tree, caused by air passing from the duodenum through the fistula into the gall bladder.

Jaundice

Scenario: abdominal pain and jaundice

A 78-year-old man is admitted with a 4-day history of increasing jaundice, dark urine, and pale stool. He also complains of right upper quadrant pain and episodes of shivery turns at home.

Fast facts—Gallstone disease (stone forming within the biliary tree)

Epidemiology

◆ M/F 1:2, 30% of population >70

◆ Risk factors include obesity, female, pregnancy, and ageing

Pathology

◆ Stone obstruction at GB neck + infection/cholecystitis

◆ Stone passing through ampulla/pancreatitis

◆ Obstruction of common bile duct + infection/cholangitis

Clinical features

◆ Recurrent right upper quadrant pain and vomiting

◆ May have pancreatitis

◆ May have jaundice, caused by stone in common bile duct

Investigations

◆ U&E, FBC, LFTs, clotting

◆ Ultrasound

◆ ERCP/magnetic resonance cholangio-pancreatography

Management

◆ Laparoscopic cholecystectomy

◆ ERCP to extract stones in the common bile duct

On examination he has a tachycardia, obvious jaundice, a dry tongue, and tenderness in the right upper quadrant.

Patients with cholangitis can be very unwell with severe sepsis and require appropriate fluid resuscitation and IV antibiotics (e.g. amoxycillin + clavulanic acid, to cover *E. coli* and *Klebsiella*). **Examination will reveal tenderness in the right upper quadrant and jaundice.**

The patient's LFTs, amylase, U&Es, and coagulation are checked. After fluid resuscitation and IV antibiotics are given an ultrasound is performed, which shows a dilated common bile duct (15 mm, rather than the normal 7 mm) with gallstones in the gall bladder and a normal looking pancreas.

LFTs confirm the obstructive jaundice and give a baseline for the severity of the jaundice. Pancreatitis is excluded by checking the serum amylase and the patient may be dehydrated, as shown by a raised urea and/or creatinine. **Blood should also be sent for virology to exclude an infective cause.**

The prothrombin time (INR) **may be raised as fat-soluble vitamin K is not absorbed in obstructive jaundice**—if the INR is raised, then the patient is given parenteral vitamin K to correct the coagulation defect, prior to any surgical procedure, to reduce the chance of bleeding.

Ultrasound of the biliary tree is the initial investigation of choice. A gallstone stuck in the common bile duct would seem to be the cause of this man's jaundice, as he has gallstones in the gall bladder, and there was no obvious mass in the head of the pancreas (carcinoma of the head of the pancreas can present with obstructive jaundice).

At this stage the patient undergoes an ERCP (see below).

ERCP reveals gallstones in the common bile duct and these are removed by cutting the sphincter at the bottom end of the bile duct (called a sphincterotomy), which opens up the bile duct and allows the stones to be pulled out of the bile duct by a basket and into the duodenum, from where they are eventually safely passed in the stool.

The history of jaundice, dark urine, and pale stool points towards obstruction of the common bile duct. Bilirubin is not passed down the bile duct (causing pale stool) and the bilirubin is deposited in tissues, including the sclera and conjunctiva, resulting in yellow pigmentation: jaundice. The raised conjugated bilirubin in the blood is excreted by the kidneys, causing dark urine. The additional symptoms of right upper quadrant pain and shivery turns (rigors—an indication of severe systemic infection) are classical for cholangitis (Charcot's triad).

If the stones cannot be removed, a stent can be inserted into the common bile duct to allow drainage of the bile past the stones. At this age (78) there is a good chance that the patient will have no further attacks of cholangitis, particularly as the lower end of the bile duct has been widened by the sphincterotomy, and cholecystectomy, to remove the source of the gallstones, is not usually indicated. Younger (usually aged <70) patients tend to undergo cholecystectomy, provided that they are otherwise fit enough.

Clinical key points in jaundice

- Ask about change in colour of the skin, urine, and stool—increasing jaundice, dark urine, and pale stool point to obstructive jaundice, which generally has a surgically treatable cause

- Ask about abdominal pain and any history of shivery turns—right upper quadrant pain, jaundice, and rigors (Charcot's triad) point to cholangitis

- Examine the patient for jaundice, and signs of right upper quadrant tenderness and possible mass. Painless jaundice and a palpable distended gall bladder is a worrying sign of possible malignant obstruction of the common bile duct (e.g. by pancreatic cancer)

- Blood should be sent for virology to exclude an infective cause

- Always check the clotting in patients with jaundice, as vitamin K is not absorbed if bile is not getting into the small bowel, leading to a prolonged INR

- The key initial investigation is a biliary ultrasound, to see whether the common bile duct is dilated and if gallstones are present. If the common bile duct is dilated then further investigations with ERCP, CT, or MRI will be required

Background: jaundice

- Jaundice is the development of a yellow green discoloration due to the accumulation of bilirubin in the skin and tissues.

- Bilirubin is one of the end products of the breakdown of haem coming from haemoglobin and myoglobin.

Bilirubin metabolism and the enterohepatic circulation

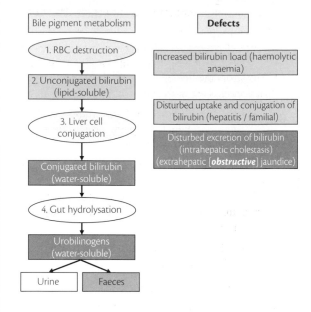

1. Following the breakdown of red blood cells in the reticuloendothelial system, haem is degraded to produce biliverdin. Biliverdin is then converted into bilirubin

2. Unconjugated bilirubin is released into the blood, tightly bound to albumin. This unconjugated bilirubin is water insoluble but lipid soluble, and consequently cannot be filtered by the glomerulus and does not appear in urine

3. Unconjugated bilirubin is taken up by hepatocytes, where it is conjugated. Conjugation makes bilirubin water soluble and, consequently, this form of bilirubin can be filtered by the glomerulus and can appear in urine. However, under normal circumstances bilirubin enters the small intestine via the biliary tract. In the lumen of the distal ileum and colon, bilirubin is hydrolysed to form unconjugated bilirubin, which is then reduced by gut bacteria to urobilinogens. Part of this is excreted in the faeces, giving the stool the characteristic brown colour. In obstructive jaundice this mechanism is interrupted and this explains why the urine is dark (due to excess conjugated bilirubin in the urine) and the stool pale (due to no bile salts in the bowel). In addition the patient may complain of itch (pruritus), which is caused by deposition of the bile salts in the skin

Classification of jaundice

The conventional classification is into three types: pre-hepatic, hepatic, and posthepatic (cholestatic) jaundice.

1. *Prehepatic*. Total serum bilirubin levels are increased but the levels of the transaminases and alkaline phosphatase are normal. The circulating serum bilirubin is largely unconjugated. The cause may be:

   ◆ overproduction of bilirubin (presentation to liver, which exceeds hepatic capacity for uptake and conjugation) as in haemolysis.

2. *Hepatic*. The jaundice usually comes on rapidly. There may be systemic upset and varying degrees of hepatic failure. Serum biochemistry shows increases in transaminases (alanine transaminase and aspartamine transaminase). The cause may be:

   ◆ hepatocellular dysfunction due to hepatitis (viral, alcohol, drugs), or cirrhosis

   ◆ hereditary: Gilberts syndrome.

3. *Posthepatic (cholestatic)*. This is due to failure of adequate amounts of bile to reach the duodenum. There is a rise in serum conjugated bilirubin and alkaline phosphatase. **The cause is usually due to obstruction of the bile duct, by either gallstones or carcinoma of the bile ducts (cholangiocarcinoma) or of the head of the pancreas.** The gallstones found in the common bile duct come from the gall bladder via the cystic duct. Primary common bile duct stones are very rare. Occasionally, the bile duct may be compressed from outwith the duct (called extrinsic compression), caused by metastatic lymph nodes enlarged at the porta hepatitis where the bile duct enters the liver or is affected by a sclerosing (tissue hardening) process within the liver, squeezing the intrahepatic bile ducts.

Approach to the diagnosis of jaundice

A careful history and physical examination with routine biochemical and haematological tests are essential. The history should include travel, family, and drug history. The urine should be tested for bilirubin and urobilinogen (see above). The place of special tests such as ultrasonography, CT, ERCP, or liver biopsy will depend on the features of the jaundice.

Obstructive jaundice

This is posthepatic or cholestatic jaundice in which there is obstruction to the flow of bile from the biliary tree into the intestines. The principal causes of this are:

◆ gallstones (choledocholithiasis), either primary (formed in the bile ducts) or more usually secondary to stone migration from the gall bladder

◆ cancer of the head of the pancreas occluding the lower end of the common bile duct

◆ cancer of the bile ducts occluding the lumen of the bile duct at the site of the tumour

◆ secondary hepatic deposits or lymph node enlargement in the porta hepatis compressing the bile duct.

Clinical presentation

The patients present with jaundice with a variable pain component. In general, obstructive jaundice caused by gallstones is accompanied by pain, while jaundice associated with malignancy is more likely to be painless. Typically, patients will have pale stools and dark urine. In some, steatorrhoea (fatty offensive stools) may be troublesome. Some patients may report fever and chills if cholangitis is present. Pruritus is a particularly distressing complaint in patients with obstructive jaundice.

Physical examination may additionally reveal an **enlarged gall bladder**, caused by the obstructed biliary tree with subsequent distension of the gall bladder (**Corvoisier's sign**) or hepatic masses.

Urine testing shows a raised bilirubin and absent urobilinogen. Serum biochemistry demonstrates markedly elevated levels of alkaline phosphatase and gamma-glutamyltranspeptidase, which remain elevated until the obstruction is removed or bypassed. The transaminases may be transiently and mildly elevated. Owing to malabsorption of the fat-soluble vitamins, a prolonged INR may be found if vitamin K stores are depleted.

Classically obstructive jaundice presents with increasing jaundice, dark urine, pale stools, and itchy skin (pruritus). 'Surgical' causes of jaundice are obstructive.

Diagnosis

Ultrasound should be the first line of investigation and may demonstrate a dilated biliary tree, gallstones, a mass in the head of the pancreas, or hepatic deposits. ERCP is extremely useful in diagnosing the cause and level of the obstruction. In addition, the bile duct can be cleared of stones or stented to allow drainage of the bile.

More recently, MRI has been adapted to provide detailed contrast imaging of the biliary and pancreatic duct in addition to providing assessment of the rest of the abdomen. Currently, MRI should be used for diagnosing the problem and ERCP should be used as a therapy (either clearing or stenting the duct). Remember that ERCP can have its problems—particularly post-ERCP pancreatitis. Laparoscopy, intraoperative contact ultrasonography, or endoscopic ultrasound may be indicated in staging patients with malignant bile duct obstruction.

Complications and their management

1. *Cholangitis.* Patients with obstructive jaundice require urgent investigation and management before bile in the obstructed biliary tree becomes infected, as cholangitis has additional morbidity and mortality.

   If cholangitis is present, the management becomes more urgent. These patients are usually seriously ill and require hydration, antibiotics, and intensive monitoring. Urgent drainage of the biliary tree is essential endoscopically or percutaneously. When cholangitis has resolved definitive treatment by surgery can be contemplated, e.g. cholecystectomy to remove the source of the gallstones.

2. *Fat-soluble vitamin malabsorption (A, D, E, K).* In general, patients should be given vitamin K parenterally to correct their coagulopathy.

3. *Hepato-renal syndrome.* Adequate hydration and the possible use of osmotic diuresis is indicated to avoid hepato-renal syndrome, which occurs when inadequately fluid resuscitated patients with jaundice develop acute renal failure. If surgery is contemplated antibiotic prophylaxis is essential.

Fast facts—Obstructive jaundice (accumulation of bilirubin)

Causes

- Gallstones in the common bile duct
- Malignant stricture of common bile duct (cholangiocarcinoma)
- Common bile duct obstruction by cancer of the head of the pancreas
- Extrinsic compression of the common bile duct by metastatic lymph nodes at the porta hepatitis

Clinical features

- Increasing jaundice, dark urine, pale stool
- Jaundice, right upper quadrant pain, and rigors/pyrexia (Charcot's triad) = cholangitis = ill patient
- Hepatomegaly or palpable gall bladder may be present

Investigations

- U&Es, FBC, LFTs, amylase, INR
- Ultrasound scan to look for gallstones and common bile duct diameter (? dilated)
- MRI/ERCP—to clear stones in common bile duct or insert stent if malignant cause for obstruction

Treatment

- IV fluids to maintain hydration
- Correct clotting abnormalities
- Antibiotics if cholangitis
- ERCP
- Consider cholecystectomy if gallstones the cause
- Consider surgery if malignant cause found

Background: liver

The liver is the largest solid organ of the body. It is situated under the right diaphragm in the right upper outer quadrant of the abdomen. Its function is many fold including: detoxification, synthetic, metabolic, and immune functions.

Conditions:

- cirrhosis
- portal hypertension
- tumours of the liver.

Cirrhosis

Cirrhosis is a diffuse process in the liver and results from the death of hepatic cells, followed by fibrosis/scarring and the conversion of normal liver architecture into structurally abnormal nodules. The condition may be associated with failure in the function of hepatic cells and interference with blood flow in the liver. This results in:

- portal hypertension and varices
- ascites
- jaundice
- hepatic encephalopathy
- ultimately hepatic failure.

Causes of cirrhosis

1. *Common*:

    ◆ alcohol.

2. *Rare*:

    ◆ viral hepatitis (B, C, D, and others)

    ◆ metabolic causes including iron overload (haemochromatosis), copper overload (Wilson's disease), cystic fibrosis

    ◆ biliary disease, including extrahepatic and intrahepatic biliary obstruction, as well as childhood biliary diseases.

Clinical features

Generalized non-specific symptoms such as fatigue, anorexia, malaise, weight loss, and muscle wasting are common. Patients may present with gastrointestinal bleeding, which may be from varices, or associated peptic ulcer disease. The bleeding may be made worse by associated thrombocytopenia, leucopenia, or impaired coagulation secondary to the liver disease itself.

Signs of portal hypertension (including ascites, splenomegaly, caput medusae) and jaundice may also be present.

Dermatological manifestations include spider telangiectasis, palmar erythema, finger clubbing, Dupuytren's contractures, gynaecomastia, and scanty body hair (the last two caused by raised oestrogen levels).

Late stage neurological features include hepatic encephalopathy (including a flapping tremor), and peripheral neuropathy.

Diagnosis

◆ *Laboratory evaluation*:

- hepatocellular damage, leading to raised levels of aminotransferases

- cholestasis (sluggish bile excretion) with raised levels of alkaline phosphatase, serum bilirubin, gamma glutamyltranspeptidase

- reduced hepatic synthetic function with low serum albumin and prolonged prothrombin time (INR)

- aetiological tests including viral serology, ceruloplasmin (Wilson's disease), alpha-1 antitrypsin level and protease inhibitor type, serum immunoglobulins, and autoantibodies: antinuclear antibodies, antimitochondrial antibodies, and antismooth muscle antibody

- screening tests for hepatocellular carcinoma: alphafetoprotein is a tumour cell marker for hepatocellular carcinoma (also called hepatoma).

◆ *Investigations*:

- abdominal ultrasound can easily detect ascites, biliary dilatation, and hepatic masses. Used in the colour Doppler mode, it can assess hepatic and portal vein patency and blood flow.

- liver biopsy—this is the 'gold standard' for the diagnosis of cirrhosis. **Every patient suspected of cirrhosis should have a liver biopsy to establish the presence of cirrhosis, aid in the determination of the aetiology of cirrhosis, and provide an assessment of the activity of cirrhosis.**

Management

◆ General management focuses on treatment of complications that arise in the setting of cirrhosis such as variceal haemorrhage, hepatic encephalopathy, ascites, and spontaneous bacterial peritonitis.

◆ Screening for hepatocellular carcinoma with serial ultrasound examinations at regular intervals, and serum alpha-fetoprotein measurement in selected patients such as those with chronic hepatitis B, C, and haemochromatosis.

◆ Liver transplantation can be considered in appropriate candidates.

Prognosis

This depends mainly on the development of cirrhosis-related complications. The Child–Pugh modification of the Child's classification is helpful in assessing survival (Table 1.4c1 and 2).

Class C has the worst outlook, though a precise prognosis for an individual patient may be difficult to predict.

TABLE 1.4c1   Child-Pugh classification of liver disease

Parameter	Numerical score		
	1	2	3
Ascites	None	Slight	Moderate/severe
Encephalopathy	None	Slight/moderate	Moderate/severe
Bilirubin (mg/dl)	<2.0	2–3	>3.0
Albumin (mg/dl)	>3.5	2.8–3.5	<2.8
Prothrombin time increased in seconds	1–3	4–6	>6.0

TABLE 1.4c2   Severity score

Total numerical score	Child–Pugh class
5–6	A
7–9	B
10–15	C

Portal hypertension

Portal hypertension, an increase in the portal venous pressure, is caused by obstruction to the portal blood flow at various sites (see Classification table 1.4d). This raised pressure is decompressed by the formation of abnormal direct connections between the portal venous and systemic venous systems (portosystemic collaterals) and dilated portal veins at the areas of portosystemic anastomoses—e.g. the lower oesophagus where the dilated veins are called oesophageal varices. These varices can also occur less commonly at the umbilicus and anus.

Classification

Just as with the classification of jaundice this scheme is based on the location of the block to portal blood flow, which is responsible for the increased pressure, and is usually divided into prehepatic, hepatic, and posthepatic causes of the portal hypertension (see Table 1.4d).

Clinical consequences of portal hypertension

* *Gastro-oesophageal varices*. Found in the lower oesophagus and the fundus of the stomach. They can be a major cause of significant or even life-threatening haematemesis.

* *Ascites*. This is an accumulation of fluid in the peritoneal cavity. This results from several factors includ-

TABLE 1.4d   Causes of portal hypertension

Prehepatic	Intrahepatic	Posthepatic
Portal vein thrombosis	All causes of cirrhosis	Hepatic vein thrombosis (Budd–Chiari syndrome)
	Chronic or acute viral hepatitis	
	Primary biliary cirrhosis (in the early stages)	
	Sarcoidosis	
	Schistosomiasis	
	Congenital hepatic fibrosis	

ing: exudate from the inflamed liver, and an abnormal production and sensitivity to various fluid retaining hormones and factors.

* *Congestive splenomegaly*. This results from an increase in the portal venous pressure causing resistance to blood flow in the splenic vein. This back pressure causes the spleen to enlarge progressively.

* *Hepatic encephalopathy*. As a result of the portal blood being diverted from the liver into the systemic circulation, hepatic detoxification is inadequate.

Management

The majority of active treatment centres around the management of the above complications. Severe variceal bleeding requires sclerotherapy (where a highly irritant liquid is injected into the varices to cause them to thrombose) or banding (where a rubber band is used to occlude the variceal vessels). The second short-term option is to compress the bleeding vessels with a balloon in the upper stomach and lower oesophagus.

The elective intervention is to create a track between the portal and systemic venous circulation. This is done by passing a percutaneous stent from the hepatic vein (entered by the internal jugular) to the portal vein through the substance of the liver. This technique is called transjugular intrahepatic portosystemic shunt (TIPSS).

Benign tumours of the liver

Hepatocellular adenoma is a rare benign proliferation of hepatocytes associated with the use of the oral contraceptive pill. Patients typically present with right upper quadrant pain. They may be single or multiple, and are usually more than 5 cm in diameter before they cause symptoms. The diagnosis can be confirmed by CT. Adenomas may rupture causing haemoperitoneum (blood in the peritoneal cavity). Treatment includes discontinuation of the oral contraceptive pill and surgical resection.

Liver malignancies
Metastatic disease

The liver is **a common site for metastases** from a variety of tumours and is usually detected on ultrasound scan or CT scan (Fig. 1.4h). **Metastases are by far the commonest form of hepatic malignancy**. The most frequent sites of origin for hepatic metastases are lung, gastrointestinal tract, breast, and genitourinary tract. Owing to the high incidence of colorectal cancer, liver metastases from these primary foci are the most commonly treated. Partial hepatic resection may be considered for metastases confined to a single hepatic lobe.

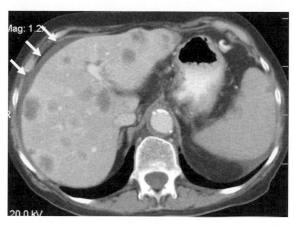

Fig 1.4h CT scan showing hepatic metastases (from a carcinoma of the pancreas) and perihepatic fluid (arrowed).

If the metastases are spread throughout the liver, then palliative treatment, such as radiofrequency ablation, 'freezing' the tumours (called cryotherapy), or chemotherapy, may be used.

Hepatocellular carcinoma (HCC—also called hepatoma)

This is one of the most common malignancies world wide due to its high incidence in the Chinese subcontinent and in sub-Saharan Africa. More common in males, a number of risk factors have been identified for this tumour: cirrhosis (of any cause); chronic hepatitis B and C; and carcinogens, e.g. aflatoxin.

- *Clinical features.* Abdominal pain (discomfort) and weight loss are the common presenting symptoms. HCC may occasionally rupture and the patient presents acutely with haemoperitoneum (blood in the peritoneal cavity). Some patients may be asymptomatic and the tumour is discovered incidentally or during screening of at-risk subjects. HCC may also be associated with non-metastatic manifestations including hypoglycaemia, hypercholesterolaemia, or feminization.

- *Diagnosis.* Ultrasound and CT are the mainstay of diagnosis, together with a raised level of serum alpha-fetoprotein, a tumour cell marker.

- *Management.* Surgical resection (partial hepatectomy) is feasible provided the patient has sufficient remaining hepatic reserve. Most patients are not amenable to surgery because of the extent of the tumour or severity of cirrhosis. In these patients, direct injection of absolute alcohol into the lesion or chemoembolization can be attempted. Liver transplantation can also be considered for young cirrhotic patients

with HCC. The outlook is generally poor with limited survival.

Cholangiocarcinoma

This is a less common tumour than HCC. It tends to occur at an older age than HCC with an equal sex distribution. The following factors have been implicated in its aetiology:

Fast facts—Liver disease (diseases of the liver)

Cirrhosis

- Caused by scarring of the liver usually resulting from alcohol consumption
- Portal hypertension

Causes

- Prehepatic
- Intrahepatic
- Posthepatic

Complications

- Gastro-oesophageal varices
- Ascites
- Congestive splenomegaly
- Hepatic encephalopathy

Investigation

- FBC, clotting studies
- LFTs
- Endoscopy (to check for varices)
- Ultrasound—diagnosis of ascites, masses, portal vein thrombosis

Management

- Management of complications
- Sclerotherapy/banding, balloon tamponade
- Transjugular intrahepatic portosystemic stent shunt (TIPSS)
- Liver transplantation

Tumours of the liver

- Metastatic disease is the commonest
- Hepatocellular and cholangiocarcinoma

◆ primary sclerosing cholangitis, and

◆ *Clonorchis sinensis* infestation.

Patients present with abdominal pain, weight loss and obstructive jaundice, and may be diagnosed by ultrasound and CT.

◆ *Management.* Both peripheral and central tumours are amenable to resection when small. Larger peripheral tumours can still be resected but the recurrence rate is very high. The jaundice caused by advanced central tumours can be palliated by stenting performed either endoscopically or percutaneously.

Lumps in the scrotum and hernias

Chapter contents

Lumps in the scrotum *73*

Scenario: painless groin swelling *73*

Background: lumps contained within the scrotum *74*

Groin hernia *75*

Scenario 1: recurrent groin swelling *75*

Scenario 2: vomiting and tender groin swelling *75*

Background: hernias *76*

Lumps in the scrotum

Scenario: painless groin swelling

A 70-year-old man presents with a 3-month history of a painless lump in the left side of the scrotum (Fig. 1.5a).

Lumps in the scrotum can be caused by a swelling in the testes, fluid around the testes, or from a swelling descending from the groin (an inguino-scrotal hernia).

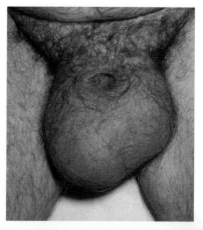

Fig 1.5a Clinical picture of a large hydrocoele (which would trans-illuminate).

> On examination you can feel the lump is contained entirely within the scrotum.

If you can feel above the lump, this implies that it is arising from within the scrotum rather than descending as with a hernia and is caused by a swelling either within the testis itself or around the testes (the tunica vaginalis).

> On further examination the testis is not palpable and is surrounded by the swelling. The swelling also trans-illuminates (i.e. you can shine a light through it).

This means that the cause of the swelling is a hydrocoele, caused by a build up of lymph between the covering of the testis (the tunical vaginalis) and the testis itself. If the swelling was separate from the testis, then it would probably be an epididymal cyst.

The commonest cause of a hydrocoele is a benign hydrocoele in the elderly (caused by failure of the lymphatic drainage within the tunica), but beware of an underlying testicular tumour in a patient under 40 years of age. **If there is any doubt, investigate with an ultrasound to examine the underlying testis.** Benign hydrocoeles can be left alone if asymptomatic, but if causing problems, they can be aspirated (they usually recur) or treated by surgery.

Clinical key points in scrotal lumps

- Lumps in the scrotum can be caused by a swelling of the testes or adjacent structures, fluid around the testes, or from a swelling descending from the groin (a hernia)

- On examination—if you can get above the lump, this means that the lump is from within the scrotum; if you cannot get above the swelling then the lump is coming from above (i.e. an inguinal hernia)

- Patients <40 years old presenting with a hydrocoele should have an ultrasound to exclude underlying testicular cancer as the key investigation. If there is a testicular cancer, then check the tumour cell markers (alpha-fetoprotein/HCG) before surgery

Background: lumps contained within the scrotum

- hydrocoele
- epididymal cyst
- varicocoele
- testicular tumour.

Examination of the scrotum is extremely simple: ask yourself two important questions:

1. Is the lump entirely within the scrotum, **can you feel normal tissue above the swelling?**—if not then it is descending from above, i.e. an inguino-scrotal hernia.

2. **If you can feel above it** (i.e. the swelling is arising from the scrotum), **can you feel the testes separate from the mass?**—if you can then it is an epididymal cyst; if not then it is a hydrocoele, or more rarely a primary tumour of the testis.

Hydrocoele

A hydrocoele is a collection of lymph fluid around the testis and within the tunica vaginalis. The majority of primary hydrocoeles slowly enlarge, are painless, and occur in men over 40. They can be left alone if asymptomatic or treated by either aspiration or surgery if symptomatic.

Surgery consists of draining the fluid and everting the sac (tonica vaginalis) to prevent further reaccumulation.

Secondary hydrocoeles are caused by underlying testicular pathology, either inflammation (orchitis) or tumour. **Be suspicious of a hydrocoele developing in an adult aged <40**—when there is doubt about the underlying testis, then an ultrasound should be performed.

Epididymal cyst

If the swelling is separate from the testis and the testis is palpably normal, then the swelling is probably an epididymal cyst (also called a spermatocoele if it contains semen), which is a small cystic swelling of the epididymis. These are benign and can be left alone unless symptomatic.

Varicocoele

This is a 'varicose vein' of the pampiniform plexus, which is commoner on the left. On examination of the scrotum it looks like a 'bag of worms'. There may be little to feel due to low pressure within the veins. Bilateral varicocoeles *may* cause subfertility. They can be left alone if asymptomatic or treated by surgery or radiological embolization.

Testicular tumour

These present as a painless lump in the scrotum. The majority (90%) are either seminoma (30–40 year age group) or teratoma (20–30 year age group). There is an increased risk in undescended testes. **The tumours spread to the para-aortic lymph nodes** (not the inguinal lymph nodes).

Investigations include a testicular ultrasound, tumour cell markers (alpha-fetoprotein, beta-HCG) **and a CT scan of the abdomen and thorax to stage lymphatic involvement and to look for metastases in the lungs.** At surgery, the testis is removed through an inguinal approach to avoid spreading the tumour to the scrotal skin lymphatics. Adjuvant therapy is with radiotherapy and chemotherapy for seminoma (survival rate 90% at 5 years) and chemotherapy for teratoma (survival rate 60–90% at 5 years).

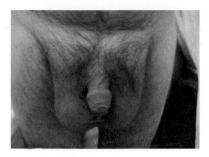

Fig 1.5b Clinical photograph of bilateral inguinal herniae (which would not trans-illuminate).

Fast facts—Scrotal lumps

Pathology

♦ Derived from scrotal structures—testis, cord, linings

Clinical features

♦ Hydrocoele may transilluminate

Investigations

♦ Ultrasound/tumour cell markers

Management

♦ Depends on pathology

NB If you cannot feel above a scrotal lump then it is probably an inguinal hernia

---

Groin hernia

Scenario 1: recurrent groin swelling

A 50-year-old man presents with a lump in the right groin (Fig. 1.5b).

The majority of hernias present as a lump in the groin. **Groin hernias are 10 times more common in men than women.**

The patient has a history of chronic obstructive pulmonary disease.

Any factor causing raised intra-abdominal pressure can lead to the development of a groin hernia, by pushing the intra-abdominal contents through the defect. **Predisposing factors include heavy lifting, chronic cough, constipation, prostatism, pregnancy, and obesity.**

The lump appears on standing but usually disappears on lying flat, although occasionally requires to be pushed in manually.

If the hernia is able to return to the abdominal cavity, it is a *reducible* **hernia. If the hernia is not able to return to the abdominal cavity then it is termed** *irreducible.*

On examination, the hernia came out above and medial to the pubic tubercle.

Inguinal hernias come out through the superficial inguinal ring, which is above and medial to the pubic tubercle. A femoral hernia comes out of the femoral canal, which is below and lateral to the pubic tubercle.

Scenario 2: vomiting and tender groin swelling

An 82-year-old lady presented with a 2-day history of abdominal pain and distension, brown foul smelling vomiting, and confusion. On examination the abdomen was tympanitic and auscultation revealed high-pitched bowel sounds.

An obstructed femoral hernia is an important cause of small bowel obstruction, particularly in the elderly thin female patient.

If the bowel becomes obstructed for whatever reason, then the proximal bowel dilates with gas and the intestinal contents, which normally pass through the bowel. This leads to a distended and tympanitic abdomen. High-pitched (or obstructive) bowel sounds are caused by active peristalsis in the dilated proximal bowel.

Gut contents that are stagnant for a period of time become partially digested by gut bacteria, leading to a brown discoloration and a foul smell (so-called faeculent vomiting, because of the colour and smell).

> Further examination revealed a 3-cm tender swelling in the right groin with surrounding erythema. The swelling was below and lateral to the pubic tubercle.

The pubic tubercle is an important landmark in the identification of groin hernia. If the hernia is below and lateral to the pubic tubercle, then it is a femoral hernia. An inguinal hernia would come out above and medial to the pubic tubercle. The fact that the hernia is tender and erythematous implies that the small bowel within the hernia is ischaemic.

> Initial treatment was by, oxygen, analgesia, the insertion of a nasogastric tube, IV fluid resuscitation, followed by emergency surgery.

ABC A nasogastric tube is passed to decompress the stomach and to avoid further vomiting and potential aspiration of vomit particularly on induction of anaesthesia. An IV drip is started as the patient will be dehydrated due to the fluid lost within the small bowel and the vomiting.

The diagnosis is a clinical one and except for cases where there is suspicion of bowel obstruction or perforation when abdominal X-ray and erect CXR are indicated imaging is not required.

As soon as possible after rehydration, the patient is taken to theatre as the potential of ischaemic bowel is a surgical emergency. If the bowel within the hernial sac is necrotic then that portion of the bowel requires resection, and the hernial defect closed. **An obstructed femoral hernia is an important cause of small bowel obstruction, particularly in the elderly thin female patient.**

Background: hernias

Definition

A hernia is defined as a 'an abnormal protrusion of a viscus with its normal body cavity'.

Clinical key points in groin hernia

- Men are affected 10 times more commonly by groin hernias than women
- Ask about a history of a reducible lump in the groin, and as to what symptoms it is causing
- Ask about possible predisposing factors, such as prostatism, constipation, chronic cough
- On examination—identify the pubic tubercle—this is the key to differentiating inguinal from femoral hernias
- Check that the hernia is reducible—if it is irreducible and there is surrounding erythema, then there is the possibility of strangulated bowel within the hernial sac, which is a surgical emergency
- An obstructed femoral hernia is an important cause of small bowel obstruction, particularly in the elderly thin female patient
- There are no key investigations required in patients with groin hernias, unless you think that the hernia is causing a bowel obstruction, in which case a plain abdominal X-ray and erect CXR (for closed loop bowel perforation) are required

Most abdominal wall hernias present as a lump, and may contain omentum, small bowel, or large bowel. The majority of hernias are *reducible* (i.e. the contents of the hernia can reduce to their normal cavity); as a hernia develops, it carries a layer of investing peritoneum, which acts as a sac. The point at which the sac comes through the abdominal wall is the *neck* of the sac. The neck is the narrowest point of the sac and may constrict the hernia contents.

If the hernia is **irreducible** (i.e. the contents cannot be reduced), then the contents (e.g. bowel) can either be *incarcerated* (when the hernia is stuck, but there is no bowel obstruction or interference with the blood supply) or become *obstructed* (the bowel within the hernia becomes obstructed) or *strangulate* (when the blood supply of the bowel is compromised and the bowel becomes ischaemic) (see flow chart). If the bowel is ischaemic, this causes an intense local inflammatory reaction and the overlying skin can become erythematous and tender. Ischaemic bowel may progress to necrosis and perforation.

Abdominal wall hernias are common and account for 10% of all surgical procedures. They come through natural openings or weak areas caused by stretching or surgical incisions. The main types of hernia that you should know about are (Fig. 1.5c):

- inguinal hernia
- femoral hernia
- para-umbilical hernia
- epigastric hernia
- incisional hernia

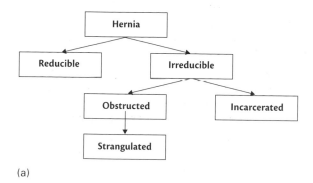

(a)

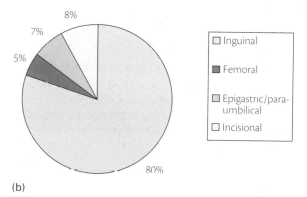

(b)

Fig 1.5c Distribution of types of hernia.

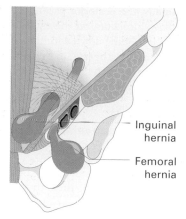

Fig 1.5d Diagram of the anatomy of the inguinal canal and femoral/inguinal hernias.

Inguinal hernias

Inguinal hernias exploit defects in the inguinal canal. They are commoner in men and can be caused by any factor that raises the intra-abdominal pressure, including coughing, constipation, heavy lifting, prostatism, pregnancy, and obesity.

There are two types of inguinal hernia: indirect and direct:

- if the defect is directly through the posterior wall of the inguinal canal (i.e. arising **medial** to the inferior epigastric artery, it is a **direct** inguinal hernia
- if the defect is through the internal inguinal ring (i.e. arising **lateral** to the inferior epigastric artery), it is an **indirect** inguinal hernia.

If the hernia is large enough then an indirect hernia can descend into the scrotum—called an inguinoscrotal hernia. They can be difficult to reduce, in view of their size.

Examination of the patient

Examine the patient standing up; look for an obvious bulge in the inguinal region. Ask the patient to cough and see whether the bulge gets bigger on coughing (i.e. raising the intra-abdominal pressure). Small hernias may only present when the patient is coughing.

Next feel for the pubic tubercle to decide the relationship of the hernia to the pubic tubercle. An inguinal hernia will come out of the superficial inguinal ring, which is above and medial to the tubercle. A femoral hernia comes out of the femoral canal, which is below and lateral to the pubic tubercle. This is the best way to identify whether the hernia is inguinal or femoral.

Then examine the patient lying down, to see whether the hernia is reducible. At this stage in the examination, you will have identified the hernia as being either inguinal or femoral and reducible or irreducible.

If the hernia is inguinal, do not attempt to decide whether it is indirect or direct. It is difficult to define whether the inguinal hernia is indirect or direct clinically and is best done at the time of operation, when you can define the relationship of the hernia to the inferior epigastric vessels.

To repeat—**the inferior epigastric vessels mark the medial boundary of the internal ring** and therefore if the hernia originates lateral to the vessels, then it is coming out through the internal ring (i.e. indirect); if it is medial to the vessels then it is a direct hernia.

Occasionally, the posterior part of the sac is formed by large bowel (caecum on the right, sigmoid on the left) or bladder sliding down with the peritoneum, and this is called a *sliding* hernia. In these cases, care must be taken at surgery with the management of the sac, to avoid damage to the bowel.

Summary of the signs

1. **Examine the patient upright**

   - if hernia descends to the scrotum, it is probably indirect

   - if they are bilateral, then they are more commonly direct

   - find the pubic tubercle

     —if above and medial to the tubercle—an **inguinal** hernia

     —if below and lateral to the tubercle—a **femoral** hernia

   - look for a cough impulse.

2. **Examine the patient lying down**

   - determine if the hernia is reducible or irreducible

   - if it is irreducible, look for signs of small bowel obstruction or strangulation (tenderness/erythema over the hernia)

   - **DON'T** try and distinguish between indirect and direct inguinal hernias clinically—it will be obvious at surgery

   - **DO** distinguish between inguinal and femoral hernias.

Treatment

The vast majority undergo surgical repair, to relieve symptoms and to prevent the possibility of complications such as obstruction or strangulation. Occasionally, a small direct inguinal hernia in an elderly patient can be left alone as they rarely cause obstruction. At surgery, the hernial sac is reduced (pushed back into the abdominal cavity) and the posterior wall of the inguinal canal is reinforced with a synthetic polypropylene mesh.

Femoral hernia

In a femoral hernia, **the defect is through the femoral canal** (bounded medially by the lacunar ligament, superiorly by the inguinal ligament, inferiorly by the pectineal ligament, and laterally by the femoral vein—Fig. 1.5d). It occurs more often in women than men (though inguinal hernias are still more common than femoral hernias in women overall). The femoral canal is narrow and thus femoral hernias are at high risk of causing bowel obstruction, and indeed commonly present in elderly women with small bowel obstruction. It is very important to look for a femoral hernia in a patient who presents with small bowel obstruction with no obvious cause.

ALL femoral hernias should be treated surgically, because of the high risk of bowel obstruction. Nowadays, the hernia can be repaired by placing a synthetic mesh 'plug' within the femoral canal.

Umbilical hernia

These are congenital in origin, may spontaneously resolve up to the age of 3, but if persistent after this, usually require surgical repair. A para-umbilical hernia (i.e. just next to the umbilicus, but not directly through it) is an acquired hernia, usually in middle-aged, obese patients and requires surgical repair, as the neck of the sac is usually narrow and at risk of strangulation.

Epigastric hernia

These usually occur in young males and are caused by a defect or tear in the linea alba. They are usually small, with a tight neck, and cause pain. Again, because of the narrow neck, these hernias require surgical repair.

Fast facts—Hernia (an abnormal protrusion of a viscus outwith its normal body cavity)

Pathology

- A congenital or acquired defect acts as a route
- Raised intra-abdominal pressure applies force to the defect

Clinical features

- Lump/swelling at the site of the hernia
- May present with incarceration, bowel obstruction, strangulation

Investigations

- No investigation is usually required

Management

- Surgical repair

Outcome

- Hernia recurrence approximately 5%
- 15% of patients may develop neurogenic pain

Incisional hernia

An incisional hernia is where the defect is through a previous abdominal surgical incision. The same definitions apply as for inguinal hernia (reducible, irreducible, obstructed, or strangulated). In addition there may be more than one defect in the previous incision, when the hernia is then *multiloculated*.

The **aetiological factors** that predispose to the development of an incisional hernia **include age, obesity, wound infection, and steroids**. Incisional hernias are repaired by direct further suturing and by inserting a mesh (usually made of polypropylene) to reinforce the abdominal wall.

Breast lumps

Chapter contents

Scenario 1: lumpy breast *81*

Scenario 2: discrete breast lump *82*

Scenario 3: multiple breast lumps *82*

Scenario 4: hot, painful breast lump *82*

Scenario 5: non-tender ill-defined breast lump *83*

Background: diseases of the breast *83*

Scenario 1: lumpy breast

> An otherwise healthy 23-year-old girl has noticed three lumpy areas in her right breast, which have persisted for the last 10 weeks. These lumps are more prominent just before her period but are less obvious afterwards.

It is important to find out any relationship to the menstrual period in patients with breast lumps/ breast pain.

> She also has discomfort in both breasts, which worsens just before her periods and disappears after menstruation. She has never been pregnant and is on the oral contraceptive pill.

Breast pain related to periods is called cyclical mastalgia and is quite common. **Breast pain is usually benign: 80% of patients can be treated by simple reassurance.**

> Clinical examination demonstrates normal breast tissue on both sides with no palpable lump at the time of examination.

Examination should include both breasts and also check for any surrounding palpable lymph nodes (in the axilla and supraclavicular). This girl probably has benign lumpy changes responding to the hormonal cycle. Breast lumps that change with the hormonal cycle are usually benign.

If the pain persists, they can be advised to wear a supportive bra, modify their dietary intake to a low fat diet, and avoid caffeine in coffee, tea, or soft drinks. If these conservative measures fail, evening primrose oil (gamma linoleic acid) is effective in one-third of women, as it has been postulated that mastalgia is due to a deficiency in essential fatty acids.

Other medications including *danazol*, *bromocriptine*, or *tamoxifen* have a role in severe persistent mastalgia, and work by altering the oestrogen levels (tamoxifen and danazol) or by acting against prolactin (bromocriptine).

Scenario 2: discrete breast lump

> An otherwise healthy 32-year-old woman has identified a 2 cm by 1 cm smooth, discrete, mobile lump in the upper outer quadrant of her right breast, which has been present for 6 weeks. Clinical examination confirms the lump.

Fibroadenoma of the breast is a benign tumour. It is well encapsulated, which separates it from the surrounding tissue. As it is very well circumscribed it 'floats' on normal breast tissue and is therefore very mobile. This lesion is also called a 'breast mouse' by the way it can be 'chased' around the breast, as they are so mobile.

> A breast ultrasound and fine needle aspiration cytology confirmed the lump as a fibroadenoma.

Ultrasound in women under 35 years and fine needle aspiration are extremely useful in the management of a breast lump.

Scenario 3: multiple breast lumps

> A 47-year-old woman identified a lump in her left breast and immediately went to her general practitioner who identified a further lump in the left breast and a third lump on the right side. These lumps are slightly tender but not associated with any skin changes.

Multiple well circumscribed lumps in the breast of middle-aged women are usually benign cysts.

> On clinical examination the three discrete, smooth lumps are identified but no local regional lymph nodes are palpable.

Triple assessment, including clinical history and examination, mammography, and complete needle aspiration of the lumps confirms that all three lumps are breast cysts.

Multiple breast cysts are usually benign and do not need further follow-up. They may recur.

Scenario 4: hot, painful breast lump

> A 43-year-old women presents with a hot, tender, red swelling in the right breast adjacent to the nipple (Fig. 1.6a). She is a smoker and this is the third episode over a period of 2 years.

Hot and tender and red implies an inflammatory episode—if the patient is not breast feeding, then the commonest cause is inflammation around the ducts (periductal mastitis), which is aggravated by smoking. If the infection is in a lactating breast (postpartum), it is usually caused by *Staphylococcus aureus* and the patient given flucloxacillin. In periductal mastitis the organism responsible can be anaerobic and the patient should be given amoxycillian–clavulinic acid.

> On examination, there is fluctuation underneath the swelling.

Fluctuation implies the presence of pus underneath. **In breast abscesses this can be treated under topical anaesthetic by aspiration with a needle.** If the infection fails to settle with needle aspiration and antibiotics, then the abscess may require to be surgically drained. Patients with recurrent infection (this is the patient's third episode) may require excision of the affected ducts (called microdochectomy) and should stop smoking.

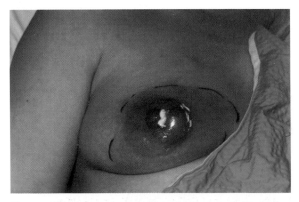

Fig 1.6a Clinical photograph showing a breast abscess with a red swollen appearance.

Clinical key points in benign breast conditions

◆ Ask about the relationship of the breast pain to the menstrual period

◆ Breast pain is usually benign, but ask about any family history of breast cancer

◆ Examine both breasts and also check for any surrounding palpable lymph nodes (in the axilla and supraclavicular)

◆ Ultrasound, mammography, and fine needle aspiration are the key investigations in the management of a breast lump

◆ A tender, red, hot breast suggests a breast abscess, which if the abscess is fluctuant is best treated by aspiration

Scenario 5: non-tender ill-defined breast lump

A 56-year-old woman noticed a non-tender 3-cm lump in her right breast while bathing. In the mirror she noted the skin was dimpled over the lump when she raised her arm (Fig. 1.6b). She is otherwise fit and well.

Skin tethering and nipple inversion associated with a painless breast lump are worrying signs, highly suggestive of cancer and are caused by fibrous contracture around the cancer. **A history of anorexia, weight loss, tiredness, and breathlessness are sinister symptoms suggesting metastatic disease.**

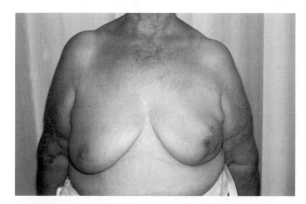

Fig 1.6b Clinical photograph of skin dimpling over breast carcinoma.

Clinical examination confirms the presence of a breast lump with skin tethering overlying it and the nipple is inverted on that side. There are palpable large lymph nodes in the axilla.

Palpable lymph nodes in the axilla are suggestive of spread (metastases) of the tumour to the nodes. Mammography (Fig. 1.6c) and fine needle aspiration cytology are undertaken and confirm the lump is a cancer. The treatment options for breast cancer depend on the stage of the cancer (how far it has spread) and staging investigations are therefore important. The patient undergoes staging investigations for metastatic disease and is then in a position to discuss the surgical and oncological options including breast cancer trials.

Clinical key points in malignant breast disease

◆ Most patients present with a painless lump in the breast

  —ask about how long they have had the lump, and any other symptoms (anorexia, weight loss, tiredness, breathlessness)

  —these are sinister symptoms suggesting metastatic disease

◆ Examine for skin tethering and nipple inversion—these are worrying signs, suggestive of cancer and are caused by fibrous contracture by the cancer

◆ Examine for palpable lymph nodes in the axilla or supraclavicular region—if present this is suggestive of spread (metastases) of the tumour to the nodes

◆ The key investigations are a 'triple assessment', including clinical, radiological (mammogram, ultrasound), and cytological (fine needle aspiration, core biopsy) assessments

Background: diseases of the breast

The breast consists of multiple ductal-lobular units, which secrete milk at times of lactation through several ducts, which converge on the nipple. It is important to know that the lymphatic drainage of the breast is mostly to the axilla, but some of the medial aspect of the breast may drain to the internal mammary nodes. Diseases of the breast, both benign and malignant, are common and are now treated by a multidisciplinary team, involving surgeons, radiologists, pathologists, specialist breast nurses, and oncologists.

Clinical conditions:

1. benign
   - fibrocystic changes/fibroadenoma
   - breast abscess
2. malignant
   - breast carcinoma.

Fibrocystic changes/fibroadenoma

Benign changes in the breast are very common, particularly in young women. Fibrocystic changes usually present as bilateral nodularity or lumpy breasts, where the lumpy areas are prominent or uncomfortable before a period and tend to disappear with time.

Fibrocystic changes, as the name suggests, are a combination of fibrosis, adenosis (epithelial hyperplasia), and cysts. These changes are caused by cyclical proliferation and involution of breast tissue.

Fibrocystic changes are benign and can be assessed by triple assessment, i.e. clinical, radiological, and cytopathological examination. If the history and examination point to fibrocystic changes alone, the patient can be reassured without surgical intervention.

Fibroadenoma also presents in young women but as a single, smooth, mobile non-tender lump, which is usually unchanged by menstruation. The fibroadenoma is a benign proliferation, which following triple assessment may be excised under local or general anaesthetic or if there is no change in size over a 6- to 12-month period of observation, and the patient wishes, may be left alone.

Breast abscess

A breast abscess presents as a hot, red, tender swelling of the breast and occurs in breast feeding mothers (where the organism is staphylococcal) and in middle-aged smokers (where the organism is anaerobic). Abscess formation may be prevented by use of appropriate antibiotics at an early stage. However, once an abscess has formed it requires surgical drainage by aspiration or incision.

Carcinoma of the breast
Incidence

Many factors have been implemented in the aetiology of breast cancer, including hormonal influences, diet, and family history. **The lifetime risk of developing breast cancer is 1 in 11 in the UK.** The incidence of breast cancer increases with age. Breast cancer is uncommon before the age of 35 and becomes progressively more

---

> ## Fast facts—Benign breast disease
>
> ### Fibroadenoma
>
> ### Clinical features
> - Age <30
> - Hard mobile painless lump
>
> ### Management
> - Excision
> - Fibrocystic changes
>
> ### Clinical features
> - Age 25–45
> - Pain/breast lump—may be worse before menstrual cycle
>
> ### Management
> - Reassurance
> - Cyst aspiration or excision of localized lesion if required
>
> ### Breast abscess
>
> ### Predisposing factors
> - Lactating breast, smoker (non-lactating)
>
> ### Clinical features
> - Swollen, hot, painful breast
>
> ### Management
> - Antibiotics
> - Drainage

common in women over the age of 64. A new breast lump in a women over the age of 45 should be considered potentially malignant until proved otherwise by triple assessment (clinical, radiological, and cytological examination).

Presentation and pathology

Clinical presentation is usually as a symptomatic lump that may be associated with skin dimpling, skin discoloration, recent nipple retraction, blood-stained nipple discharge, or rarely symptoms of metastatic disease (bone pain, breathlessness, or nausea).

The histological type is invasive ductal carcinoma in 80% of women. The breast screening programme, which in the UK targets women aged 50–70, aims to detect small cancers (which have a better prognosis) and ductal carcinoma in situ, a pre-invasive condition, which can also be surgically cured.

Assessment and examination

Clinical assessment of breast cancer includes a history of the presenting problem, hormonal and gynaecological history, family history (present in 10% of women with breast cancer), and other relevant medical/surgical history. The examination of the breast, for which male doctors should be chaperoned, involves inspection for changes in contour, skin colour or nipple retraction, palpation of each breast in turn, and palpation of the local/regional lymph nodes of the axilla, supraclavicular and infraclavicular fossa, and cervical region.

Investigations

Investigations for carcinoma of the breast include radiology and cytopathology. Bilateral two view mam-

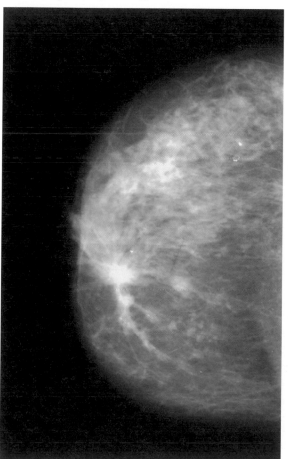

Fig 1.6c Mammogram of breast carcinoma with an area of increased shadowing but a poorly defined edge.

mography of both breasts is required for all women with a suspected breast cancer (Fig. 1.6c). The quality of the image is often better in women over the age of 35. Under this age breast ultrasound may be more useful. Aspiration from the lump with a fine bore needle will yield material for cytology examination on which a diagnosis of a cancer may be made.

Following diagnosis of breast cancer staging investigations include full blood count, blood biochemistry, liver function tests, and chest X-ray. The aims of these tests are to identify disease distant from the breast and to establish the general health of the patient. For large or advanced cancers and in women with symptoms suggestive of metastatic bone disease, a liver ultrasound and isotope bone scan for liver and bone metastases, respectively, are useful.

Treatment

Treatment of breast cancer follows on from diagnosis and staging with discussion from a multidisciplinary team (surgeon, oncologist, pathologist, radiologist, nurse specialist) and with the patient and her family. Options include surgery, radiotherapy, endocrine therapy, and/or chemotherapy.

Surgical treatment may be wide local excision (lumpectomy) if the cancer is less than 4 cm and the breast of reasonable size or mastectomy if the lump is larger than 4 cm, or if there is multifocal disease, or if the patient prefers.

Axilliary node clearance or axillary node sampling (sentinel node or four node sampling) provides evidence of metastatic spread to the axillary lymph nodes, which has implications for prognosis (the more nodes involved the worse prognosis) and for the selection of additional treatment. In addition the cancer is tested for the presence of oestrogen receptors and the tumours subdivided into oestrogen receptor positive and negative—this has important implications for prognosis and adjuvant therapy (see below).

Following surgery breast irradiation after wide local excision/lumpectomy is required to reduce the chance of disease recurrence in the remaining breast.

Adjuvant therapy (protective treatment for the future) can be oophorectomy for premenopausal women where the tumour is hormone receptor positive, or tamoxifen for all age groups if the tumour is oestrogen receptor positive.

Chemotherapy is given to women with axillary node involvement particularly if they are oestrogen receptor negative.

Some cancers present at an advanced stage and are inoperable. The use of antihormonal therapy, chemo-

Fast facts—Malignant breast disease

The lifetime risk of developing breast cancer is 1 in 11 in the UK

Aetiology

- Strong family history
- Early menarche, late menopause
- Nulliparous

Pathology

- Ductal carcinoma
- Spreads via lymphatics (lung, liver, bone, brain, adrenals)

Clinical features

- Painless breast lump
- Nipple retraction, skin tethering
- Palpable axillary nodes

Diagnosis

By 'triple assessment'—clinical, radiological, and pathological assessment.

Staging

To demonstrate the extent of disease.

Treatment

Breast surgery + radiotherapy for loco-regional disease control, chemotherapy, and/or anti-endocrine treatment for systemic disease control of oestrogen receptor positive disease.

Prognosis

Eighty per cent 5-year survival, 60% 10-year survival overall, but depends on axillary node metastases, tumour size and histology, oestrogen receptor status, and the treatment given.

therapy, or radiotherapy techniques to reduce the local disease and provide good palliation.

For breast cancer the outcome depends on the following factors:

- presence of the number of axillary lymph node metastases (more = worse)
- size of the primary tumour (big = worse)
- tumour histology (higher grade = worse)
- histological tumour type
- hormone receptor status (oestrogen receptor positive tumours have a better prognosis)
- the treatment the patient receives.

Lumps in the neck and thyroid gland

Chapter contents

Lumps in the neck 87

Scenario 1: hoarse voice and painless neck lump 87

Background: lumps in the neck 88

Thyroid 91

Scenario 1: painless thyroid swelling 91

Scenario 2: diffuse thyroid swelling 92

Scenario 3: weight loss and irritability 93

Background: thyroid 94

Lumps in the neck

Scenario 1: hoarse voice and painless neck lump

A 58-year-old man presents with a lump in the right side of the neck (anterior to sternocleidomastoid). It has been present for 6 weeks and is painless.

The commonest cause of a lump in the neck is lymphadenopathy (85%). A painful lymph node usually denotes an inflammatory reaction (i.e. an infective cause).

He admits to recent hoarseness and a non-productive cough over the last 3 months.

Ask about general symptoms including dyspnoea, cough, hoarseness, and any systemic upset, such as malaise, cachexia, and weight loss. These symptoms may point to a primary cause of the lymphadenopathy.

On examination the 2 cm lump is firm, craggy, and fixed.

Examine the neck for lymphadenopathy (submental, submandibular, cervical). If present, examine for generalized lymphadenopathy (axillary, inguinal) and splenomegaly. This is because we want to know whether the lymph node is caused by a haematological disorder (when there is a problem that affects many lymph nodes, i.e. generalized lymphadenopathy) or whether the nodes are only located in the neck, when they are far more likely to be caused by a local or regional problem, i.e. localized/regional lymphadenopathy.

> Examination revealed a solitary fixed lymph node in the cervical chain, with no generalized lymphadenopathy.

Having found only a local cervical problem, the next step is to find the underlying cause.

Routine investigations for a lymph node in the cervical chain include an otolaryngology examination (**examine the larynx and pharynx for a possible primary site, and to check the vocal cords, in view of the hoarseness**), and a CXR, to look for possible primary sites of malignancy.

The lymph node in the neck was biopsied by fine needle aspiration (FNA), which demonstrates metastatic adenocarcinoma.

> ENT examination revealed a right vocal cord palsy.

This may have been caused by infiltration of the recurrent laryngeal nerve by tumour. This leads to the right vocal cord being paralysed with subsequent non-apposition of the cords on speech, leading to hoarseness.

> CXR showed a mass in the right upper lobe, consistent with a primary bronchogenic carcinoma (Fig 1.7a).

The extent of the bronchogenic carcinoma can be delineated with a CT scan of the chest.

Background: lumps in the neck

Patients commonly present with a lump in the neck, with the commonest cause being infective cervical lymphadenopathy (from, for example, tonsillitis or viral infection). However, there are many conditions that can present with a swelling in the neck and it is important to divide the neck into three areas to have a better understanding of where the potential swellings are arising from—these three areas are the **anterior triangle**, **posterior triangle**, and **midline** (Fig 1.7b):

- *anterior triangle*—this is bounded by the mandible superiorly, midline medially, and the anterior border of sternocleidomastoid laterally

- *posterior triangle*—this is bounded by the posterior border of sternocleidomastoid anteriorly, the anterior border of trapezius laterally, and the clavicle inferiorly

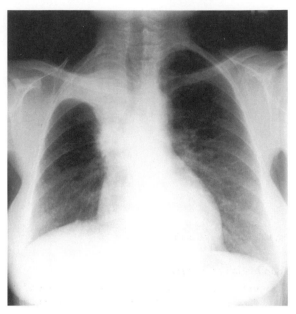

Fig 1.7a Plain chest X-ray of a bronchogenic carcinoma with right upper lobe collapse.

Clinical key points in neck lumps (lymph nodes)

- Ask about any associated symptoms (e.g. dysphagia may point to oesophageal cancer with lymph node metastasis, night sweats can be associated with lymphoma)

- On examination, if a lymph node is found, check whether it is solitary, several localized to one area, or generalized (other areas in the body affected)

- If there is generalized lymphadenopathy, check for enlarged liver/spleen, and think about haematological causes (such as lymphoma)

- If there is solitary or localized lymph nodes then the key investigations are an ENT examination (to look for possible primary tumours, e.g. larynx, pharynx), a CXR (to look for a possible primary lung tumour), and an FNA of the lymph node(s), to get cytology

- If there is generalized lymphadenopathy, then the key investigations are a lymph node biopsy and a staging CT of the chest and abdomen (to see which groups of lymph nodes are affected)

- *midline*—this is the anterior area of the neck, between the two anterior triangles, from the submental region superiorly, to the manubrium inferiorly.

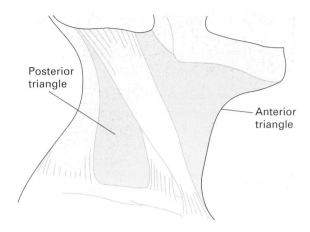

Fig 1.7b Diagram of triangles of the neck.

Examination of the neck

Examine the patient with the neck partly extended. Look for deformities, skin changes (pigmentation, rashes), and obvious swellings. Pay particular attention to the lymph nodes, thyroid, and the salivary glands. When defining a lump, comment on its position, size, shape, mobility (e.g. the thyroid moves with swallowing) the consistency, and whether there is associated lymphadenopathy.

Midline swellings

The important questions to ask to differentiate between midline swellings are:

◆ **Does it move on swallowing?**—if it does then it is the thyroid (see section on thyroid)

◆ **Does it move on sticking out the tongue?**—if it does then it is a thyroglossal cyst

◆ *If the swelling does not move on swallowing or sticking out the tongue, then it is probably a dermoid cyst.*

Definition

A thyroglossal cyst is a cyst arising in any part of the thyroglossal tract, which extends from the back of the

TABLE 1.7a Causes of lumps in the neck

Midline	Anterior triangle	Posterior triangle
Thyroid	Lymph nodes	Lymph nodes
Thyroglossal cyst	Salivary glands	Cystic hygroma
Dermoid cyst	Branchial cyst	
{-------------Sebaceous cyst, lipoma-------------}		

Common problems such as sebaceous cysts and lipomas can also be found anywhere in the neck.

tongue (foramen caecum) to the thyroid. The connection to the back of the tongue explains why **a thyroglossal cyst moves on sticking out the tongue.** They usually present in teenage years, and if symptomatic are best excised. If the swelling in the midline does not move with swallowing or sticking out the tongue, then it is a *dermoid cyst, which is an embryological cyst that can be excised if symptomatic.*

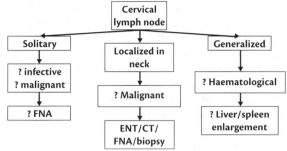

Anterior triangle swellings: lymph nodes

Lymphadenopathy accounts for 85% of all swellings in the neck. There are three main causes of cervical lymphadenopathy—infective, malignant, and haematological (leukaemia/lymphoma), and a history should be taken to differentiate between the causes—systemic symptoms such as fever, weight loss, or sweats point to a potential infective or haematological cause. Specific symptoms, such as hoarseness (caused by a vocal cord palsy), cough, or dyspnoea point to a potentially malignant cause, while a history of recent travel abroad, a recent immigrant, or a sore throat point to an infective cause.

Examination

Always examine from behind the patient and have a routine so that you remember to examine all groups of lymph nodes (start at submental, submandibular, then the cervical chain and the supraclavicular region and finish with the posterior triangle and pre- and post-auricular lymph nodes).

On examination, you need to find out whether the lymph node is:

◆ solitary (i.e. no other lymph nodes involved), localized to the neck (i.e. involving a group of lymph nodes in the neck but nowhere else in the body)

◆ part of a generalized process involving other lymph nodes (e.g. inguinal or axillary) in which case you should also examine for hepatosplenomegaly as the liver and spleen can be involved in a haematological or infective disorder

- the position of the lymph nodes involved may point to a specific site, for example gastric carcinoma may metastasize to the left supraclavicular region (*called Virchow's node or Troisier's sign*).

Investigation

The investigation of generalized lymphadenopathy should be done by a haematologist but may include lymph node biopsy and bone marrow aspiration to establish a diagnosis.

Cervical lymph nodes (either localized or solitary) should be investigated by CXR (to look for a primary lung carcinoma), and ENT opinion (to assess the vocal cord if the patient is hoarse and to examine the larynx and pharynx for a possible primary).

It is also important to establish a cytological diagnosis of the lymph node, which is best done by either FNA, which can be done at presentation to the clinic, or an open lymph node biopsy.

Anterior triangle swellings: salivary glands

Both the **submandibular** and **parotid** glands can present as swellings in the anterior triangle of the neck.

The commonest causes of swellings of the salivary glands are stones in the duct (causing blockage of the duct and swelling of the gland), benign tumours of the gland, or infection (e.g. mumps or parotitis).

Stones are more common in the submandibular duct than the parotid because the submandibular gland is mucus-secreting. **Remember to examine the mouth** and to feel the duct in the floor of the mouth for stones. If the stone blocks the duct, this leads to a build up of secretions within the gland, which causes pain and swelling of the gland. X-rays of the floor of the mouth will show calcified stones.

The treatment is to excise the stone from the duct or excision of the gland. Benign tumours of the salivary glands (called pleomorphic adenomas) are more common in the parotid gland and can be diagnosed by FNA. **Always examine for a facial nerve palsy with parotid tumours**, as malignant tumours of the parotid gland can invade the facial nerve.

Anterior triangle swellings: branchial cyst

This is a rare embryological cyst, which usually presents in early adolescence with a cystic swelling (said to feel like a 'half-filled hot water bottle') in the upper part of the anterior triangle. On FNA, pus-like material is obtained, which contains cholesterol crystals, because the lining of the cyst contains sebaceous glands. These cysts get secondarily infected or can fistulate (branchial fistula) and are best treated by excision.

Posterior triangle: lymph nodes

Lymphadenopathy is the commonest cause of a swelling in the posterior triangle and is treated as for lymph nodes in the anterior triangle.

Posterior triangle: cystic hygroma

These rare swellings present in early childhood and are a type of lymphangioma (tumour of the lymphatic vessels). As such they are filled with lymphatic fluid, which gives it a characteristic sign of being **transilluminable** (i.e. you can shine a light through the fluid filling the swelling). They can grow large and cause pressure symptoms. They can also occur in the axilla and groin.

Fast facts—Neck lumps

Pathology

- The majority of neck swellings are lymph nodes
- The commonest causes of salivary gland swelling are:
  —stones in the duct
  —benign tumours of the gland
  —infection (e.g. mumps)
- Generalized lymphadenopathy = ? a haematological cause (check for enlarged liver/spleen)

Clinical features

- Are there lymph nodes swollen in other parts of the body?
- With a parotid swelling always examine for weakness in the facial nerve as this may indicate that the swelling is malignant
- Always examine inside the mouth in patients with salivary gland swellings

Investigations

- FNA/lymph node biopsy
- CXR
- ENT opinion

Management

- Depends on pathology

Thyroid

Scenario 1: painless thyroid swelling

> A 45-year-old female presents with a painless lump in the right side of the neck (Fig 1.7c). The lump has been present for 6 months. She has had no change in her voice, or breathing, or swallowing difficulties.

Solitary thyroid nodules are common (5% of the population) and predominantly affect females. **Only 5% of these nodules are malignant and the aim is to differentiate between benign nodules** (i.e. not requiring surgery) and malignant nodules (i.e. requiring surgery). If the patient is aged <16 years or >60 years, the incidence of malignancy is higher. **Hoarseness may be a sign of malignancy with involvement of the recurrent laryngeal nerve. Breathing or swallowing problems relate to the nodule pressing on the trachea or oesophagus, and do not necessarily point to malignancy.**

> There is no family history of thyroid problems or previous neck irradiation.

Benign generalized swellings of the thyroid (**goitre**) may be familial. Previous neck irradiation in childhood may predispose to thyroid malignancy.

> On examination there is a smooth 4 × 3 cm mass in the right side of the neck. There is no palpable lymphadenopathy. The trachea is not deviated.

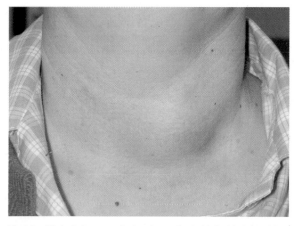

Fig 1.7c Clinical photograph showing unilateral left-sided thyroid lump.

A mass that is hard and irregular is suggestive (but not diagnostic of) malignancy. Surrounding lymphadenopathy is suspicious for papillary thyroid carcinoma. Often, thyroid nodules can be large enough to cause deviation of the trachea; if significant enough, this can lead to tracheal compression and stridor (a low-pitched crowing sound on inspiration).

> *Investigations*: thyroid-stimulating hormone (TSH)—1.71 mU/l (normal = 0.4–4 mU/l); FNA—compatible with follicular neoplasm.

There are two essential investigations in the management of a solitary thyroid nodule.

- **What is the patient's thyroid status** (normal, over- or underactive)—check the TSH. If the TSH is elevated the patient is hypothyroid; if suppressed, the patient is thyrotoxic.

- **To assess the cells in the nodule by FNA**—this will tell whether the nodule is benign, suspicious, or malignant. If the FNA is benign, the nodule can be observed and the FNA repeated in 6 months. If the report is suspicious or malignant then surgery is required. A report of follicular neoplasm is regarded as suspicious (cannot differentiate between malignant and benign) and therefore surgery is required (thyroid lobectomy).

Clinical key points in solitary thyroid nodules

- Most thyroid nodules (95%) are benign and asymptomatic

- Ask about any family history of thyroid cancer, or previous radiotherapy to the neck (which can predispose to thyroid cancer)

- Ask about any history of hoarseness (indicating possible infiltration of the recurrent laryngeal nerve by cancer)

- On examination assess the size of the thyroid nodule and check that there is only one palpable nodule—if there are several nodules then it may be a benign multinodular goitre

- Also examine for surrounding lymph nodes in the neck

- The two key investigations are TSH and FNA

Scenario 2: diffuse thyroid swelling

A 75-year-old man presents to his GP with a 3-year history of an increasing swelling in his neck (Fig 1.7d). Over the last 3 months he had noticed occasional difficulty in breathing (dyspnoea) and over the last month, difficulty in swallowing his food (dysphagia).

Examination of the neck revealed a large thyroid swelling (moves on swallowing) with several nodules palpable within the thyroid—this is called a multinodular goitre.

A **multinodular goitre develops slowly over a period of years**. The cause of a multinodular goitre is largely unknown. **If large enough, a multinodular goitre can compress the trachea, leading to dyspnoea or stridor** (a low-pitched crowing noise heard on inspiration) or compress the oesophagus, leading to dysphagia. They are more common in women and are usually euthyroid (non-toxic multinodular goitre), although occasionally they can produce excess thyroxine (toxic multinodular goitre).

As with a solitary thyroid lump **the key investigations are TSH and FNA** of the dominant nodule. A CT scan is useful to assess retrosternal extension and tracheal compression.

CT scan of the neck revealed bilateral multiple nodules within the thyroid, with retrosternal extension of the right lobe and tracheal deviation to the left with significant tracheal compression (Fig 1.7e).

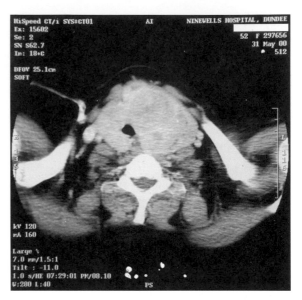

Fig 1.7e CT scan of thyroid mass causing severe tracheal compression.

A CT scan of the neck is an excellent method of delineating the extent of the goitre and to assess the degree of tracheal deviation and compression.

The patient was treated by thyroidectomy.

Surgery is indicated in patients with multinodular goitre if they have compressive symptoms (either on the trachea or the oesophagus). Occasionally, a goitre can be removed for cosmetic reasons.

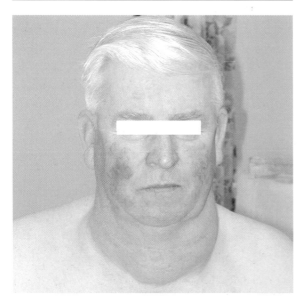

Fig 1.7d Clinical photograph showing a thyroid goitre.

Clinical key points in multinodular goitre

♦ A goitre is a swelling of the thyroid—multinodular goitres are usually long-standing and can impinge on the trachea, leading to narrowing and stridor

♦ Ask about any history of choking, problems with swallowing, difficulty in lying flat (these may indicate that the trachea or oesophagus are being compressed by the goitre)

♦ The key investigations are TSH and FNA of the dominant nodule. A CT scan is useful to assess retrosternal extension and tracheal compression

Scenario 3: weight loss and irritability

> A 25-year-old female presents to her GP with a 3-month history of weight loss, irritability, intolerance of heat, and sweating. Routine blood tests showed a suppressed TSH (<0.03 mU/l).

The thyroid gland produces the hormone thyroxine, which is responsible for the maintenance of the basal metabolic rate. In this case the patient is producing an excess of thyroxine (hyperthyroidism), which has suppressed the TSH by a negative feedback loop on the anterior pituitary. **The commonest cause of hyperthyroidism is an autoimmune disorder called Graves' disease**. Most commonly affected are females (M/F 1:5) between the ages of 20 and 40.

> On examination, a tachycardia, a goitre, and bulging eyes were noted.

An increased sympathetic activity is caused by the excess thyroid hormone production, leading to a fast pulse, sweating, and a resting tremor. The autoimmune response in the thyroid gland leads to swelling and inflammation within the gland, causing a smooth, uniform goitre.

Exophthalmos (bulging, staring eyes—Fig 1.7f) is caused by an autoimmune response in the extraocular muscles, where there is an antigen similar to the TSH receptor. This causes swelling and oedema of the muscles. Less marked signs of ophthalmopathy include bloodshot eyes (called chemosis), periorbital oedema, and upper and lower eyelid retraction. Thyroid eye disease only occurs in patients with Graves' disease.

The key investigations are the TSH (which will be suppressed in thyrotoxicosis) and the TRAb (thyroid hormone receptor antibodies—which can be raised in Graves' disease).

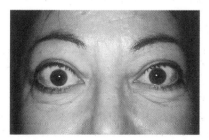

Fig 1.7f Exophthalmos with lid retraction showing the white sclera above the iris.

> The patient was initially treated with carbimazole.

Carbimazole is an antithyroid drug, which inhibits thyroid hormone synthesis and is the initial treatment of choice in patients with thyrotoxicosis. In addition, if the patient has symptoms of excess sympathetic activity (e.g. excess sweating, hand tremor), they can be given a beta-blocker, such as propranolol.

> Two weeks later, the patient developed a sore throat.

Carbimazole has potential side-effects, including rashes and a low white cell count (neutropenia), leading to an increased susceptibility to infection. All patients should be warned to report to their GP immediately if they develop a sore throat. If the patient does develop a neutropenia, then the carbimazole is stopped and the patient switched to propylthiouracil, another antithyroid drug.

Once the patient is made euthyroid (normal thyroid activity) then **the patient may require further treat-**

Clinical key points in thyrotoxicosis

- Graves' disease is the commonest cause of an overactive thyroid (hyperthyroidism)

- Ask about weight loss, irritability, and tremor, as these can be caused by the excess thyroid hormone production, leading to an increased sympathetic activity

- Ask about a family history of thyrotoxicosis or recent pregnancy (which can bring on thyrotoxicosis)

- On examination check for excess sweating, tachycardia, and resting tremor. Look for a goitre and listen for a bruit over the thyroid

- Examine for exophthalmos (bulging, staring eyes). This is caused by an autoimmune response in the extraocular muscles, where there is an antigen similar to the TSH receptor

- The key investigations are the TSH (which will be suppressed in thyrotoxicosis) and the TRAb (which can be raised in Graves' disease)

- Thyrotoxicosis is treated initially with antithyroid drugs. Definitive (long-term) treatment is by either radioactive iodine or thyroidectomy (removal of the thyroid gland)

ment with either radioactive iodine or surgery to suppress thyroid activity in the long term.

Background: thyroid

The thyroid is a midline neck organ, situated anterior to the trachea, which consists of two lobes joined in the middle by the isthmus. It secretes the hormones thyroxine (T4) and triiodothyronine (T3), which act as a metabolic thermostat. Examine the thyroid by standing behind the patient with both hands on the thyroid. A normal sized thyroid is not palpable.

Examination

Feel whether the gland is uniformly enlarged (a goitre), has one single lump (a solitary thyroid nodule), or more than one lump (a multinodular goitre). Ask the patient to swallow (with a glass of water); **if the lump moves on swallowing**, then it is in the thyroid, as the thyroid is attached to the larynx by the pre-tracheal fascia. Examine for cervical lymphadenopathy, as thyroid carcinomas can spread to the local lymph nodes. Also examine the trachea and check for tracheal deviation, as large thyroid nodules can shift the trachea. Listen to the voice for hoarseness (a sign of potential malignancy, caused by local infiltration of the recurrent laryngeal nerve, which passes close to the thyroid).

Signs in thyroid disease

Patients who have an overactive thyroid (hyperthyroid) have an **increased metabolic rate** and classically present with a **fine tremor of the hands**, **fast pulse rate**, and **increased sweating**. They can also develop **eye signs**, such as periorbital oedema, chemosis (red, injected sclera), lid retraction (when the sclera is visible either above or below the iris), or obviously protruding eyeballs (called proptosis or exophthalmos). The eye signs are caused by an autoimmune reaction in the eye muscles **and are found only in autoimmune hyperthyroidism (called Graves' disease—see pp. 95–96)**.

Conversely, patients with an underactive thyroid have a **decreased metabolic rate**, and present with **mental slowness, cold extremities, dry skin, and coarse hair**. Primary hypothyroidism is usually caused by autoimmune thyroiditis (Hashimoto's thyroiditis), when antibodies are raised against the enzyme thyroid peroxidase, which is essential for the production of thyroxine. Hashimoto's thyroiditis shows a familial predisposition, in keeping with a lot of autoimmune diseases.

Thyroid conditions

Thyroid disease from the surgical point of view presents most commonly as:

- a lump or lumps in the thyroid—solitary thyroid nodule or multinodular goitre

- hyperthyroidism (thyrotoxicosis).

Solitary thyroid nodule

Five per cent of the population can be affected (women more than men), but only 5% are malignant (95% are benign). The aim of investigations is to check the thyroid status (check the TSH) and to differentiate benign causes from malignant causes.

The current mainstay of investigations is FNA.

Thyroid nodules are investigated by checking the function of the thyroid (check the TSH) and by checking the cells of the nodule (by FNA). FNA is good for discriminating between benign and malignant nodules.

Radioisotope scans and thyroid ultrasound are relatively unhelpful in discriminating between benign and malignant nodules.

Most nodules are benign. Benign nodules (e.g. thyroid cysts, colloid nodule) do not need surgery and can be reviewed at 12 months and the FNA repeated.

Thyroid cancers generally have a good prognosis. Malignant nodules are most commonly caused by **differentiated thyroid carcinomas**, the main types of which are **papillary carcinoma** (80%) and **follicular carcinoma**. Papillary carcinoma occurs in younger patients (20–40 years) and spreads by lymphatic invasion to the local cervical lymph nodes. It generally carries a good prognosis (80% survival at 20 years). Follicular carcinoma occurs in an older age group (40–60 years) and spreads by the bloodstream to the bones and lungs. It carries a slightly poorer prognosis (70% at 5 years).

Thyroid cancers are treated by surgery (thyroidectomy) and radioactive iodine. The treatment of differentiated carcinoma is usually total thyroidectomy, followed by thyroxine therapy (to suppress the TSH) and radioactive iodine (which may be taken up by occult metastases).

Undifferentiated carcinoma (anaplastic carcinoma) is extremely uncommon and not particularly amenable to treatment by either surgery or radiotherapy—most patients are dead within a year.

Thyroid **lymphoma** usually develops on a background of autoimmune thyroiditis (Hashimoto's thyroiditis in elderly women). It can be treated by a combination of surgery, radiotherapy, and chemotherapy.

Fast facts—Thyroid goitre (an enlargement of the thyroid for any reason)

Causes

- Physiological—increase in size due to increased need for thyroxine (puberty/pregnancy)
- Iodine deficiency—$\downarrow$ T4, $\uparrow$ TSH, $\uparrow$ gland size
- Primary hyperthyroidism—goitre and thyrotoxicosis due to circulating immunoglobulins
- Multinodular goitre

Solitary thyroid nodule

- 5% of females have a solitary thyroid nodule
- 95% benign (colloid nodule, cyst)
- 5% malignant (mostly papillary, follicular)

Examination

- Check whether nodule moves on swallowing (i.e. in the thyroid)
- Check for cervical lymphadenopathy
- Check for hoarseness (? recurrent laryngeal nerve palsy)

Investigations

- TSH
- FNA

Management

- Observe with repeat FNA in 12 months if benign on FNA
- Thyroid lobectomy if suspicious or malignant on FNA

Multinodular goitre

- Multiple degenerative nodules in thyroid
  - —can extend to beneath the sternum (retrosternal) and narrow the trachea
  - —can become toxic

Examination

- Check for trachea deviation/retrosternal extension

Investigations

- TSH
- FNA (of dominant nodule)
- CT scan (to assess tracheal narrowing)

Management

- Thyroidectomy if retrosternal or tracheal compression or for cosmetic reasons
- Thyroidectomy or radioactive iodine if toxic

Thyroid cancer

- Papillary (80% of thyroid cancers)—usually age 20–40; metastasis to lymph nodes; excellent prognosis
- Follicular—usually age 30–50; metastasis via blood; good prognosis

Management

- Thyroidectomy and radioactive iodine

Multinodular goitre

This is essentially a swelling of the thyroid with more than one nodule. A multinodular goitre can be toxic (i.e. producing an excess of thyroxine), but most are non-toxic. The risk of malignancy in a dominant nodule in multinodular goitre is similar to a solitary nodule (i.e. 5%). Surgery is reserved for toxic multinodular goitre, cosmetic reasons, or if the goitre is compromising the trachea or oesophagus.

Hyperthyroidism (thyrotoxicosis)

The symptoms of an overactive thyroid (**hyperthyroidism**) include irritability, heat intolerance, increased appetite, decreased weight, and sweating. These are all signs of an increase in the basal metabolic rate (controlled by the thyroid). In hyperthyroidism, the TSH is suppressed by either a high free thyroxine (T4) or T3 level in the blood. The causes of hyperthyroidism include

- **Graves' disease** (an autoimmune disease with an antibody raised against the TSH receptor—TRAb). **Graves' disease is the commonest cause of an overactive thyroid**
- **toxic multinodular goitre**

• **solitary toxic adenoma**—when there is a single nodule in the thyroid, which is overactive.

All three causes can be initially treated by antithyroid drugs (carbimazole and propylthiouracil) and a beta-blocker if symptomatic. **An overactive thyroid is treated initially by carbimazole to stop the gland being overactive.**

Definitive treatment is by either surgery or radioactive iodine. Graves' disease can be treated in the long term by either radioactive iodine or thyroidectomy. Toxic multinodular goitre can be treated by either radioactive iodine or near total thyroidectomy and solitary toxic adenoma is treated by thyroid lobectomy or radioactive iodine.

Following total thyroidectomy, patients require thyroxine treatment (as they have no more endogenous supply) while most patients (95%) undergoing thyroid lobectomy do not require thyroxine (as the contralateral thyroid lobe supplies enough thyroxine).

The main complications to remember are damage to the recurrent laryngeal nerve leading to a palsy (1% of cases), damage to the parathyroid glands leading to hypocalcaemia (5% of cases), which is usually transient, and wound haematoma leading to laryngeal oedema and stridor.

Fast facts—Hyperthyroidism (overactive thyroid gland)

Causes

• Graves' disease (± thyroid eye disease)

• Toxic multinodular goitre

• Solitary toxic nodule

Examination

• Check for fast pulse, sweating, tremor

• Check for eye signs in Graves' disease

• Listen for thyroid bruit in Graves' disease

NB: Thyroid eye disease only occurs in patients with Graves' disease.

Investigations

• TSH/free T4/T3

• FNA if dominant nodule present

• Thyroid antibodies (TRAb)

Management

• Antithyroid drugs initially (e.g. carbimazole—beware of ↓ white cells)

• Total thyroidectomy or radioactive iodine if Graves' disease or toxic multinodular goitre

• Thyroid lobectomy or radioactive iodine if solitary toxic nodule

Vascular conditions

Chapter contents

Chronic arterial occlusive disease 97

Scenario 1: pain in the leg with walking 97

Scenario 2: pain in the foot at night 98

Scenario 3: sudden painful numb foot 99

Scenario 4: sudden weakness of the right hand 99

Background: arterial disease 100

Abdominal aortic aneurysm 110

Scenario 1: sudden abdominal pain and collapse 110

Background: peripheral arterial aneurysms 111

Venous disorders 112

Scenario 1: uncomplicated varicose veins 112

Scenario 2: chronic recurrent leg ulcer 113

Background: chronic venous disease 115

Chronic arterial occlusive disease

Scenario 1: pain in the leg with walking

> A 76-year-old male retired postman presents with pain in the left leg after walking 150 metres. This initially starts in the calf and then rises to the thigh and buttock.

'Intermittent claudication' is pain in muscle (calf, thigh, buttock) only associated with exercise and resolves quickly (less than 5 minutes) with stopping walking. It does not occur at rest.

Exercise requires the delivery of more oxygen as the muscle fibres perform more work. This is achieved by delivering more blood (200–400%) by increasing the output of the heart.

In patients with peripheral vascular disease this increase in blood delivery is impeded or prevented by narrowing (stenosis) or blockage (occlusions) of the arteries leading to the exercising muscle (usually the calves). The muscle therefore receives less oxygen than it requires and due to muscle ischaemia becomes increasingly painful forcing the sufferer to stop. The blood requirement and blood delivery become matched as the muscle rests and the pain disappears. The disease causing this is nearly always atherosclerosis.

> There is a history of smoking and a previous coronary artery bypass for angina. The patient also receives medication for hypertension.

Smoking, hypertension, diabetes, and elevated serum cholesterol (>5.0 mmol/l) are the modifiable risk factors for the development and progression of vascular disease. In an individual with evidence of vascular disease the disease will progress unless the patient stops smoking, has his/her hypertension, diabetes, and serum cholesterol checked and treated.

The presence of coronary artery disease serves to emphasize that peripheral arterial occlusive disease is part of a body-wide disease affecting large and medium sized arteries. The patient may also have suffered a cerebrovascular accident (CVA).

> On examination the patient appears healthy. The patient may have undiagnosed hypertension and an abnormal pulse (atrial fibrillation or bradycardia due to heart block or medication).

As the vascular disease may affect all parts of the vascular tree so myocardial ischaemia leading to atrial fibrillation or any other arrythmia is possible.

Peripheral pulses should be examined along with indications of chronic ischaemia (muscle wasting, loss of hair, venous guttering, ulceration at pressure points). The patient should also be examined for aortic aneurysms as up to 1 in 10 patients presenting with intermittent claudication may also have an aortic aneurysm.

> The patient has easily palpable femoral pulses on both sides. All other pulses are absent below this.

The commonest site for a significant arterial stenosis or occlusion in patients with intermittent claudication is in the distal superficial femoral artery in the lower third of the thigh. Therefore, the patient's femoral pulse is present but the popliteal pulse behind the knee and the ankle pulses (dorsalis pedis and posterior tibial) are absent. As the disease affects the whole arterial tree, it is common for the other leg to be also affected.

> The patient's ankle brachial pressure index (ABPI) is 0.6 on the left and 0.75 on the right.

The key investigations are to measure the ABPI and an angiogram if intervention is being contemplated.

Scenario 2: pain in the foot at night

> An 80-year-old-man presents with a 2-week history of severe pain in the foot at night. The pain wakes him from sleep. He finds walking round eases the pain.

The history of night pain waking the patient from sleep is classical for ischaemic rest pain. Rest pain is pain generated by nerve end ischaemia. The blood supply to the toes is so poor that when the feet are raised in bed the loss of the extra push from gravity plus the reduction of the cardiac output during sleep causes the difference, rendering the nerve roots ischaemic.

Walking about allows the addition of gravity and an increase in cardiac output to increase the perfusion pressure to an adequate level.

> On examination the affected foot has gangrene of the tip of the great toe (Fig. 1.8a).

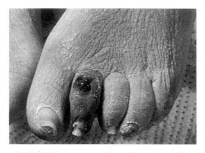

Fig 1.8a Clinical photograph showing toe gangrene from ischaemia.

Clinical key points in chronic peripheral arterial occlusive disease

- Ask about pain in the legs—'intermittent claudication' is pain in muscle (calf, thigh, buttock), which occurs with walking and resolves quickly (less than 5 minutes) when walking stops

- Ask about predisposing factors—e.g. smoking (90% of patients with vascular disease smoke), diabetes, hypertension, raised cholesterol

- Ask about rest pain—this is continuous pain felt distally in the toes and feet—it is made worse when lying flat; rest pain is pain generated by nerve end ischaemia

- On examination, check for all the peripheral pulses and listen for bruits. Look for signs of peripheral vascular disease (muscle wasting, loss of hair, venous guttering)

- Look for ischaemic ulcers—these tend to occur at the site of pressure points, e.g. the heel

- The key investigations are to measure the ABPI and an angiogram

Ulcers in ischaemia tend to occur at the site of pressure points usually exacerbated by ill-fitting shoes (medial and lateral borders of the foot, the tips of the toes, and the heel).

Scenario 3: sudden painful numb foot

A 65-year-old woman presents with a 2-hour history of initially severe pain in the foot, which developed into numbness and an inability for the leg to support her weight.

The history of acute foot/leg pain that rapidly progresses to numbness is classical for acute limb ischaemia. The patient may also notice the foot is pale or even white.

She has a history of atrial fibrillation.

Ninety per cent of emboli have a cardiac source (e.g. arrhythmia, valvular heart disease, prosthetic heart valves, mural thrombus post-myocardial infarction). This clot can then move into the systemic circulation (embolus) usually impacting at bifurcations (e.g. carotid, aortic, iliac, femoral) where the cross-sectional area of the downstream vessel becomes suddenly less. The emboli can therefore cause other vascular catastrophes such as strokes or intestinal ischaemia.

The formation of clot within the heart is prevented by anticoagulation (warfarin).

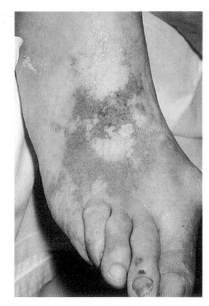

Fig 1.8b Fixed skin mottling of irreversible ischaemia.

On examination the limb has the classic 'five Ps'.

There are actually six 'Ps':

1. pain

2. pallor (no blood getting to the limb so it looks pale)

3. pulselessness

4. paraesthesia (due to nerve ischaemia)

5. paralysis (due to muscle ischaemia), and

6. 'perishing' cold (due to lack of blood warming the limb).

Limb viability is a product of depth of ischaemia and time. The total warm ischaemic time (time till cell death at room temperature) is between 4 and 6 hours. Not all episodes of acute limb ischaemia render the limb totally ischaemic. Increasing severity of ischaemia can be mapped by examination (Table 1.8a).

Scenario 4: sudden weakness of the right hand

A 65-year-old man presents with a 2-hour history of weakness of his right hand and an inability to speak.

The history of an acute neurological event (loss of speech, unilateral visual disturbance, motor or sensory loss) indicates a cerebrovascular event. The

TABLE 1.8a Findings in acute limb ischaemia interpretation

Findings	
Sensation intact	Foot salvageable, can await investigation and treatment
Calf muscle normal	
Paraesthesia of toes	Foot salvageable may wait for investigations, but needs regular review
Calf muscle normal	
Totally numb foot	Borderline limb survival (needs to be in theatre)
Tender calf muscle	
Fixed skin mottling	Too late, limb lost (Fig. 1.8b)
'Woody' calf muscle	
Unable to move foot	

Investigation may not be required but an angiogram may reveal important information concerning pre-existing arterial disease and the exact site of the emboli.

Clinical key points in acute limb ischaemia

- Ask about pain in the foot or leg(s). Usually there is sudden onset, coldness of the limb. This may rapidly progress to decreased sensation and an inability to move the leg

- Examination will show a pale/'white' leg that feels cold. Check for sensory and motor deficit

- A full cardiovascular history, examination, and ECG should be performed as 90% of emboli have a cardiac source (arrhythmia, valvular heart disease, prosthetic heart valves, mural thrombus post-myocardial infarction)

- Investigation may not be required but an angiogram may reveal important information concerning pre-existing arterial disease and the exact site of the emboli

patient's symptoms of right hand and speech indicate a left cerebral hemisphere event.

> He is already recovering by the time he is seen. He admits to a previous episode of visual disturbance in the left eye.

This is a short-term event (<24 hours) and can be classified as a transient ischaemic accident (TIA). The previous history of an episode of left eye visual disturbance points to *amaurosis fugax* (temporary blindness) and gives further evidence that the left carotid artery may be the common source for emboli.

> On examination there is minimal weakness in the grip of the left hand and slight slurring of speech. His pulse is regular.

Remember that emboli of cardiac origin can cause ischaemic neurological events. A regular pulse makes this unlikely, but an ECG is required.

> A duplex scan confirms the presence of an 80% stenosis of the left internal carotid artery and a normal right carotid artery.

Duplex scan is the investigation of choice. This confirms the presence of significant carotid artery disease (a lesion >70% stenosis). There are clear indications for a carotid endarterectomy in this individual. **The patient should be prescribed antiplatelet therapy**

(aspirin), **and risk factors should be investigated (smoking, glucose, cholesterol)** and potentially listed for surgery.

Clinical key points in carotid artery disease

- There is usually a history of an acute neurological event, loss of speech, unilateral visual disturbance, motor or sensory loss

- If symptoms last <24 hours they can be classified as a TIA

- A full cardiovascular history, examination, and ECG should be performed as emboli of cardiac origin can cause ischaemic neurological events

- Bloods should be taken for risk factor assessment (glucose, cholesterol), and the patient prescribed aspirin

- The key investigations are duplex scan of the carotid arteries and CT scan of the brain (to exclude a haemorrhage)

Background: arterial disease (Fig. 1.8c)

Knowledge of basic arterial anatomy is important; a diagrammatic representation is shown below.

The pattern of lower limb occlusive arterial disease is divided into three areas:

- aorto-iliac
- femoro-popliteal, and
- distal.

The commonest site of stenosis/occlusion is the adductor hiatus in the femoro-popliteal segment.

Vascular disease affecting the lower limb rarely exists in isolation. Peripheral vascular disease is only one manifestation of the body-wide effects of atherosclerotic disease—the tip of a vascular iceberg. Of those patients undergoing major vascular reconstruction:

- 10% have had a previous CVA
- 10% have had a previous episode of cardiac failure
- 20% have had a previous myocardial infarction
- 60% have an abnormal ECG.

A third of patients presenting with arterial disease have severe coronary artery disease. It is, therefore, vitally important to look for a history of angina, cardiac failure, arrhythmias, myocardial infarction, and CVAs.

Fig 1.8c Diagram of lower limb arterial tree.

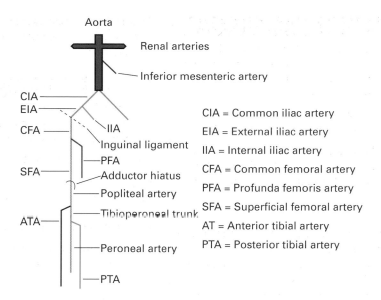

CIA = Common iliac artery

EIA = External iliac artery

IIA = Internal iliac artery

CFA = Common femoral artery

PFA = Profunda femoris artery

SFA = Superficial femoral artery

AT = Anterior tibial artery

PTA = Posterior tibial artery

Chronic peripheral arterial occlusive disease

History

There is up to a fourfold difference in blood requirement between resting and active muscle. The blood supply can be restricted by a narrowing or a blockage of a lower limb artery. When a required increase in blood supply is not delivered, this results in **ischaemic muscle pain**. This pain with exercise is termed *intermittent claudication*. The pain is cramping **brought on by exercise** and **relieved quickly by rest (<5 minutes)**. The symptom usually occurs at the same distance (sooner if going uphill). The site of the pain is related to the level of block (e.g. calf claudication usually results from superficial femoral artery stenosis/occlusion, thigh/buttock claudication from aorto-iliac artery stenosis/occlusion).

If the blood supply is even worse then the patient develops *rest pain*. This is **ischaemic skin pain** affecting the most distal part of the leg **the toes and foot**. This is due to there being insufficient blood supply at rest resulting in ischaemic nerve endings. The pain usually occurs at night, due to the foot being elevated in

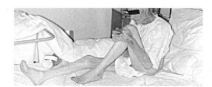

Fig 1.8d Patient with rest pain, the foot is drawn up (which can result in a fixed flexion deformity of the hip and knee), the foot is cherry red.

bed and a reduction in cardiac output with sleep, forcing the patient to hang the foot out of bed or to get up and walk around (Fig. 1.8d)

Risk factors

Risk factors impact on not only the development and future progression of the disease but also through associated diseases.

♦ *Smoking* is one of the most important contributing factors to arterial disease. Smoking also results in chronic obstructive airways disease, which may reduce exercise tolerance through shortness of breath, and may increase the risks of any surgical procedure but decrease the benefit by limiting the individual's exercise tolerance.

♦ *Diabetes* increases the incidence of peripheral arterial disease by 10- to 20-fold and the risk of limb amputation by 50-fold. Diabetes may also produce chronic renal failure, peripheral neuropathy, and blindness.

♦ *Hypertension* is often associated with cardiac, cerebrovascular, and renal disease.

♦ Other important factors are a past history of **previous amputations, deep vein thrombosis (DVT), pulmonary embolism, coagulation abnormalities, hyperlipidaemias**, and **other medication** such as aspirin, anticoagulants, and cardiac drugs (e.g. β-blockers).

Physical examination

♦ *General examination* is very important in the vascular patient with particular reference to the cardiac and respiratory systems.

- *Inspect* the extremities for paleness (due to less blood in the limb), cyanosis (due to sluggish circulation and extraction of more oxygen), redness (due to pooling of blood in capillaries dilated by ischaemia), ulceration and gangrene (due to insufficient blood to maintain skin viability), temperature (due to a reduction in the warming effect of blood), and varicosities. **Trophic changes** such as loss of hair, shiny skin, muscle wasting, and thickened toenails should also be sought. Veins on the dorsal aspect of the foot may also be 'guttered'. This is a product of insufficient blood in the vein to hold them open. The whole leg and foot should be thoroughly examined, especially the heels. This requires the foot to be lifted.

- *Palpation* of the extremities for temperature differences and diminished distal limb sensation. Capillary refilling time should also be assessed. This involves pressing on the pads of the great toes to produce blanching then release the pressure—normally the colour should fully return within **2 seconds** (i.e. the time it takes to say 'capillary refilling').

- *Peripheral pulses*, which includes bilateral carotid, radial, femoral, popliteal, dorsalis pedis, and posterior tibial, should be palpated. Some assessment of the character of the vessel can also be made (e.g. calcified, dilated). Listening for carotid, renal/aortic, iliac, common, and superficial femoral **bruit** is important.

- *Oedema* is not a direct indication of ischaemia, but can be a sign of rest pain, which causes the patient to sleep in a chair thereby causing positional-dependent oedema of the affected limb.

- *Buerger's sign* involves elevating the foot to approximately 30°, significantly underperfused feet become pale as the simple addition of the extra gravitational effect overcomes the perfusion pressure. With time the foot may also become painful, paraesthetic, or even numb.

The foot is then placed dependent over the edge of the bed, if there has been significant capillary ischaemia (a potent cause of vasodilation) the foot should then become very red due to pooling of blood within the capillaries. If the vasodilation is profound the blood pools for longer allowing more of the oxygen to be removed and the foot becomes a darker red reflecting the colour of deoxygenated haemoglobin.

Investigations

The patient's blood pressure is checked as untreated hypertension will accelerate the course of the disease. Random blood glucose, cholesterol, and a full blood count are performed to exclude diabetes, raised cholesterol, polycythaemia, and thrombocythaemia, which if present will also accelerate the course of the disease. **All modifiable risk factors should be treated aggressively**.

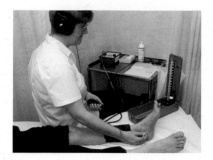

Fig 1.8e ABPI being performed.

Non-invasive investigations **are the first line as they carry minimal risk and patient discomfort**.

The standard first investigation is Doppler evaluation of the ABPI (Fig. 1.8e). ABPI is the ankle Doppler systolic pressure/brachial Doppler systolic pressure. This is the return of the Doppler systolic signal on letting a blood pressure cuff down slowly. Calcified vessels (particularly in diabetics and patients with renal failure) may give misleading readings or the signal may even be impossible to obliterate.

Colour duplex scanning is a more advanced form of ultrasound, which combines standard ultrasound scanning with 'on-screen' Doppler data concerning the vessel that is being examined. Velocity data are represented as a change in colour: the lighter the colour the faster the velocity. As arterial stenoses cause a dramatic increase in blood velocity this can be picked up easily on the ultrasound picture (Fig. 1.8f1, 1.8f2). Colour duplex is particularly used to assess the severity of carotid stenoses and to follow up lower limb bypass grafts looking for stenoses developing in the graft or native arteries.

Invasive investigations as the name implies involves 'invasion' of the body and therefore usually some discomfort and a small risk.

TABLE 1.8b ABPI and symptoms		
ABPI	**Non-diabetic**	**Diabetic**
1	'Normal'	'Normal'
0.6–0.8	Claudication	Rest pain
0.3–0.6	Rest pain	Gangrene
0.0–0.3	Gangrene	

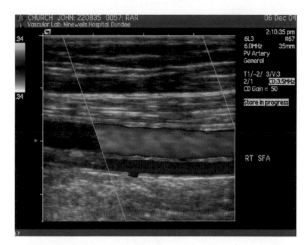

Fig 1.8f1 Duplex scan of normal artery.

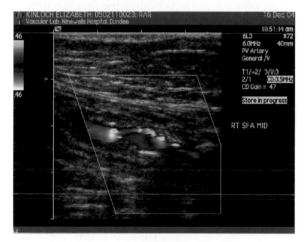

Fig 1.8f2 Duplex scan of a diseased artery showing an irregular vessel and turbulent flow as shown by the diffuse colours.

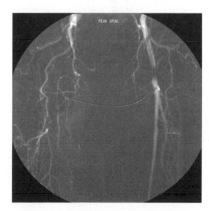

Fig 1.8g Angiogram of arterial disease with occlusion of the superficial femoral arteries.

Angiography involves direct puncture of an artery (usually the femoral, but rarely in certain circumstances the aorta or brachial artery). A fine catheter is introduced from the groin into the aorta and radio-opaque dye is injected while X-rays are taken (Fig. 1.8g). This gives a luminal 'road-map', showing occlusions or stenoses, but no information about the wall of the vessel.

Management

The management of non-disabling claudication revolves around the management of the risk factors. Overall the risk of amputation is about 1% per year. In smokers, this is 2% per year and in those who give up smoking is near to 0%. **Patients must, if at all possible, give up smoking.** As mentioned above, diabetes, a raised cholesterol, hypertension, polycythaemia, and increased clotting risk should all be aggressively managed.

Alongside the treatment of the presenting symptom is the management of the arterial tree. **Antiplatelet drugs (aspirin) reduce the incidence of myocardial infarction and stroke** as does reduction of the patient's cholesterol. Encouraging exercise also has a beneficial effect both in terms of walking distance and general cardiac fitness.

In disabling claudication (as judged by the patient) and critical limb ischaemia the options are limited. **Balloon angioplasty with or without a stent (a metal cage tube) can open up narrowed arteries.** The success of this intervention is very dependent on the site and nature of the lesion being treated. Angioplasty of iliac arteries is very successful (90% of arteries open at 1 year) while angioplasty of the superficial femoral artery is much less so (50% of arteries open at 1 year).

Surgery consists of either cleaning out a vessel (e.g. common femoral endarterectomy) for a short lesion or performing a bypass (e.g. femoro-popliteal bypass) for a longer lesion and carries significant risks (see Issue of

TABLE 1.8c Bypass procedures and patency rates

Bypass procedure	1-year patency rate
Aortobifemoral bypass	90
Femoro-above knee popliteal bypass (vein)	80
Femoro-above knee popliteal bypass (prosthetic)	70
Femoro-below knee popliteal bypass (vein)	70
Femoro-below knee popliteal bypass (prosthetic)	50

consent, p. 132). **The results of bypass surgery are also dependent on the site and the nature of the bypass used** (native vein or prosthetic (plastic) bypass).

In a number of cases no form of reconstruction/limb salvage is possible. In this event amputation is the only intervention left (see Table 1.8c).

Amputation

Amputation is always something that patient and clinician hope to avoid. It can, however, be an extremely positive treatment and may in some circumstances be the best alternative even when there are other options.

It can, when the patient is properly counselled and the operation appropriately done, turn a patient's life around. Chronic arterial disease can result in patients being unable to leave the house and being socially cut off, being unable to sleep because of rest pain, feel continuously unwell due to the effects of ulceration, and be emotionally isolated due to a sense of helplessness and hopelessness.

An amputation (particularly a below-knee amputation) can turn round this situation completely, with the patient becoming fully mobile, able to get out and meet people, get a full night's sleep, and feel well. The biggest barrier to this is the emotional response to the thought of amputation.

Clinical features

An amputation should be considered for two broad reasons:

1. A *lethal limb*—where the patient's life is at risk if the limb is retained:

    ◆ the limb is dead due to dense ischaemia

    ◆ there is gas gangrene

    ◆ there is a malignant condition (osteogenic sarcoma).

2. A *detrimental limb*—where the limb is useless and is detrimental to the patient:

    ◆ the limb is intractably painful (e.g. rest pain)

    ◆ the limb is causing the patient to feel unwell with no prospect of improvement (e.g. arterial or gross venous ulceration).

Investigation

Amputation must be performed through skin with enough blood supply to allow wound healing. This is invariably much higher than the site of the problem. The vast majority of amputations are performed either just below the knee or just above. **The chances of the**

TABLE 1.8d Rehabilitation to full independence following amputation	
Level	**All patients**
Unilateral below knee	66%
Unilateral above knee	36%
Bilateral below knee or below knee and above knee	45%
Bilateral above knee	11%

patient mobilizing on a prosthetic limb are very dependent on the level of the amputation.

The level of the amputation may be clinically obvious by the nature of the problem but a failed amputation with a further amputation at a higher level is a disaster for the patient and their emotional and physical well-being.

There are tests available to help guide the decision about the level, thermography, skin blood flow assessment, and Doppler pressure.

Management

Except in emergency amputation the patient requires counselling with the run-up to an amputation and the input from physiotherapy, rehabilitation medicine, occupational therapy, and clinicians.

The major levels for amputation are (Fig. 1.8h1, 1.8h2):

◆ digital—toe or toes

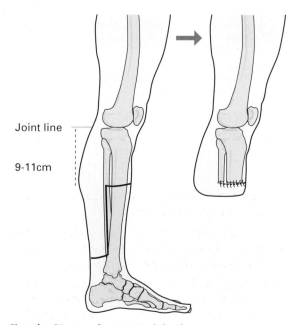

Joint line

9-11cm

Fig 1.8h1 Diagram of amputation below knee.

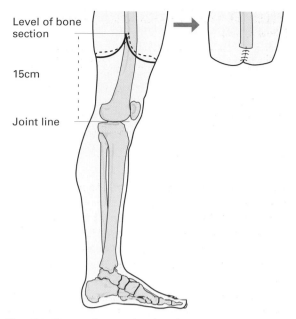

Fig 1.8h2 Diagram of amputation above knee.

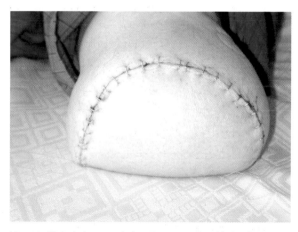

Fig 1.8i Clinical photograph showing a completed below knee amputation.

♦ transmetatarsal, which preserves the ankle joint and allows mobility with a modified ordinary shoe

♦ below knee, which preserves the knee joint and allows the fitting of a lightweight prosthesis and an excellent chance of full mobility (Fig. 1.8i)

♦ above knee, which requires a heavy, more difficult to use prosthetic limb. This can result in more elderly patients depending on a wheelchair for mobility but allow weight transfer.

Fast facts—Chronic peripheral arterial disease (chronic interruption of blood supply to a limb)

Aetiology

♦ Atherosclerosis

Risk factors

♦ Smoking

♦ Hypertension

♦ Diabetes

♦ Hyperlipidaemia

Clinical features

♦ Intermittent claudication

♦ Rest pain

♦ Ulceration and gangrene

Investigations

♦ ABPI

♦ Duplex scanning

♦ Angiography

Management

♦ Stop smoking

♦ Control other risk factors

  —reduce lipids/cholesterol

  —treat hypertension

  —control diabetes

♦ Aspirin

♦ Angioplasty

♦ Bypass surgery

♦ Amputation

Prognosis

♦ Stop smoking—limb loss at 5 years: almost 0%

♦ Continue smoking—limb loss at 5 years: 10%

Acute limb ischaemia

Acute limb ischaemia is due to the sudden loss of blood supply to a limb. It has two major causes: (1) **acute thrombosis of a pre-existing arterial stenosis** (acute thrombosis of popliteal aneurysms can also occur), and (2) acute arterial occlusion due to an **embolus**.

Emboli from the heart generally have two origins: mural thrombus due to laying down of thrombus either at a site of myocardial infarction or along the wall of a non-contractile left atrium (atrial fibrillation). The second site of cardiac origin is thrombus deposited on diseased valves (rheumatic fever or prosthetic valves).

Acute ischaemia can also be associated with trauma, but this is relatively uncommon.

Clinical features

Presentation of acute limb ischaemia is classically with the six 'Ps'.

1. *Painful* (due to skin and muscle ischaemia). A past history of claudication is important as this indicates thrombosis of a pre-existing lesion (usually superficial femoral artery) rather than an embolus as the cause.

2. *Pallor* (due to a lack of blood). This is only initially, as the foot/leg will soon become mottled. If there is no blanching then there is small vessel thrombosis and the ischaemia is probably irreversible (i.e. the leg is lost).

3. *Pulseless* (due to no arterial input to the limb). It is important to assess the other leg as the strong presence of all its pulses is an indication of a probable embolus as pre-existing arterial disease is likely to be bilateral.

4. *Paraesthetic* (due to sensory nerve ischaemia) is a symptom of a severe degree of ischaemia, particularly if it extends to the lower leg. Diabetics can have a pre-existing peripheral neuropathy that can mask this change.

5. *Paralysed* (due to muscle ischaemia) is again a sign of severe ischaemia and an indication of early intervention and revascularization.

6. *Perished with cold* (due to not being heated up by the input of warm blood).

Management

Treatment of patients with acute limb ischaemia centres around the cause (e.g. myocardial infarction) and the acute limb ischaemia itself. Therefore, general investigations of a FBC, U&Es, and ECG are essential.

Non-operative treatment is only appropriate if the limb is not in immediate jeopardy of being lost (i.e. there is no calf muscle paralysis or lower leg paraesthesia—see clinical scenario (3)). The patient is initially treated with heparin to prevent further propagation of thrombus, which may occlude vital collaterals.

Thrombolysis using streptokinase or tissue plasminogen activator to dissolve (lyse) the thrombus/embolus is now the commonest form of treatment. A catheter is placed in the artery into the clot and the tissue plasminogen activator is slowly instilled. If an underlying stenosis is identified as the cause of the episode this can be dilated using angioplasty balloons (see Treatment of chronic limb ischaemia, p. 103).

Operative treatment

Surgical embolectomy consists of opening the artery and passing a balloon catheter to the other side of the embolus. The balloon at the tip of the catheter is inflated and the catheter retrieved, the balloon drags the occluding thrombus out to the opening in the artery where it is picked out.

The amputation rate following surgical embolectomy is 15–20% with 25% of patients dying. Death is due to the cause of the problem (i.e. myocardial infarction) rather than the procedure itself.

Occasionally, particularly when there has been a prolonged period of muscle ischaemia, a compartment syndrome may develop. This can be difficult to diagnose. Classically, the muscle becomes painful and very hard due to swelling in its fascial compartment. If the patient is likely to develop (long history of ischaemic paralysis) or has developed compartment syndrome a **fasciotomy** is required (Fig. 1.8j). In this the deep investing fascia covering the muscle compartments of the lower leg is surgically opened along its full length (i.e. knee to ankle). This releases the raised pressure within the compartment by allowing the muscle to bulge out.

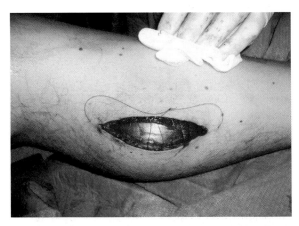

Fig 1.8j Short fasciotomy with subcutaneous division of the deep fascia.

Following treatment of whatever nature the patient is formally anticoagulated with warfarin to prevent further thrombosis or potential embolus formation.

The outcome of acute ischaemia depends on three factors—the general state of the patient, the duration of the ischaemia, and the level (i.e. aortic occlusion is worse than iliac is worse than femoral, etc.).

Diabetic foot

Three elements comprise the pathophysiology of the 'diabetic foot': angiopathy, neuropathy, and infection.

1. Diabetic *angiopathy* takes two significant forms:
   - microangiopathy affects arterioles and capillaries and is responsible for the renal, ophthalmic, and neurological complications of the disease. It does not have a significant role in diabetic foot disease
   - diabetics have a significantly higher incidence of large vessel vascular disease. This in turn accounts for the ischaemic element of diabetic foot problems (contribution to ulceration and poor healing).

2. Diabetic *neuropathy* affects sensory, motor, and autonomic nerves:
   - the reduced sensation can result in undetected trauma, leading to infection
   - the motor component causes the small muscles of the feet to alter the pressure distribution across the sole of the foot leading to areas of abnormally high pressure, which causes ulceration
   - the autonomic component affects the sympathetic nerves reducing sweating with drying and cracking of the skin.

3. The third element is *infection*. Bacteria enter the skin through ulcers or cracks. The blood supply may be poor due to arterial disease. Once the infection becomes established deep intra-foot abscesses develop.

Clinical features (Fig. 1.8k1, 1.8k2)
The diabetic foot, therefore, presents as part of a spectrum with a greater or lesser combination of the above

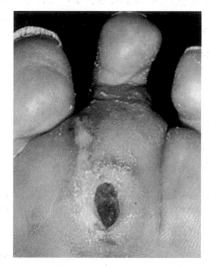

Fig 1.8k1 Clinical photograph showing diabetic foot: a penetrating ulcer at a pressure point.

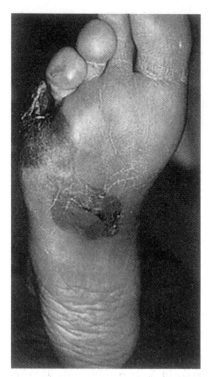

Fig 1.8k2 Gangrenous fifth toe due to abscess formation within the foot.

features. A patient presenting with a predominantly neuropathic foot exhibits a sensory deficit with plantar ulceration. The pedal pulses are present.

With a neuroischaemic foot the features may include ulcers over the borders of the foot or between the toes. Toe gangrene may be the product of digital artery thrombosis secondary to infection or a more profound global ischaemia due to proximal large artery occlusion (superficial femoral and tibial arteries).

The bacteria involved in infection are usually staphylococci, streptococci, and anaerobic bacteria. If neglected, gas gangrene may occur.

Investigation

Identification of osteomyelitis is important. MRI is the best investigation, but plain X-ray and radio-isotope bone scan have a supportive role.

Doppler pressure assessment is unreliable, as the arteries are uncompressible by the blood pressure cuff.

Management

Prevention is by far the most important aspect of the care of the patient with a neuropathic/neuroischaemic foot. The foot should be cared for and the term 'foot at risk' is useful to get across the concept of how precarious the well-being of the foot is.

If ulceration and infection occur the single most significant issue is the presence of a palpable ankle pulse. If a pulse is present debridement (occasionally quite extensive) and antibiotics will settle the problem in most cases. If there is no pulse and the problem has an ischaemic element limb loss (amputation) becomes more likely. An angiogram and some form of revascularization (usually bypass graft) will probably be necessary to save the leg.

Fast facts—Diabetic foot (damaged foot due to ischaemia and/or neuropathy in diabetes)

Pathophysiology

- Neuropathy
- Ischaemia
- Infection

Clinical features

- Neuropathy
  - —insensate foot
  - —pressure area ulceration
- Ischaemia—trophic skin changes
- Infection
- —osteomyelitis
- —soft tissue with very rapid progression

Investigations

- ABPIs may be unreliable
- MRI/X-ray/radio-isotope bone scan—of foot for osteomyelitis
- Angiography

Management

- Prevention
  - —inspect feet
  - —correctly fitted footwear
- Treat infection aggressively
  - —antibiotics
  - —surgical debridement
- Bypass surgery for limb salvage

Carotid artery disease

Stroke is a major problem world-wide. One cause is embolization from a narrowing (stenosis) of the origin of the internal carotid artery caused by atheroma.

Clinical features

Many people with carotid artery disease are asymptomatic. Once symptoms develop it is usually due to platelet emboli from the atheromatous plaque. The emboli can cause a number of symptoms.

- *amaurosis fugax*: transient visual disturbance/loss in the eye on the same side as the stenosis. It is classically described as a 'curtain coming down' on the vision from one eye

- *TIA*: transient (<24 hours) contralateral focal neurological deficit, usually motor weakness, sensory loss, or speech-related receptive or expressive dysphasia), the latter if the symptomatic carotid is on the dominant side (usually left in a right-handed patient)

- *CVA*: a neurological deficit lasting more than 24 hours. This may have been preceded by a TIA or amaurosis fugax.

Investigation

All patients with a history of focal neurological events should undergo a duplex scan (Fig. 1.8l). This allows a non-invasive assessment of the state of the carotid arteries. The key issue is the presence of an internal carotid artery stenosis (>70% stenosis).

A CT scan of the brain should be performed in patients with an established stroke to rule out a haemorrhage as this would contraindicate a carotid endarterectomy (Fig. 1.8m, 1.8n).

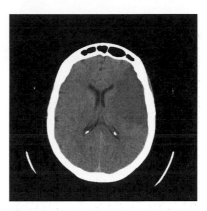

Fig 1.8m CT scan showing cerebral infarct with the darker infarcted are on the left.

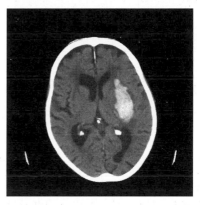

Fig 1.8n CT scan of cerebral haemorrhage shown by the white patch.

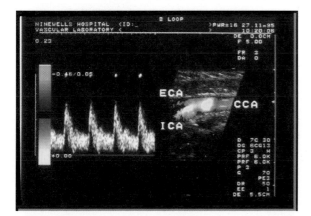

Fig 1.8l Duplex scan of a normal carotid artery, the velocity profile on the left and the colour image on the right.

Management

With the identification of carotid artery disease general cardiovascular risk reduction should be instituted (stop smoking, diagnose and treat diabetes, hypertension, hyperlipidaemia).

Specific medical therapy revolves around antiplatelet therapy (aspirin, aspirin and dipyridamole, and clopidogrel). These produce a degree of inactivation of platelets and therefore less chance of platelet adhesion to and embolization from the carotid atheromatous plaque.

Surgical therapy consists of carotid endarterectomy. This involves the opening of the carotid artery and removal of the atheromatous lining. With this operation there is a 5% chance of perioperative stroke or death.

Aetiology

- Atherosclerosis

Risk factors

- Smoking
- Hypertension
- Diabetes
- Hyperlipidaemia

Pathophysiology

- Embolization from carotid artery disease
- Reduction of flow

Clinical features

- Contralateral motor/sensory deficit
- Speech-related deficit
- Ipsilateral eye signs (amaurosis fugax)

Investigations

- Duplex scanning
- CT scan—identify infarct (not haemorrhage)

Management

- Stop smoking
- Control risk factors
  - —stop smoking
  - —reduce lipid
  - —treat hypertension
  - —control diabetes
- Antiplatelet agents—aspirin/dipyridamole/clopidogrel
- Carotid endarterectomy—>70% stenosis with symptoms

Prognosis

- Carotid endarterectomy has a 5% perioperative stroke/death risk

Abdominal aortic aneurysm

Scenario 1: sudden abdominal pain and collapse

> A 75-year-old-man presents with history of collapse associated with sudden onset of severe back pain.

A history of sudden collapse with abdominal or back pain in patients over the age of 50 must raise the possibility of a ruptured aortic aneurysm until proved otherwise.

> On examination his pulse is 60/min, but with a blood pressure of 80/40.

A low blood pressure indicates circulatory collapse. In a young patient the pulse would be expected to rise before the blood pressure falls. However, in the elderly there is not infrequently an inability to mount the usual compensatory mechanisms. This may be due to ischaemic heart disease (this is a worrying sign, the patient's heart may not be able to cope with the severe insult to which it is being subject), or medication (β-blockers), which prevent any tachycardia as part of its cardiac sparing action.

> On examination of the abdomen there is an obvious large pulsatile mass in the central abdomen.

The diagnosis may be fairly obvious if the abdomen is examined and there is an obvious aortic aneurysm in a shocked patient. The patient should be transferred directly to the operating theatre.

Sometimes things are not so clear cut. Two investigations are available to help. These both may involve a

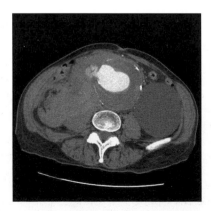

Fig 1.80 CT scan of ruptured aortic aneurysm with white contrast leaking from the aortic lumen surrounded by soft tissue shadow haematoma.

growing degree of delay, something that a shocked elderly patient may not be able to afford.

- **an ultrasound of the abdomen will diagnose an abdominal aortic aneurysm, but it will not reliably diagnose rupture**

- **a CT scan will diagnose both an aneurysm and whether it has ruptured but this involves significant delay in a haemodynamically unstable patient (Fig. 1.8o).**

Bloods should be sent urgently for FBC, U&Es, and cross-match 6 units of blood with platelets and clotting factors.

Clinical key points in abdominal aortic aneurysm

- Always think of a ruptured aortic aneurysm in sudden collapse with abdominal or back pain in patients >50 years

- The diagnosis may be fairly obvious on abdominal examination when there is an obvious aortic aneurysm in a shocked patient

- Bloods should be sent urgently for FBC, U&Es, and cross-match 6 units of blood with platelets and clotting factors

- If the presence of an aneurysm is in doubt an ultrasound of the abdomen will diagnose an abdominal aortic aneurysm, but it will not reliably diagnose rupture

- A CT scan will diagnose both an aneurysm and whether it has ruptured but this may involve dangerous delay in a haemodynamically unstable patient

---

Background: peripheral arterial aneurysms

Abdominal aortic aneurysm

Abdominal aortic aneurysm arises below the renal arteries in 95% of cases. Pathology reveals a very thin-walled dilated aorta containing laminated mural thrombus with a lumen through the thrombus not much larger than normal.

Aortic aneurysms can be familial, they are more common in males and are associated with hypertension (40%), with severe coronary artery disease (30%), and other peripheral aneurysms (20%).

The **natural history** of aortic aneurysms follows the **law of Laplace**, which simply translated states: **the bigger the transverse diameter of the aneurysm the faster it grows.**

The size of the aneurysm also indicates the risk of rupture, the larger the aneurysm the bigger the chance of rupture. A 5-cm aortic aneurysm has about a 5% chance of rupturing per year and an 8-cm aortic aneurysm about 15%.

The usual presentation of aneurysms is as an asymptomatic pulsatile abdominal mass, in 50% of cases, detected either by physical examination, or on abdominal X-ray, or abdominal ultrasound scan.

Symptoms from aneurysms can either be as abdominal or back pain. **More dramatically an aneurysm can present by rupturing**, which usually results in sudden abdominal or back pain, collapse, shock, and probably most frequently death.

Investigation

1. *Ultrasound scanning* is used in the investigation and diagnosis of aortic aneurysms. This shows a 2-D black and white picture of the structure under examination (Fig. 1.8p). In the case of aortic aneurysms it can diagnose and size the aorta but it is poor for diagnosing rupture.

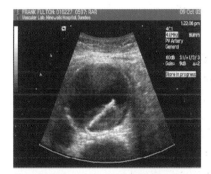

Fig 1.8p Ultrasound of circular aortic aneurysm.

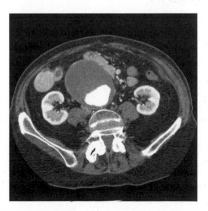

Fig 1.8q CT scan of aortic aneurysm using contrast which emphasizes that the blood only runs in part of the vessel the rest occupied by luminal thrombus.

2. *Angiography*, because of thrombus lining the inside of the aneurysm (*mural thrombus*) is very inaccurate in measuring aneurysm size, though it is used to visualize the distal circulation (because of coexisting occlusive arterial disease) and the upper limit of the aneurysm (i.e. the relationship to the renal arteries).

Fast facts—Abdominal aortic aneurysm (localized dilatation of the abdominal aorta)

Risk factors

- Smoking
- Hypertension

Pathology

- Increase in size is related to aneurysm size
- Risk of rupture is related to aneurysm size
- Mural thrombus within the aneurysm may embolize

Clinical features

- Asymptomatic, incidental finding
- Symptomatic—back pain, abdominal discomfort
- Rupture—sudden pain, collapse, death

Investigations

- Ultrasound scan to diagnose
- CT scan to evaluate extent—renal/iliac artery involvement
- Angiogram—to assess for endovascular repair

Management

- Surgical repair if >5.5–6 cm in diameter
- Endovascular repair for certain patients
- Protect the oesophagus
  —alginates
- Ruptured abdominal aortic aneurysms require immediate repair

Prognosis

- Perioperative mortality
  —elective: 5%
  —acute symptomatic: 15%
  —rupture: 50%

---

3. *CT scan* can be used, but it has no real advantage over ultrasound, except when used to diagnose aneurysm rupture, the relationship of the aneurysm to the renal arteries, or an inflammatory aneurysm (Fig. 1.8q). (An inflammatory aneurysm is a rare type (5%) in which the aortic wall is grossly thickened due to inflammation and fibrosis. These can cause severe back and abdominal pain in the absence of rupture.)

Management

Treatment of aneurysm is dependent on size and symptoms. Presently, unless the patient is severely medically disabled, any aneurysm over 5.5 cm is repaired electively.

In patients with abdominal pain and a tender aneurysm the aneurysm is repaired urgently (within 24 hours).

Finally, a ruptured aneurysm is the ultimate surgical emergency. **The real task of the clinician is to identify patients with an aortic aneurysm and repair the aneurysm electively.**

The operation consists of inserting a prosthetic graft within the aneurysm sac connecting normal upper aorta to normal distal aorta or iliac arteries, either at open surgery or as a combined radiological/surgical procedure (endovascular repair).

Popliteal artery aneurysm

About 10% of patients with an aortic aneurysm have a popliteal aneurysm and visa versa. The condition also tends to be bilateral.

A popliteal aneurysm rarely ruptures but much more commonly thromboses. It should therefore be borne in mind with cases of acute limb ischaemia.

The aneurysm is at risk of blocking when it gets to 2.5–3.5 cm in diameter. If it does then the chances of limb loss are about 35%.

It is repaired by tying off the popliteal aneurysm and performing an arterial bypass graft.

Venous disorders

Scenario 1: uncomplicated varicose veins

A 39-year-old female teacher presents to her GP with varicose veins. The veins first appeared during her second pregnancy. Her legs have become uncomfortable and sore particularly after prolonged standing. She complains of one episode of localized redness and tenderness over one of the calf veins.

Patients presenting with varicose veins tend to be female, though there is actually no difference in incidence between males and females. There is an association with a history of childbirth, the prevalence of varicose veins increasing with the number of pregnancies.

Standing as opposed to walking causes the highest intraluminal pressure. Occupations that involve a lot of standing are more likely to cause people to complain of discomfort with varicose veins rather than cause the problem itself.

The veins may become locally tender due to inflammation of the superficial veins (**thrombophlebitis**). The varicose veins may cause **failure of the venous drainage of the leg (chronic venous insufficiency), which may lead to skin ulceration or discoloration around the ankle.**

> There is no history of DVT, pulmonary embolism, or major leg fracture.

The past history is important as an underlying deep vein occlusion following a DVT is very important. This may follow a leg fracture (there is a high incidence of DVT with a fractured femur). Varicose veins in the presence of a deep vein occlusion may act as the pathway to get blood out of the leg. If there is any doubt about the patency of the deep veins then some form of investigation is required (e.g. ascending venogram or duplex ultrasound examination of the deep veins).

> The patient reports that her mother also had varicose veins.

As varicose veins are common (40% of the population) it is impossible to say whether a family predisposition to varicose veins really exists.

> On examination the patient appears healthy. There are no abnormal findings except for the affected leg. There is a cord-like vein passing medially from the groin to just below the level of the knee where it branches into two and passes down the anteromedial and medial aspect of the lower leg. The veins below the knee are distended and tortuous. Tapping the long saphenous vein below the groin can be felt at the level of the knee.

The long saphenous vein, which drains into the deep veins at the groin, is the commonest vein involved. The long saphenous vein passes down the medial aspect of the thigh and medial to the knee. A palpable tap transmitted from the upper thigh to the level of the knee means there is a column of standing blood within the vein with incompetent valves.

The veins are distended and tortuous due to a high intraluminal pressure. With increased intraluminal pressure the veins lengthen becoming tortuous and dilated, like a thin party balloon when it is blown up.

> The patient lies flat, the leg is held up emptying the veins and a tourniquet applied at the mid-thigh. Patient then stands and the state of the varicose veins is noted. The tourniquet is then released and again the state of the veins noted.

This is Trendelenberg's test. Control of the varicose veins by the tourniquet with their reappearance on release means that the abnormal connection between the deep and superficial veins lies above the tourniquet. Failure to control the veins implies that the prime site of deep-to-superficial valvular incompetence is below the tourniquet.

If there is any doubt about the origin of the veins (long or short saphenous) or the patency of the deep veins then duplex ultrasound is required.

Clinical key points in varicose veins

- Patients presenting with varicose veins tend to be female

- Ask about skin ulceration or discoloration around the ankle, episodes of thrombophlebitis, or leg discomfort

- A history of DVT as underlying deep vein occlusion is significant

- The legs should be examined to map the extent and origin of the varicose veins. The long saphenous vein that drains into the femoral vein at the groin is the commonest vein involved

- If there is any doubt about the origin of the veins (long or short saphenous) or the patency of the deep veins then duplex ultrasound is required

---

Scenario 2: chronic recurrent leg ulcer

> A 55-year-old female presents to her GP with a 6-month history of a leg ulcer (Fig. 1.8r). The ulcer is on the medial side of the lower leg just above the medial malleolus.

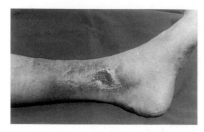

Fig 1.8r Clinical photograph showing a chronic venous ulcer.

This description is **characteristic of a chronic venous ulcer with a relapsing course**.

> There is history of DVT following childbirth 25 years previously.

A past history of DVT is important as this may be the underlying cause either due to deep venous obstruction or deep venous reflux due to valve destruction. Ulceration may follow up to 30 years after the event. Deep and/or superficial venous problems that lead to a failure of venous drainage with secondary effects is termed chronic venous insufficiency.

> The patient reports that the leg becomes increasingly uncomfortable as the day progresses. She gets relief by putting the leg up on a foot stool.

With poor venous drainage from a limb it will tend to retain interstitial fluid with an upright position, this in turn will make the leg feel heavy and uncomfortable. Elevating the leg will counteract this.

> On inspection of the leg there are gross varicose veins. The skin round the ulcer is thickened and has a brown discoloration.

As the effects of chronic venous insufficiency progress there is damage to the skin with subcutaneous fibrosis, and pigmentation due to red cell breakdown in the tissues. This is termed lipodermatosclerosis.

> The ankle pulses are easily palpable.

Although the clinical picture is of chronic venous insufficiency the state of the arterial circulation is as important. The absence of ankle pulses would require a further assessment with ABPI measurement.

A poorly perfused limb (ABPI <0.5) would suggest that the ulcer is unlikely to heal without improvement in arterial blood supply.

An ABPI <0.8 would contraindicate the use of compression therapy. Compression therapy is the mainstay of conservative management.

> A duplex scan shows no evidence of deep venous occlusion or valvular dysfunction. There is, however, gross long saphenous vein incompetence.

Duplex scan is the investigation of choice as it will give anatomical and functional information.
The treatment of chronic venous ulceration is graduated compression. This is by four-layer bandaging with the greatest compression at the ankle reducing as the bandage rises up the leg. This improves venous function and allows healing to occur.

The presence of isolated superficial venous incompetence (varicose veins) indicates that if the patient is fit then a simple varicose vein operation may well reduce the likelihood of the ulcer returning once healed. There is no evidence that healing will be quickened by surgery.

If the picture had been isolated deep venous problems then the only management available would have been graduated compression.

The presence of significant arterial disease (ABPI <0.8) would contraindicate compression therapy as the arterial perfusion pressure would be less and on occasion gangrene has resulted.

Clinical key points in chronic venous ulceration

- The history is usually one of relapsing leg ulceration potentially over many years. Ask about varicose veins and if there has been a DVT

- On examination the ulcer is usually above the medial malleolus but can become circumferential. The surrounding skin can be damaged with subcutaneous fibrosis, pigmentation (lipodermatosclerosis), and acute inflammation

- The key investigation is a duplex scan

- The treatment of chronic venous ulceration is graduated compression (significant arterial disease would contraindicate compression therapy—ABPI <0.8). Operative treatment on varicose veins may reduce the chances of recurrence after the ulcer has healed

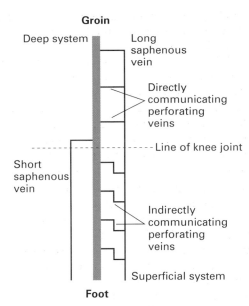

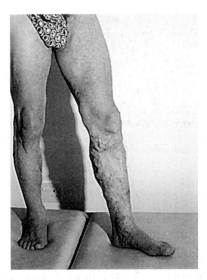

Fig 1.8t Clinical photograph showing dilated tortuous varicose veins, a product of high venous pressure within the superficial veins.

Fig 1.8s Diagram of venous drainage of the leg, blood returning to the heart by passing superficial to deep and bottom to top, allowing the muscle pump to act on the deep veins.

Background: chronic venous disease

There are two parallel venous drainage systems within the leg: the superficial and the deep veins. Blood travels from superficial to deep (via the perforating veins) then from distal to proximal (Fig. 1.8s).

The blood is propelled from distal-to-proximal by the combination of plantar and muscle pumps. The plantar pump works by compression of a plexus of veins in the sole of the foot during walking. The muscle pumps work by external compression of the deep veins as part of their resting and active muscle tone.

The second essential part of the system is the presence of venous valves. These valves prevent reflux of blood in distal and superficial directions. Hence the need for blood to pass to the deep veins for the muscle pump to act on the veins. Failure of these valves accounts for the majority of lower limb venous disease either by allowing a high deep venous pressure to be transmitted to the unsupported superficial system (varicose veins) or by preventing efficient passage of blood out of the leg (chronic venous insufficiency).

DVT and pulmonary embolism are dealt with in Section 2 (p. 189).

Varicose veins
Aetiology

Primary varicose veins appear to have a strong familial pattern (but as the condition is so common it is difficult to prove) and present more often in women (though the incidence in the sexes is probably the same). There is usually incompetence of the highest long saphenous vein valve (the sapheno-femoral valve) along with other long saphenous vein or perforating vein valves. This allows the transmission of pressure from the deep into the superficial system. This superficial venous hypertension results in dilated tortuous superficial veins (varicose veins) (Fig. 1.8t).

Secondary varicose veins are a product of deep venous obstruction following a previous DVT. This causes a marked increase of deep venous pressure in an attempt to push blood up the leg against the obstruction, overcoming the perforating vein valves. This allows blood to pass around the obstruction.

If there is any suggestion of a previous ipsilateral DVT (fractured leg, previous anticoagulant therapy) further investigation by duplex scan is required as the removal of the varicose veins may cause chronic venous insufficiency.

Clinical features

Presentation of patients with varicose veins is most commonly with displeasure at the cosmetic appearance, intermixed with tiredness and heaviness of the legs, or infrequently with skin ulceration or its precursors (dry, itchy, and thickened skin).

The patient is assessed using Trendelenburg's test. This involves raising the leg to empty the veins and applying a high thigh tourniquet. If the veins do not refill rapidly then the majority of the blood is entering via the sapheno-femoral junction (release of the tourniquet should produce rapid filling). If the veins fill rapidly then the problem is with the perforator veins.

Fast facts—Varicose veins (prominent, dilated tortuous superficial veins)

Epidemiology

- M/F = 1:1, 40–50% of adult population

Aetiology

- Primary/post-pregnancy
- Secondary to DVT

Pathology

- Superficial vein valve failure

Clinical features

- Uncomplicated
  - —asymptomatic/cosmetic
  - —dull ache, heavy legs

Complicated

- —superficial thrombophlebitis
- —bleeding
- —eczema, ulceration

Investigation

- Handheld Doppler
- Duplex scanning

Management

- Support stockings
- Surgery
  - —sapheno-femoral (high) ligation
  - —long saphenous vein thigh stripping
  - —local avulsions

Outcome

- Correctly managed varicose veins should give a durable result

Investigation

The investigation of choice is duplex scanning. This allows the identification of the precise site of venous incompetence. It is particularly useful in assessing the short saphenous vein (10% of cases), which drains into the popliteal vein somewhere round the popliteal fossa. It also allows assessment of the deep veins to rule out a previous DVT, the presence of which may contra-indicate surgery.

Treatment

The first step is by simple compression stockings, which apply a gradient of pressure from the ankle upward (there is probably no indication to apply stockings above the knee).

Alternatively varicose veins can be surgically removed with sapheno-femoral junction ligation, thigh long saphenous vein stripping, and local avulsions. The sapheno-femoral junction ligation prevents pressure transmission from the deep to superficial systems. The stripping prevents the same situation occurring again with the directly communicating thigh perforating veins. Local avulsions remove the below-knee perforating vein connections and the varicose veins themselves.

The patient's varicosities are marked prior to operation (as they disappear when the patient lies down on the operating table). The leg is bandaged at the end of the procedure to prevent bruising. The patient is encouraged to take daily walks for about a month after the operation.

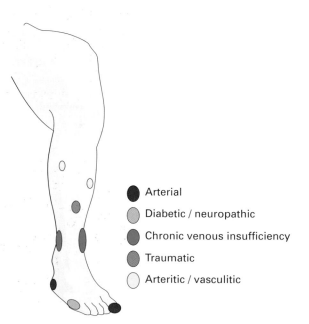

Arterial
Diabetic / neuropathic
Chronic venous insufficiency
Traumatic
Arteritic / vasculitic

Fig 1.8u Diagram of distribution of types of leg ulcer.

Chronic leg ulceration

There are a number of causes of chronic leg ulceration, which can exist either in isolation or combination (Fig. 1.8u):

♦ venous

♦ ⬦

♦ ⬦

♦ traumatic

♦ arteritis

♦ neoplastic.

1. **Chronic venous ulcers are associated with a past history of venous disease** (i.e. DVT or varicose ⬦s) producing chronic venous insufficiency.

   ⬦ronic venous insufficiency is a failure of ⬦quate venous drainage of the leg either due

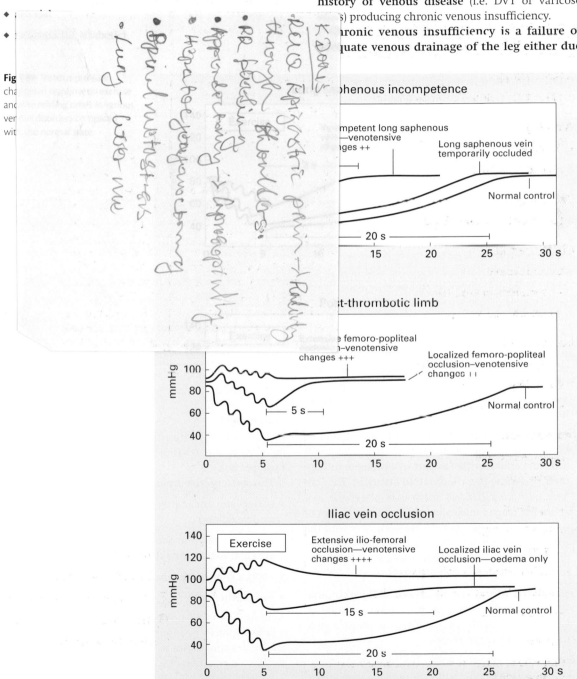

Fig ⬦ ⬦
cha ⬦
and ⬦
ver ⬦
wit ⬦

⬦henous incompetence

⬦mpetent long saphenous
⬦—venotensive
⬦ges ++

Long saphenous vein
temporarily occluded

Normal control

20 s

15   20   25   30 s

⬦st-thrombotic limb

⬦e femoro-popliteal
⬦—venotensive
changes +++

Localized femoro-popliteal
occlusion—venotensive
changes ⬦

Normal control

mmHg 100
       80
       60
       40

5 s

20 s

0   5   10   15   20   25   30 s

Iliac vein occlusion

mmHg 140
       120
       100
       80
       60
       40

Exercise

Extensive ilio-femoral
occlusion—venotensive
changes ++++

Localized iliac vein
occlusion—oedema only

Normal control

15 s

20 s

0   5   10   15   20   25   30 s

to obstruction of the deep system by post-thrombotic scarring and/or by valvular failure of deep and superficial systems either in combination or singly.

At its worst it produces 'varicose ulceration', classically just above the ankles. The same area can be affected by brown pigmentation (due to haemosiderin deposits), skin thickening (lipodermatosclerosis) and dry skin (varicose eczema) (Fig. 1.8m).

2. **Chronic arterial insufficiency produces ulceration due to skin ischaemia at areas of pressure.**

   The ulcers are as distal as possible in the limb, usually outer edges of great and little toes, tip of great toe, and at the heel. There is likely to be a past history of smoking and intermittent claudication. The ulcer will be painful particularly in bed at night (see Rest pain).

3. **Neuropathic ulcers occur in association with diseases of the nervous system, which result in sensory loss. The commonest cause is diabetes.**

   The ulcer results from unappreciated repeated injury or pressure. It is therefore painless and is situated at the site of such damage (i.e. sole of the foot, heel). As arterial disease is common in diabetics the ulcer may be neuroischaemic in origin showing features of both (i.e. distal but painless).

4. **Traumatic ulcers are likely to occur where there is subcutaneous bone (i.e. the shin).** There is no cushioning of the skin by underlying muscle. The commonest example is the pretibial ulcer in which a triangular skin flap is raised and undergoes necrosis.

5. **Arteritis ulcers are the result of a local loss of blood supply due to inflammation of the small arteries ('endarteritis') as part of a collagen inflammatory disease (i.e. rheumatoid arthritis).** They are 'normal' looking ulcers in strange places (i.e. not above the medial malleolus, not distal, not at sites of pressure or trauma). As they are associated with the collagen inflammatory diseases the patient may have other features, such as arthritis or Raynaud's phenomenon (cold-induced digital vasospasm).

6. **Neoplastic ulcers are squamous cell carcinoma.** They exhibit the neoplastic feature such as a raised base with a variable surface. They are unusual looking ulcers in strange places.

Investigation

The history and examination should give very strong pointers.

Volumetry/photoplethysmography allows an assessment of venous function. Both methods depend on exercise-induced venous emptying and tracing the rate of return to the resting state.

The state of both the superficial and deep venous systems can be delineated by one or more of the following: duplex scanning, venography, and volumetry/photoplethysmography (Fig. 1.8v).

Three venous states can exist:

- superficial venous incompetence either primary or due to recurrent varicose veins following previous surgery
- deep venous incompetence due to primary valvular failure or following recanalization after a DVT
- deep venous occlusion due to a previous DVT.

This is aimed at delineating the state of both the superficial and deep systems by duplex scanning.

The arterial circulation can be assessed by Doppler examination (see Arterial investigation above under Background: arterial disease, p. 100), with angiography being reserved for those cases with significant arterial disease (i.e. ABPI <0.8).

The neurological state can be assessed by soft touch examination with cotton-wool as part of the neurological examination. The presence of diabetes may already be known or if in doubt tested for by a fasting blood glucose.

The presence of collagen inflammatory disease is based on the history and the presence of specific autoantibodies (antinuclear factor, rheumatoid factor).

Management

In the vast majority this will be venous. The treatment in these cases is to reduce any superficial venous hypertension.

The **conservative treatment** can be summarized:

- correct any underlying general disorders (i.e. obesity, cardiac failure)
- apply dressings to the limb to protect the healing area and soak up any slough
- apply a compression bandage in four layers
- elevate the limb.

Antibiotics should not be used unless there is a systemic response to infection or local cellulitis. Local antibiotics should not be used. A positive bacteriology swab is a normal finding.

Surgical treatment is indicated if there is a significant element of superficial system incompetence. This should be treated by excision of the superficial venous system (as in varicose vein operations).

Venous ulcers may also have an element of arterial insufficiency; if the ABPI (see Arterial investigation, p. 102) is less than 0.8 then compression bandaging is contraindicated without arterial reconstruction either by angioplasty or reconstruction.

Fast facts—Chronic leg ulcer (ulceration of the leg due to failure of venous drainage, arterial inflow, or neuropathy)

Epidemiology

- M<F, common, affecting up to 5% of adults over the age of 60

Aetiology

- Majority (85%)—venous in origin, arterial insufficiency (10%), neuropathy, trauma, arteritis, and neoplasia are significant causes

Pathology

- Failure of venous drainage (deep and/or superficial venous) system
- Failure of arterial inflow due to arterial disease
- Loss of protective sensation leading to recurrent trauma at pressure points

Clinical features

- Site, symptoms, and associated features are dependent on underlying cause

Investigations

- Handheld continuous wave Doppler
- Duplex scanning
- ABPI
- Plethysmography (photoplethysmography)

Management

- Dressings and compression in the majority
- Superficial venous surgery, arterial reconstruction when indicated

Outcome

- In the case of simple superficial venous surgery the outlook is good

---

As there is likely to continue to be a predisposition to ulceration once the ulcer is closed the patient should continue to wear a below-knee support stocking that has been professionally sized and fitted.

The treatment of **arterial** ulcers is the same as the treatment for critical limb ischaemia.

The treatment of **neuropathic** ulcers revolves around protecting the area and the foot. This may involve orthotic ('surgical') shoes and foot surgery designed to move the pressure areas away from the ulcer site. The best treatment is prevention in the 'at-risk' population by careful foot care (i.e. specialist fitted footwear, professional chiropody, and constant foot inspection). These actions rather than medical intervention prevent most amputations in the 'at-risk' group.

Neoplastic ulcers or ulcers that are suspicious should be biopsied for confirmation and if positive excised or treated with radiotherapy.

Lymphatic disease

The lymphatic system transports tissue fluid—lymph (cells, protein, and water)—from the intercellular space to the bloodstream via lymphatic vessels.

Lymphoedema is a swelling of a part of the body caused by the accumulation of lymph in the interstitial spaces secondary to a fault in the lymphatic system, which can be divided into primary and secondary lymphoedema.

1. **Primary lymphoedema** may present at any age. Eighty per cent of cases start before the age of 35 years.

2. **Secondary lymphoedema** is much more common and involves other disease processes:

   - *malignant disease* involving the lymphatic drainage (i.e. inguinal or axillary nodes)

   - *surgery* due to dissection of regional nodes (i.e. inguinal or axillary nodes)

   - *radiation damage* (particularly in conjunction with surgery)

   - *infection* either recurrent pyogenic infection (*Staphylococcus* or beta-haemolytic streptococci), or in Africa or India due to *Wucheria bancrofti* (filariasis).

Clinical features

The history is of usually painless swelling, but may be associated with recurrent cellulitis and ulceration.

On examination the affected limbs should be inspected for the level of oedema and the presence of ulceration or fissuring and venous disease. **It is vital to**

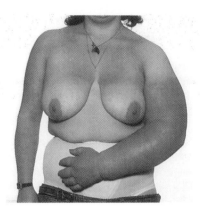

Fig 1.8w Lymphoedema of the arm with gross swelling (compare with the other side). In this case it is due to lymphatic scarring secondary to radiotherapy to the axilla as part of the treatment for breast cancer.

separate out primary and secondary lymphoedema, by careful inspection of regional lymph nodes, pelvis, and abdomen for malignancy. In the upper limb there is usually a history of axillary clearance for breast cancer and/or radiotherapy to the axilla (Fig. 1.8w).

Investigation

This should be related to aetiology with abdominal and pelvic ultrasound, CT scanning, and venous duplex. Specific investigation is by isotope lymphography, 70% of cases are due to *hypoplasia* (fewer and smaller lymphatics than normal).

Treatment

Treatment is usually conservative with care of foot hygiene, the use of graduated elastic stockings and pneumatic compression in the lower limb. In the upper limb it is aimed towards prevention of infection (wearing rubber gloves, gardening gloves) and skin care to reduce progression.

Operative interventions are rarely performed and usually entail excision of swollen tissue.

Outcome

Complications of lymphoedema include recurrent infection via fissures, leg ulceration (rare, but slow to heal), lymph leak (following trauma), and, finally, lymphosarcoma (very rare and invariably fatal).

Fast facts—Lymphoedema (swollen limb due to a failure of lymph drainage)

Aetiology

- Primary—defined by age when lymphoedema develops
- Secondary
  —malignant obstruction
  —surgery
  —radiotherapy

Clinical features

- Painless swelling
- Associated with recurrent infection

Investigations

- CT/ultrasound looking for the cause
- Isotope lymphography to define nature

Management

- Skin care/protection
- Compression

Outcome

- Symptoms can be controlled but the condition is not cured

Perioperative care

Chapter contents

Preoperative assessment, investigation, and premedication 122

Scenario 1: preoperative elective varicose vein surgery 122

Scenario 2: preoperative hernia repair in elderly man 122

Scenario 3: preoperative elective cholecystectomy in a patient with diabetes 123

Scenario 4: preoperative emergency appendicectomy 124

Background: preoperative care 125

Issues of consent 132

Scenario: consent for carotid endarterectomy 132

Background: consent 132

Anaesthesia and sedation 133

Scenario 1: general anaesthesia for a varicose vein operation 133

Scenario 2: spinal anaesthesia for an inguinal hernia repair 135

Scenario 3: anaesthesia, muscle relaxation, and analgesia for a laparoscopic cholecystectomy 136

Scenario 4: rapid sequence induction for an emergency laparotomy 137

Background: anaesthesia 138

Background: postoperative care 142

Fluid management 145

Scenario: fluid regimen following an uncomplicated laparotomy 145

Background: fluid management 145

Transfusion and blood products 148

Scenario 1: perioperative blood transfusion 148

Scenario 2: unanticipated intraoperative blood loss 149

Background: transfusion and blood products 149

Nutrition 152

Scenario: preoperative chronic malnutrition 152

Background: surgical nutrition 153

Preoperative assessment, investigation, and premedication

Scenario 1: preoperative elective varicose vein surgery

> A 39-year-old lady is on the next day's operating list to have bilateral varicose vein surgery. She is fit and healthy, on no medication, a non-smoker, and has never had an anaesthetic before.

The patient is visited preoperatively by the anaesthetist, to ensure that the patient is in an optimal condition for anaesthesia.

It allows the anaesthetist to reassure the patient and to discuss with her the choices for anaesthesia and postoperative analgesia. Any preoperative investigations should be based on history and examination and should only be performed if they can provide information that will influence the patient's perioperative care.

> This lady has no past history of note and specifically has no cardiac or respiratory symptoms. Physical examination is unremarkable.

In this case the preoperative visit is likely to be largely for reassurance and to discuss options for anaesthesia and analgesia. 'Routine' investigations, e.g. U&Es, ECG, and CXR will be extremely unlikely to provide information that will alter the perioperative management. However, women of child-bearing age may be anaemic and, therefore, the haemoglobin (Hb) concentration may be measured.

A decision regarding the need for prophylaxis against deep venous thrombosis and pulmonary embolism (DVT/PE) is also made. **Lower limb surgery is associated with an increased incidence of DVT** and this risk is exacerbated by other findings, e.g. obesity, malignancy, past history of thrombosis, and use of the combined oral contraceptive pill. Patients may require mechanical methods of thromboprophylaxis or the use of subcutaneous heparin during the perioperative period, depending on their level of risk.

> This lady has thus been fully assessed and is fit for surgery but is anxious about anaesthesia and the operation in general.

The anaesthetist will explain the various anaesthetic techniques that could be used for the proposed surgery (see under Anaesthesia, p. 133), and what the preferred option of both anaesthetist and patient might be. The need for pharmacological premedication ('premed') is also assessed. The commonest reason for premedication is to allay anxiety. This is usually achieved with a short- or medium-acting benzodiazepine, e.g. *temazepam*, *lorazepam*.

> This patient is prescribed 20 mg *temazepam*, which she is to receive 1 hour before surgery. The patient and anaesthetist have agreed on general anaesthesia.

Prior to receiving the premedication any anxieties about the upcoming surgery that the patient may have should be addressed by the surgeon and informed consent obtained. The **side of surgery should be marked** and in the case of varicose veins the veins themselves should be marked, as they will disappear with the patient lying on the operating table.

Scenario 2: preoperative hernia repair in elderly man

> A 70-year-old man is on the list to have repair of a left inguinal hernia. He has a history of a myocardial infarction 3 years ago. Since then he has had angina and is also on treatment for hypertension. He has been a smoker for over 50 years and is prone to chest infections.

In this case it is important to establish the severity of both his cardiac and respiratory disease. Asking about his exercise tolerance (what he can manage—shopping, stairs, etc.) gives a good indication of functional reserve and how the patient is likely to cope with the stresses of surgery and anaesthesia.

> The patient experiences angina rarely and only in association with unusual exercise (he is able to play a round of golf and usually does not have to use his anti-anginal *GTN* spray). He takes a regular long-acting *nitrate* and a *calcium channel blocker* for his angina. His hypertension is well controlled by a *thiazide* diuretic.

Attention must also be given to ensuring that hypertension is adequately treated, as poorly controlled BP is a risk factor for perioperative stroke and myocardial infarction.

An active respiratory tract infection should also be ruled out as this may worsen after surgery and anaesthesia and compromise recovery.

> He always has a morning cough, which at present is productive of clear sputum and he is able to lie flat without becoming short of breath.

A note of any medications the patient is receiving should be made, as some drugs may interact with those given during anaesthesia. A history of any previous anaesthetics should also be sought.

This patient's cardiac disease is well controlled and at the present time his chest appears to be in good condition.

The anaesthetist decides which drugs the patient should continue to receive over the perioperative period. In general, most drugs should be given on the day of surgery. This is especially true of cardiac and respiratory drugs where rebound worsening of symptoms can occur if they are stopped suddenly. Exceptions may be diuretics (uncomfortable for the patient as their bladder fills up) and hypoglycaemic agents (see p. 127 for management of diabetics).

Further investigations may provide useful information in this case. In the elderly, Hb concentration should be estimated to check for undiagnosed anaemia, as occult blood loss is not uncommon.

This man is receiving a diuretic and should therefore have his U&Es assessed. This is to check that his sodium and potassium are within normal limits, and may also show evidence of any renal impairment, secondary to hypertension.

An ECG may show evidence of his old myocardial infarction and of any left ventricular hypertrophy associated with his hypertension, and can be compared with old ECGs looking for new changes.

Patients who have cardiac or respiratory disease should also have a CXR performed. In this case left ventricular hypertrophy due to hypertension may be seen or evidence of emphysema in a long time smoker. However, if a patient's disease is stable and they have had a CXR within the last 2 years, a further X-ray is not required.

> This patient has stable, well-controlled cardiac and respiratory disease, and is fit for the proposed surgery.

Having established that the patient is in optimal medical condition, decisions regarding premedication can be taken. He is prescribed all his usual medications on the morning of surgery except his diuretic.

The need for an anxiolytic is dependent on the patient himself, although in general it is best to avoid anxiety in patients with cardiac disease, as the resultant sympathetic activity increases heart rate, BP, and myocardial work. In this case, he is to receive 10 mg temazepam 1 hour prior to surgery.

The anaesthetist will then discuss with the patient the type of anaesthesia he will receive. For this procedure, both general and regional anaesthetic techniques would be suitable. The use of a regional anaesthetic technique, e.g. spinal or epidural, may confer a benefit, due to reduced cardiovascular and respiratory complications.

Scenario 3: preoperative elective cholecystectomy in a patient with diabetes

> A 25-year-old woman who has been an insulin-dependent diabetic for 10 years requires laparoscopic cholecystectomy.

The preoperative visit in this instance allows the anaesthetist to ascertain if the patient has any of the complications associated with diabetes. Diabetes is a multisystem disorder and can lead to nephropathy, sensory, motor, and autonomic neuropathy, as well as retinopathy and vascular disease. In general these complications appear to be related to duration of the disease and how well it is controlled.

Diabetic patients are also more prone to infection after surgery and again this may be related to the degree of diabetic control. If diabetes is poorly controlled prior to elective surgery, time should be taken to improve control, even if surgery has to be postponed, to allow a period of stabilization on a new regimen.

> This women has well-controlled diabetes and is reviewed regularly at the diabetic clinic. She takes insulin twice daily but is on no other medications.

Further investigation of this patient would risk obtaining FBC (increased incidence of infection), U&Es (renal impairment due to diabetic nephropathy), and blood glucose. The preoperative visit also enables the anaesthetist to discuss perioperative diabetic management with the patient.

For all but the most minor surgery, insulin-dependent diabetics require that their normal regimen be replaced with an infusion of insulin, dextrose, and potassium until they resume a normal oral intake. These infusions can be given in a variety of ways, the commonest being a 'GKI' (glucose–potassium–insulin) regimen. This involves setting up an infusion of 10% dextrose to run at 100 ml per hour. To this is added short-acting *insulin*, the dose depending on the value of the patient's blood glucose, e.g. if blood glucose is 10 mmol/l then 10 iu of soluble *insulin* is added to the bag, if 14 mmol/l then 14 iu of insulin is added and so on. Potassium must also be added as it is driven intracellularly by insulin, and hypokalaemia can result. It is usual practice to add 10 mmol of potassium to each 500 ml of 10% dextrose. This regimen has the in-built safety feature that insulin and dextrose are administered through the same infusion and so overdose of one without the other is unlikely (assuming all drug additions are carefully made and checked).

This regimen may be unsuitable for the very brittle diabetic, in those who are hyperglycaemic to start with, and in those with renal impairment. In these situations separate infusions of 5% dextrose and potassium (or normal saline depending on starting blood glucose) and soluble insulin (1 iu/ml) using a sliding scale to determine the amount of insulin required may be used.

Both regimens require hourly blood glucose readings to be carried out in order to avoid both hyper- and hypoglycaemia. This is usually done by pricking the finger and blood drop stick testing. In the perioperative period, hypoglycaemia is extremely dangerous and can lead to permanent brain damage if symptoms go unrecognized, or are masked by general anaesthesia.

TABLE 2.1a Sliding scale insulin regimen	
Blood glucose reading	**Insulin infusion* (units/hour)**
>22	5.0+ call doctor
14.1–22	4.0
10.1–14	3.0
7.1–10	2.0
4.1–7	1.0
<4	0.5+ call doctor

*5% Dextrose infused at 100 ml/hour AND IV actrapid insulin 50 iu in 50 ml 0.9% saline. If blood glucose is >14 mmol/l, 0.9% saline should be substituted for 5% dextrose.

> In this case an infusion of dextrose, *insulin*, and potassium can be commenced on the morning of surgery at the time of premedication with *temazepam* 20 mg. She is also given 150 mg of ranitidine (an H_2 agonist)—to reduce gastric acid secretion, as diabetics may have delayed gastric emptying. General anaesthesia is required for this type of procedure and thromboprophylaxis should be given as there is an increased incidence of DVT with laparoscopic surgery. This can be given intraoperatively after discussion with the surgeon.

Scenario 4: preoperative emergency appendicectomy

> A 35-year-old man has been admitted with a 48-hour history of abdominal pain and vomiting. The surgeon wishes to take him to theatre, with a presumed diagnosis of appendicitis.

In the emergency situation, the same information that is required for assessment of elective cases must be obtained. There may, however, be very limited time in which to take a history, perform an examination, and get the results of all relevant investigations before the patient must go to theatre.

In very sick patients information may have to be obtained from a relative or friend. It is also the case that extra investigations may have to be requested, in view of the acute physiological upset being experienced by the patient. However, appropriate assessment and investigation must be performed in order to ensure patient safety.

> This man is normally fit, healthy, and on no medications. He has never had an anaesthetic before and is not aware of any problems with anaesthetics running in the family. He has been unwell for about 48 hours with frequent vomiting and has been unable to eat for 24 hours, although he has managed some fluid intake.

If this patient were presenting for elective surgery it is likely that he would require no further investigations. However, in this case he has a history of gastrointestinal upset and therefore a number of tests are required preoperatively.

A history of vomiting raises the possibility of metabolic disturbance, U&Es should be obtained. Patients with prolonged vomiting may become hypokalaemic and hypochloraemic as well as being dehydrated (elevated urea). Any imbalance should be corrected with IV fluids before theatre.

In addition, patients with appendicitis may be toxic and a FBC should be taken to establish if there is a raised white cell count.

> In this case apart from a white cell count of 14×10^9/l, all investigations were normal and the surgeons confirmed their intention to perform an appendicectomy.

It is often difficult to predict when patients having emergency surgery will be called to the operating theatre. For this reason, premedication with an anxiolytic agent is usually omitted. **However, there is no reason to withhold analgesia** for those patients whose underlying condition is painful. In this case the use of an opiate (narcotic) analgesic may be necessary before surgery. IV fluids should be commenced on the preoperative surgical ward in order to provide ongoing maintenance fluids, while the patient is continuing to fast and to replace previous losses.

In this case, the patient arrives in theatre to undergo an emergency appendicectomy under general anaesthesia. He has received 10 mg of *morphine* intramuscularly for pain 45 minutes prior to arriving in theatre and is now comfortable. Since his admission to hospital he has received 750 ml of normal saline intravenously and no longer feels thirsty.

Clinical key points in preoperative care

- A full history and examination should be performed in all preoperative patients, as age and comorbidity influence the effects of anaesthesia and surgery on recovery

- Concomitant diseases such as cardiorespiratory problems, and diabetes should be optimized prior to elective surgery

- Preoperative investigation (FBC, U&Es, CXR, ECG) should be requested where indicated and results checked

- In emergency patients, analgesia should NOT be withheld before surgery if required

- The side of surgery should be marked (e.g. varicose veins, breast, and hernia surgery)

- DVT prophylaxis should be prescribed when indicated

Background: preoperative care

There are a number of issues in the patient's journey of care towards an operation. These must be addressed in order for an operation to occur in a safe, controlled environment. Failure to do so is unsafe and uncontrolled.

- preoperative assessment
- premedication
- preoperative prophylaxis
- consent.

Preoperative assessment

As part of the preoperative assessment of patients, anaesthetists read the case notes (especially admission notes and previous anaesthetic records) and any correspondence concerning the patient.

Anaesthetists are particularly concerned about intercurrent cardiac and respiratory disease, as these are the two systems under most strain during anaesthesia and surgery. On reviewing the patient at the preoperative visit, the anaesthetist asks about any pre-existing conditions, how well the symptoms are controlled and what medications they take. This enables the anaesthetist to decide whether the patient is in an optimal condition prior to surgery and will also alert to any potential drug interactions with anaesthetic agents, e.g. *monoamine oxidase inhibitors* (MAOI), which can interact with anaesthetics to cause severe hypertension.

A history of drug allergy is also sought, including to topical preparations (e.g. betadine) and latex.

It is important to ask about previous anaesthetic experiences especially if an adverse event occurred, e.g. difficult intubation, postoperative nausea and vomiting, anaphylaxis, and if there is a family history of reactions to anaesthesia.

A number of inherited conditions can cause serious anaesthetic problems e.g. malignant hyperpyrexia, plasma cholinesterase deficiency, and acute intermittent porphyria. Screening tests can be performed on those with a family history of a reaction.

The patient's cardiorespiratory system is assessed and the upper airways examined, to predict those patients where difficulty might be expected in maintaining airways or achieving endotracheal intubation.

Cardiovascular disease

A specific cardiovascular assessment must identify and quantify:

- *Angina*—how often it occurs and precipitating factors. Angina of increasing frequency, or occurring on minimal exercise, or at rest is unstable and carries a high risk of perioperative myocardial infarction. The medications taken to treat angina should also be documented.

- *Past history of myocardial infarction* has a significant impact on the risk of postoperative myocardial infarction. Non-urgent cases will normally only be anaesthetized 6 months after a myocardial infarction. The precise risk is also dependent on the nature of the surgery and other risk factors that may be present (Table 2.1b).

- *Evidence of heart failure.* If the patient suffers from shortness of breath especially when lying flat (orthop-

TABLE 2.1b   Risk of perioperative MI

Time since myocardial infarction	Reinfarction risk (%)
0–3 months	4–40
4–6 months	2–15
>6 months	1.5–6

noea) or wakes up with breathlessness during the night (paroxysmal nocturnal dyspnoea), this should be documented. The presence of any leg oedema, or of their sacral area if confined to bed, may also suggest heart failure. Medications to treat cardiac failure must also be documented.

◆ *Presence and nature of cardiac arrhythmias.* Some arrhythmias need only be documented and no further action taken, e.g. long-standing atrial fibrillation with a controlled ventricular rate. In some cases, e.g. complete heart block, a cardiological opinion will be required and a pacemaker inserted prior to anaesthesia and surgery. If the patient already has a pacemaker *in situ*, this should undergo a check prior to anaesthesia to ensure it is working normally.

◆ *Nature and severity of heart murmurs.* If a murmur is a new finding it may require investigation before surgery, usually by echocardiography, in order to quantify the extent of valvular disease and how well the heart is compensating.

◆ *Hypertension.* If this is a new finding it should be established with serial readings whether it is a manifestation of short-term anxiety. In these cases the patient is usually normotensive but due to anxiety related to hospital admission and being treated by doctors the BP readings are elevated ('white coat hypertension'). If BP fails to settle it may represent an undiagnosed condition that requires assessment and treatment before surgery can be undertaken. Uncontrolled hypertension leads to an increased risk of perioperative stroke and myocardial infarction.

Up to 40% of patients will have their hypertension inadequately treated and, therefore, the adequacy of current treatment should be established. Also check for any end-organ damage as a result of high BP (left ventricular hypertrophy or renal failure).

   Patients with a history of cardiovascular disease will require some simple investigations. As a minimum an ECG should be performed and blood taken for FBC (to check they are not anaemic) and U&Es (to ensure nor-

Fast facts—Cardiovascular assessment

History

◆ Angina

◆ History of myocardial infarction

◆ Heart failure

◆ Arrhythmia

◆ Heart murmur

◆ Hypertension

Examination

◆ Pulse, BP, cardiorespiratory system

Investigation

◆ ECG

◆ FBC

◆ U&Es

◆ Creatinine

◆ CXR

◆ Assessment of left ventricular function

   —echocardiography

   —cardiac radio-isotope study

mal values of sodium and potassium, which if high or low can predispose to arrhythmias, and a normal creatinine level as a check for renal function). In addition, if a CXR has not been performed in the last 2 years or if symptoms have deteriorated in recent times, one should be performed on this admission. Where major surgery is being proposed it may be necessary to arrange some further tests of cardiac function, e.g. echocardiography or a myocardial perfusion scan.

Respiratory disease

To help gauge the severity of respiratory problems a careful history should elucidate:

◆ Shortness of breath—and specifically its relationship to activity or its occurrence at rest or when lying flat (this may suggest a cardiac cause).

◆ The presence of cough—and if this is productive the nature of any sputum.

◆ The presence of asthma—and any precipitating factors (including non-steroidal anti-inflammatory drugs (NSAIDs)). The treatments being taken for asthma

---

Fast facts—Respiratory assessment

History

- Shortness of breath
- Cough
- Asthma/wheeze
- Upper respiratory tract infection
- Smoking

Examination

- Respiratory system

Investigation

- Pulse oximetry
- CXR
- May need arterial blood gas (if respiratory condition is borderline)
- May need pulmonary function tests (if respiratory condition is borderline)

---

should also be documented as well as ascertaining how well their symptoms are normally controlled. Operation should be postponed during periods of exacerbation of the condition.

- If there is any acute respiratory tract infection (upper or lower) as this increases the likelihood of perioperative respiratory complications. Patients with active chest infection or colds should have their routine surgery postponed until they are fit.

- Smoking habit—smokers have a high incidence of cardiovascular and respiratory disease. They also are likely to have laryngeal irritability, increasing the chance of coughing and laryngospasm during induction and reversal of anaesthesia.

Other conditions

A number of other conditions exist to which the anaesthetist should be alerted:

1. *Diabetes*: careful control is required over the perioperative period to avoid both **hyper-** and hypoglycaemia.

2. *Gastro-oesophageal reflux*: risk of aspiration of gastric contents during anaesthesia.

3. *Rheumatoid arthritis*: patients may have unstable cervical vertebrae (possibly leading to cervical spine

injury during intubation), respiratory problems (pulmonary fibrosis), and joint deformities, which make venous access difficult.

4. *Liver disease*: patients may be confused, coagulopathic, and will require reduced doses of some drugs to prevent toxicity.

5. *Renal impairment*: some drugs are contraindicated (*suxamethonium*), whereas those that are excreted by the kidneys should be used with care and in lower dosage, to avoid prolonged effects.

There is little to be gained from performing routine investigations in all patients presenting for surgery.

Ideally an investigation should only be carried out if there is a reasonable likelihood of it revealing an abnormal result that may influence the perioperative course. In some cases, the anaesthetist may decide from history and examination that more specialized investigation or opinion is required to ensure that the patient is in the best possible condition prior to surgery, e.g. assessment of left ventricular function and pulmonary function tests. This may necessitate the patient having their surgery postponed until the results of the tests are available.

Summary

The preoperative assessment is a form of risk assessment to ensure that:

- the patient is in optimal medical condition for surgery and anaesthesia
- the benefits of surgery outweigh the risks associ-

Fast facts—Preoperative care

- Each patient is unique and therefore care must be tailored to the individual
- Routine use of laboratory tests on all patients is wasteful
- Careful assessment of the cardiorespiratory systems is important in all patients requiring anaesthesia and surgery
- A history of previous anaesthetic experiences may alert to potential problems
- A number of medical conditions exist which can affect anaesthetic management. These should be elicited and their management documented
- Concurrent drug use should be clearly documented

ated with intercurrent disease and anaesthesia and surgery.

This ensures that likely complications can be predicted and steps for avoidance taken in order that the patient receives the most appropriate perioperative care.

Premedication

The prescription of premedication is the final component of the preoperative visit.

Premedication refers to the administration of drugs 1–2 hours prior to the induction of anaesthesia. **The main aim of premedication is usually seen as allaying anxiety.** Short-acting *benzodiazepines* such as *temazepam* can be prescribed, but for many patients talking to the anaesthetist, surgeon, and nursing team is sufficient anxiolysis.

Other reasons to premedicate patients include:

- prophylaxis of the complications of anaesthesia (e.g. vagal overactivity, aspiration of gastric contents)
- prophylaxis of the complications of surgery (e.g. infection, thromboembolism)
- analgesia in painful conditions (e.g. emergency surgery)
- continued management of intercurrent disease.

Certain types of surgery are associated with vagal stimulation, which can lead to bradycardias. Antimuscarinic drugs can be given as premedication to prevent this complication, e.g. in ophthalmic surgery, laparoscopy, and in very young babies requiring surgery.

The traditional intramuscular injection of opiates (e.g. morphine) as part of premedication has largely been displaced by IV administration at induction of anaesthesia, with further doses titrated during the surgical procedure. However, especially in the emergency situation where the patient is in pain, analgesia including opiates should be given before surgery. Analgesic agents such as the NSAIDs can be given prior to surgery or during the procedure as part of a 'balanced anaesthetic technique' (see Anaesthesia on p. 133).

It is accepted that most drugs patients may be receiving for the management of intercurrent disease should be continued into the perioperative period (by alternate route if necessary, i.e. intravenously). This is especially true for drugs used to control cardiac disease and hypertension where rebound worsening of symptoms can occur if drugs are stopped precipitously.

Some drugs, e.g. *monoamine oxidase inhibitors*, *warfarin*, *clopidogrel*, should be discontinued for a period of time prior to surgery although other treatments should be instituted. The combined oral contraceptive pill, HRT

Fast facts—Premedication (summary)

- Reducing anxiety is often the reason for premedication
- Continued management of intercurrent medical disease is vital in the preparation of patients for surgery

(hormone replacement therapy) and other contraceptive measures should be stopped 6 weeks prior to major surgery.

A small number of drugs, e.g. corticosteroids, will require increased dosage perioperatively while others will require almost constant administration, e.g. *insulin*. Hospitals often have their own guidelines for the management of the diabetic patient undergoing surgery and the doctor has a duty to be aware of them.

Risk of aspiration of gastric contents

Aspiration of gastric contents is a potentially life-threatening complication of anaesthesia. Unconscious patients under general anaesthesia no longer have a protective gag mechanism that under normal circumstances protects the patient from aspiration. Aspiration can cause a mild bronchial and alveolar inflammatory response or more severe reactions with scarring (fibrosis) and adult respiratory distress syndrome and possibly death.

Those at most risk include:

- pregnant women
- patients with diabetes
- patients with a history of gastro-oesophageal reflux or hiatus hernia
- patients having emergency surgery where an empty stomach cannot be guaranteed (not fasted, small bowel obstruction, 'acute abdomen').

In these groups of patients mechanical methods such as passing a nasogastric tube can be attempted to empty the stomach. In some, the use of pharmacological agents is prescribed prior to theatre in order to raise the pH of gastric contents so that they are less damaging if aspirated into the lungs. Proton pump inhibitors (e.g. *omeprazole*) or H_2 receptor antagonists (e.g. *ranitidine*) and simple antacids may be used.

Fasting preoperatively reduces gastric volume and the risk of aspiration. It is normal to fast patients for 6 hours for solids and 2–4 hours for liquids.

In patients where there is a high risk of aspiration, a rapid sequence induction of anaesthesia is performed.

This involves preoxygenating the patient and applying pressure on the cricoid cartilage, in order to occlude the upper oesophagus just as consciousness is lost. An endotracheal tube is then passed and the larynx sealed before cricoid pressure is released.

Preoperative prophylaxis

Prophylaxis against deep venous thrombosis/pulmonary embolism

Patients undergoing surgery are at risk of developing a DVT. The likely risk can be assessed preoperatively and appropriate measures taken to reduce the risk of this complication.

Certain conditions are associated with a higher risk of developing a DVT and pulmonary embolus in the perioperative period:

+ obesity

+ malignancy

+ extensive pelvic/abdominal surgery

+ sepsis

+ past history of DVT

+ concurrent use of the combined oral contraceptive pill/pregnancy

+ thrombophilia.

A number of methods are available, mechanical and pharmacological, to try to prevent the occurrence of DVT. The choice of prophylaxis is graded with the level of risk (low, moderate, and high) of the patient developing a DVT and/or pulmonary embolus (Table 2.1c).

+ *Elastic compression stockings (TEDs)* (Fig. 2.1a). These should be considered in all patients requiring surgery

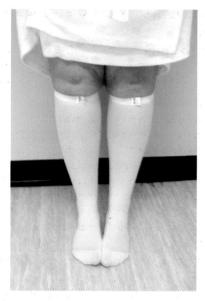

Fig 2.1a Elastic compression stockings as part of DVT prophylaxis.

except those with arterial disease in whom they can contribute to limb ischaemia and occasionally lead to amputation. They should be of an appropriate size for the patient, as if too short they impede rather than improve venous return.

+ *Pneumatic compression stockings.* Where the risk of DVT is high but the risk of increased intraoperative bleeding due to anticoagulants is unacceptable, e.g. neurosurgery, these may be suitable. The legs are put in a plastic stocking which is inflated and deflated in sequence throughout surgery, squeezing the calves, and improving venous blood flow.

TABLE 2.1c   Management of DVT prophylaxis

Group		Prophylaxis
Low risk	Minor surgery or trauma	Early mobilization, TEDs
	Major surgery in patients <40 years old	
	Minor medical illness	
Moderate risk	Major trauma, burns, or medical illness	Early mobilization, and either graduated compression stockings (TEDs) or subcutaneous unfractionated miniheparin 5000 IU twice daily or LMWH once daily
	Major surgery in patients >40 years	
	Minor surgery in patients with additional risk factors	
	Patients with inflammatory bowel disease	
High risk	Major cancer, pelvic, and lower limb joint surgery Those undergoing surgery or suffering illness associated with previous venous thromboembolism or thrombophilia	Early mobilization, TEDs, subcutaneous miniheparin or LMWH, and mechanical calf compression

◆ *Anticoagulation.* Either as low dose unfractionated heparin (*Mini-Hep*), which is given by subcutaneous injection two or three times daily, or low molecular weight heparins (LMWH) (e.g. *dalteparin, enoxaparin*) given once daily also by subcutaneous injection. Before prescribing either of these drugs, thought should be given to the type of anaesthetic the patient is to receive. If a regional anaesthetic technique (epidural or spinal) is to be performed, administration of unfractionated heparin within 4 hours or low molecular weight heparin within 12 hours of anaesthesia leads to an increased (and unacceptable) risk of bleeding within the epidural space. In this situation the heparin should be withheld until 1–2 hours after the regional block has been performed.

Many hospitals have their own guidelines for the prevention of DVT/PE and these should always be consulted.

For summary see Table 2.1c.

Antibiotic prophylaxis

The infection of a surgical wound is a relatively common event. Approximately 1 in 40 (2.5%) of all surgical wounds become infected.

The risk can be reduced. No surgical wound is sterile, but under normal circumstances the body's immune system will protect the patient if the bacterial count is kept low. This protection will be adversely affected where the blood supply is poor and in an immunocompromised patient (e.g. AIDS, cancer).

Clean wounds with no other risk factors have a very low incidence of wound infection, while contaminated wounds (e.g. with bowel contents) may have a 1 in 3 chance of infection (Table 2.1d).

This surgical site infection also includes infection in body cavities (e.g. subphrenic abscess), bones, and joints. When an implant or prosthetic device (e.g. hip joint, vascular bypass graft) is inserted this increases the risk of infection as a lower bacterial inoculation is required. The device may also become infected, with usually disastrous results. The bacteria adhere to the device and can become resistant to antibiotics.

The duration of surgery is also associated with an increased risk of wound infection. A further factor that increases the risk of wound infection is the general health of the patient where any ongoing limiting condition (e.g. cardiac, respiratory, diabetes) is detrimental.

The goals of antibiotic prophylaxis are to:

◆ reduce the incidence of surgical site infection

◆ minimize adverse events.

A number of measures can reduce the risk of surgical wound infection:

◆ local—skin cleansing ('skin prep'), operating room air cleaning, risk-reducing behaviour (washing hands), protective clothing, and masks

◆ antibiotic prophylaxis.

The value of antibiotic prophylaxis is related to the impact of local surgical site infection. In colorectal surgery prophylaxis reduces mortality, while in orthopaedic joint replacement surgery it reduces long-term morbidity. In the majority of operations prophylaxis reduces short-term morbidity. Wound infection prolongs hospital stay and its prevention allows undelayed discharge and earlier return to work.

Antibiotic prophylaxis is not recommended for all operations (e.g. clean ENT surgery).

The antibiotic used should cover expected pathogens and is best decided locally. The antibiotic prophylaxis should be administered immediately before or during the surgical procedure.

The risks of antibiotic prophylaxis include:

◆ the promotion of antibiotic resistance (though this is minimal with prophylaxis regimens that do not extend beyond 24 hours)

◆ increasing the number of cases of *Clostridium difficile* infection (colitis; *C. difficile* infection prolongs hospital stay and increases overall morbidity and mortality)

◆ the risk of allergic reactions to antibiotics.

It is therefore important that the simple things such as hand washing are strictly observed before and between patients to minimize cross-infection and its potentially disastrous consequences (Fig. 2.1b).

TABLE 2.1d   Incidence of wound infection by contamination without antibiotic prophylaxis

Type of wound	Definition	Examples	Incidence of wound infection (%)
Clean	No contamination	Hernia repair, breast surgery	1–5
Clean-contaminated	Minimal contamination	Cholecystectomy, prostatectomy	5–10
Contaminated	Significant contamination	Elective gut surgery	10–20
Dirty	Infection present	Abscess, bowel perforation	20–40

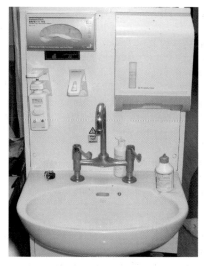

Fig 2.1b Hand washing is extremely important.

Prevention of pressure sores

Pressure sores are a product of prolonged and un-relieved pressure, usually on a prominent site (Fig. 2.1c). The common sites are:

- the heels
- the skin overlying the sacrum, (with the patient lying on their back), and
- the greater trochanter of the femur (with the patient lying on their side.

The tissue infarcts (the skin or the tissue immediately next to the bony prominence) and a large ulcer or sub-cutaneous cavity is formed. The unrelieved pressure produces localized ischaemia by squeezing blood out of the tissue.

All patients who are immobile are at risk. This particularly includes:

- the unconscious
- those with spinal cord injuries
- patients who are unable to move due to injury (e.g. fractured neck of femur)
- patients with an amputation, and
- those with reduced sensation after epidural or spinal anaesthesia.

Most pressure sores are preventable by regularly moving the position of those at risk and caring and protecting the skin at sites of concern.

Prevention of chest infection

Patients at risk of chest infection due to a pre-existing problem (smoking, chronic pulmonary disease) and those whose surgery will predispose them to chest

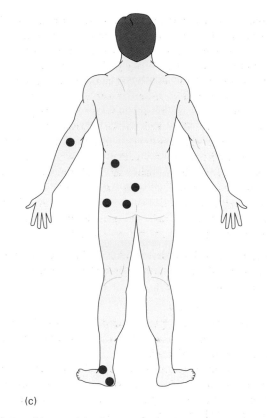

(c)

Fig 2.1c Diagram of sites for pressure sore.

problems (i.e. thoracic and upper abdominal operations) should receive special attention.

The patient should be encouraged to optimize their respiratory status before elective surgery by stopping smoking (though doing this immediately before surgery may actually make matters worse), and the use of medication such as bronchodilators and possibly steroid inhalers. Perioperative physiotherapy and incentive spirometry (blowing into a tube to make a ball rise or spin) can improve respiratory performance.

The type of anaesthetic and postoperative analgesia is important, as epidural anaesthesia will provide pain relief to allow pain-free coughing and breathing exercises. Bronchodilators if already used should be continued into the postoperative period and may have a role in the postoperative management of the respiratory tract.

Protection against HIV and hepatitis B

The risk of health workers contacting HIV and hepatitis from patients is very low, but the consequences are huge. The risk is related to body fluids (blood, saliva, faeces, urine), not with general social contact.

Most instances relate to sharp injuries contaminated with infected fluids (needlestick). As prevention is much more preferable to treatment, care of sharp instruments is vital.

The overall risk of contracting the disease is very much higher with hepatitis, and the risk of contracting HIV is greater with patients who have AIDS rather than being HIV positive.

All health-care workers should be vaccinated against hepatitis B, confirmed by serology. Only care will protect against HIV with scrupulous handling of sharps in all patient care areas (operating theatre, wards, and clinics).

Once infected with HIV or hepatitis B a health-care worker has an ethical obligation to give up patient contact which might risk transmission of the virus.

Fast facts—Prophylaxis

- Prophylaxis is a method of reducing (though rarely abolishing) the risk of an adverse clinical event

- The risk of DVT/PE varies according to circumstance, the level of DVT/PE prophylaxis is graded against the risk

- No surgical wound is completely sterile. Active measures are required to minimize the risk of frank infection

- Health-care worker behaviour is a very powerful factor both for the patient and self-protection

Issues of consent

Scenario: consent for carotid endarterectomy

A 72-year-old man is due to undergo a right carotid endarterectomy.

The patient will have had the reasons for and risks of the operation explained by the surgeon in the outpatient clinic. A decision will have been made to proceed; nevertheless, the nature and risks of the procedure must be fully explained. **It is the responsibility of the clinician obtaining the consent to be familiar with the risks related to the operation.** If they are not they cannot obtain consent.

A simple description of the operation is given with emphasis on what the patient should expect to see and feel.

The position and size of any incisions are explained along with the degree of pain with emphasis on the measures that will be taken to reduce pain.

Any direct consequences of the operation should be discussed, including scarring, bruising, disability, and numbness.

Any potential complications should also be covered with some indication of the likelihood of any severe complication and death.

The patient is informed that the risk of stroke or death with carotid endarterectomy is approximately 5% or 1 in 20.

Other less disabling or significant complications are also covered.

The potential for hypoglossal nerve injury producing usually temporary problems with speech and laryngeal nerve injury, which may affect the quality of the voice, is specifically mentioned.

A note is made in the medical records containing the substance of the discussion and the consent form is signed and witnessed.

Clinical key points in consent

- It is the responsibility of the clinician obtaining the consent to be familiar with the risks related to the operation

- Any direct consequences of the operation should be discussed

- Any potential complications should also be covered with some indication of the likelihood of any severe complication and death

- A note is made in the medical records containing the substance of the discussion and the consent form is signed and witnessed

Background: consent

In recent times, matters of consent in relation to medical treatment have achieved a high profile with the public. The General Medical Council has issued guidelines for doctors seeking consent from patients outlining what is good practice.

A number of medico-legal issues surround the obtaining and giving of consent. There is a difference between obtaining consent from a patient and ensuring that they are aware of the material risks involved in a given procedure or treatment. Failure to obtain consent may lead to a claim of assault, while failure to explain all the material risks can constitute a breach of duty and lead to a claim for compensation with respect to side-effects or complications, even if the procedure was conducted properly.

Patients have a right to information about their condition and the options for treatment. This information helps them to make a decision on whether they will consent to investigation or treatment. **All competent adults have a right to give or withhold consent to examination, investigation, or treatment.** The information a patient requires to help them make a decision may include:

◆ details of diagnosis and prognosis with and without treatment

◆ likelihood of treatment being successful

◆ what they are likely to experience during treatment, including common and serious side-effects

◆ who will be providing the treatment.

It is important also to bring to the patient's attention the possibility of other problems emerging during treatment, perhaps when the patient is unconscious, and whether they would be happy for any necessary procedure to be carried out at that time, or whether they would prefer to give further thought before proceeding.

Ideally, the doctor performing a procedure or giving treatment should obtain the patient's consent. Often this process is begun in an outpatient clinic when the surgeon discusses the pros and cons of surgery with the patient. However, it is often delegated to staff in training to obtain written consent for a procedure once the patient is admitted to hospital. Trainee staff have a duty to ensure they have sufficient knowledge of the planned procedure and likely risks, in order to give the patient enough information on which to base their decision to consent.

Consent may be implied, e.g. patient compliance with a procedure such as venepuncture. However, co-operation should not be taken as an indication that the patient understands fully all the risks.

In situations where the treatment or procedure carries significant risks, the **express consent** of the patient should be obtained either **orally or in writing**. If express consent is given orally, documentation should be made in the notes as to the nature of the information given to the patient and the extent of their consent. When express consent is given in writing on a specific form, it may still be useful to ensure that the specific information given and likely risks discussed are also outlined in the case notes.

Wherever possible, consent should be obtained before the proposed procedure and before any sedative drugs have been administered. **In an emergency** where consent cannot be obtained either because of the life-threatening nature of the emergency and the patient's condition, **medical treatment to save life can be provided.** Advance directives (Living Will), if known about, should be respected.

Finally, it is what the patient understands that is important, not what the doctor has told and documented. It is vital to get the patient to tell the doctor what they understand and not simply to list the procedure and risks.

Fast facts—Consent

◆ Consent revolves around the patient's understanding not the information they have been given

◆ All significant risks should be explained and documented (significance is the patient's judgement)

◆ The patient's signature on a consent form is important but not the be all and end all

◆ If the patient is incapable and a guardian is unavailable acting in the best interests of the patient takes precedence

---

Anaesthesia and sedation

Scenario 1: general anaesthesia for a varicose vein operation

A fit 39-year-old lady is to undergo bilateral varicose vein surgery under general anaesthesia. She received a benzodiazepine premedication 1 hour before coming to the anaesthetic room and is calm and relaxed. On arrival in the anaesthetic room, monitoring of the patient's cardiovascular and respiratory systems commence.

This monitoring as a minimum should include:

◆ pulse oximetry

◆ non-invasive BP measurement

◆ ECG monitoring

◆ capnography (expired CO_2 monitoring).

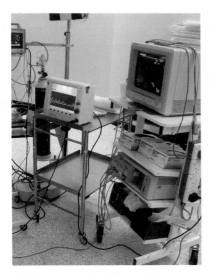

Fig 2.1d Anaesthetic monitoring stack.

These continue throughout induction, the intraoperative, and the immediate postoperative periods (Fig. 2.1d).

> Once monitoring has begun, IV access is obtained by inserting a cannula into a hand or forearm vein on the non-dominant side.

Having secured **IV access** and commenced monitoring, only now can anaesthesia be safely induced.

> In this case anaesthesia is induced with an IV induction agent (*propofol*).

The dose of *propofol* is titrated to effect (usually 2–3 mg/kg).

Anaesthesia can be thought of as a **triad of sleep, relaxation, and analgesia**. Although anaesthetic agents can provide this triad when given alone, it is common to use non-anaesthetic agents (to supplement the anaesthetics) for specific purposes (analgesia and muscle relaxation) in order to minimize adverse effects. The anaesthetist chooses the drugs to be used in a given patient depending on the individual, any medical conditions they may have and the surgical procedure to be carried out.

Loss of consciousness occurs in approximately one arm–brain circulation time (30–60 seconds—the time taken for the drug to travel from the injection site in the arm to the brain) and will last for approximately 2–3 minutes. There is no surgical requirement for

muscle relaxation, neuromuscular blocking drugs are not administered, but anaesthesia itself causes a reduction in muscle tone, which can lead to airway obstruction.

> The patient's airways are protected by using the head tilt, chin lift, jaw thrust manoeuvre (*see resuscitation*), and a laryngeal mask airway is passed.

The **airways must be protected** during anaesthesia. A laryngeal airway is one of many types of airway equipment used by anaesthetists to ensure the airway remains patent during anaesthesia. Others include face masks, oropharyngeal (Guedel) airways, nasopharyngeal airways, and endotracheal tubes.

> During this procedure the patient breathes spontaneously and anaesthesia is maintained after IV induction using an inhalational technique, with the patient spontaneously breathing in the anaesthetic. A mixture of oxygen-enriched air is used to carry 1–2% isoflurane from the anaesthetic machine through the breathing circuit to the patient.

It would also be possible to maintain anaesthesia using a total IV technique with *propofol* given as a continuous infusion.

> Analgesia for the procedure and into the postoperative period is provided by an IV dose of an opioid agent.

In this case 50–100 µg of *fentanyl* (medium duration of action) or 5–10 mg *morphine* (long duration of action) would be suitable.

> In addition a non-steroidal drug is given to improve analgesia through a synergistic action with opioids.

50–100 mg *diclofenac* can be given rectally (specific consent for this should be obtained preoperatively). The surgeon can also be asked to infiltrate larger wounds with local anaesthetic at the end of the procedure.

> As the surgical procedure nears completion, the anaesthetic agents are turned off, and the patient breathes 100% oxygen.

It is not possible to use a specific antagonist to reverse the effects of anaesthesia, which wears off when the concentration of anaesthetic agent in the brain falls below a certain level. This occurs when the lungs have eliminated sufficient anaesthetic, as only minimal metabolism of the inhalational agents takes place.

> The patient awakening from anaesthesia should be placed in the recovery position and looked after in a recovery area by trained staff until their protective airway reflexes return, they are cardiovascularly stable, pain free, and can return to a normal ward.

Scenario 2: spinal anaesthesia for an inguinal hernia repair

> A 70-year-old man with a history of hypertension, ischaemic heart disease, and recurrent chest infections is to undergo elective repair of a left inguinal hernia. He has received all his normal drugs prior to surgery as well as a benzodiazepine premedication. At the preoperative visit by the anaesthetist it was agreed that the procedure would be carried out using a regional anaesthetic technique, with sedation if required.

For certain types of surgery the use of a regional anaesthetic technique alone can provide analgesia and muscle relaxation for the duration of surgery. Benefits include:

- in patients with respiratory disease avoiding the depressant effects of general anaesthesia may lead to fewer postoperative respiratory complications
- in those with a history of ischaemic heart disease there may be a reduction in perioperative myocardial ischaemia associated with regional techniques.

Some examples of regional anaesthetic techniques include: ring block for finger or toe surgery, brachial plexus block for hand and arm surgery, and spinal or epidural anaesthesia for leg or lower abdominal surgery.

> This man is to have repair of an inguinal hernia, which requires anaesthesia of the lower abdominal wall. His operation can be performed under spinal anaesthesia.

Before commencing any anaesthetic, regional or general, IV access and routine monitoring should be secured (see Scenario 1 on p. 133).

For spinal injection the patient is positioned either sitting, or in a lateral flexed position in order to open up the intervertebral spaces.

A special long, thin, 'spinal' needle is inserted under full aseptic conditions into the subarachnoid space at the level of L3 or lower (below the level at which the spinal cord ends in order to minimize the risk of damage to it). Correct placement is confirmed by the flow of cerebrospinal fluid (CSF) through the needle.

A small volume of local anaesthetic is then injected (2–3 ml *bupivacaine*). The onset of anaesthesia is rapid due to its action on the nerve roots as they cross the subarachnoid space.

> The patient reports warm heavy legs and by testing temperature receptors, with an ethyl chloride spray, the level of the block is assessed to be satisfactory for the surgical part of the operation to start.

As well as pain fibres, all fibres including temperature, touch, proprioception (position sense), autonomic, and motor nerves are anaesthetized. Usually the patient first notices a warm feeling in their legs and buttocks followed rapidly by paraesthesia (tingling), then anaesthesia and 'heavy legs' as the full effect is seen.

A check must be made that the level of the block is adequate for the surgery to be performed, in this case about T8 (up to xiphisternum and down to the toes) would suffice. This is done by testing sensation to cold (using ethyl chloride spray or ice cubes) over the patient's legs and abdomen.

> During the operation a constant check of the patient's well-being is made with special attention to the BP and ECG monitor.

As the sympathetic outflow from the spinal cord occurs from T1 to L2, the autonomic block produced by spinal anaesthesia leads to blockade of sympathetic nerves. This causes vaso- and venodilatation, and can lead to hypotension (decreased venous return and lowered peripheral resistance) especially if the patient is sedated or volume depleted (e.g. due to dehydration or blood loss).

If the block spreads even higher it can lead to blockade of the sympathetic outflow to the heart (T1–T4), producing hypotension and bradycardia. The patient must be closely monitored and the anaesthetist must have measures available to treat these side-effects should they occur.

Hypotension can occur at any time and will be exacerbated in those who are volume depleted whether due to dehydration or blood loss. It remains important to consider other causes of hypotension in those having spinal anaesthesia, e.g. blood loss, myocardial ischaemia. Treatment of hypotension due to sympathetic blockade includes administering oxygen, elevating the feet to augment venous return, giving vasopressors (usually *ephedrine* or *methuruminol*), and providing IV fluid to restore circulating volume.

> At the end of the procedure the patient is given a simple analgesic timed to cover the spinal anaesthetic wearing off.

The duration of spinal anaesthesia is in the order of 2–4 hours, although the analgesia obtained can be prolonged by the addition of opioid drugs to the local anaesthetic injection.

As the effect of the spinal injection wears off, it is important to ensure that the patient can receive other methods of analgesia. For hernia repair it is likely that the patient will require an opioid drug postoperatively and this can be supplemented with simple analgesics (e.g. *paracetamol*) and non-steroidals taken orally.

> In the early postoperative period the patient becomes increasingly uncomfortable due to acute urinary retention and a urinary catheter is passed to decompress the bladder.

A cause of discomfort in the postoperative period after spinal anaesthesia is urinary retention. This is related to sacral nerve block and the use of fluid to prevent and treat hypotension. To limit this complication in the elderly, IV fluids should be used sparingly with the judicious use of vasopressors to treat hypotension.

An important complication of spinal anaesthesia is postdural puncture headache, caused by leakage of CSF through the dural puncture hole. The headache is characteristically related to posture, being worse on standing, and can be extremely incapacitating.

The patient should be prescribed regular analgesia and fluid intake should be maximized, the headache is self-limiting but this can take several days. If the patient does not respond rapidly to simple measures they can be offered an 'epidural blood patch', which attempts to seal the hole in the dura and prevent further leakage of CSF by injecting some of the patient's own blood into the area as a biological patch.

Scenario 3: anaesthesia, muscle relaxation, and analgesia for a laparoscopic cholecystectomy

> An otherwise fit 25-year-old lady with long-standing insulin-dependent diabetes requires general anaesthesia for laparoscopic cholecystectomy. She had an infusion of dextrose, insulin, and potassium commenced on the morning of surgery and her blood glucose level is within normal limits. She received a benzodiazepine premedication as well as an H_2 antagonist due to the possibility of delayed gastric emptying, due to her diabetes.

Patients with diabetes require specific management in all but the simplest and shortest operations. As before, IV access and monitoring should be established prior to induction of anaesthesia.

> The patient receives an IV induction with *propofol* and after checking that manual ventilation of the patient is possible, a non-depolarizing muscle relaxant (*atracurium* 0.5 mg/kg) is given. The anaesthetist continues to manually ventilate the patient until the onset of muscle relaxation sufficient for intubation (90–180 seconds). The anaesthetist uses a laryngoscope to view the larynx and to guide placement of an endotracheal tube through the vocal cords into the trachea.

During laparoscopic surgery there is a requirement for profound muscle relaxation to facilitate surgery. It is therefore modern practice to administer a specific neuromuscular blocking agent, to intubate the patient's trachea, and to mechanically ventilate the lungs.

> Anaesthesia is maintained with a mixture of oxygen—enriched air and the anaesthetic agent *isoflurane* (1%) delivered to the patient by a mechanical ventilator, while analgesia is provided using IV increments of *morphine* 2 mg.

The patient requires both anaesthesia and analgesia during the operation.

> At the end of surgery the anaesthetic gases are stopped and the patient is ventilated with 100% oxygen. A mixture of *neostigmine* (acetyl cholinesterase inhibitor) and *glycopyrrolate* (antimuscarinic agent) is given to reverse neuromuscular blockade and to prevent unwanted parasympathetic stimulation.

Ventilation with 100% oxygen helps flush the inhalational agent from the patient and aids more rapid recovery. The muscle relaxation required to perform the surgery needs to be completely reversed to prevent any residual effects on postoperative breathing.

> Once the patient is breathing spontaneously she is placed into the recovery position and the endotracheal tube removed.

Like all patients recovering from anaesthesia, she should be looked after by a recovery nurse in a dedicated recovery area until return of all her protective reflexes.

Scenario 4: rapid sequence induction for an emergency laparotomy

> A previously healthy 35-year-old man arrives in theatre for an emergency appendicectomy. He has an IV infusion of saline in progress and is comfortable having recently received an injection of *morphine* for analgesia.

Although in this case IV access already exists, it is important to check that the drip runs freely and does not cause pain, before using it to inject anaesthetic agents. As in elective surgery all monitoring should be commenced prior to induction of anaesthesia.

In this case the patient has been vomiting, has been in pain, and has received opioid analgesia. He therefore cannot be guaranteed to have an empty stomach and is at risk of regurgitation during induction and recovery from anaesthesia. In order to minimize the risk of aspiration of stomach contents into the lungs he requires to have a **rapid sequence induction.**

> The anaesthetist ensures the trolley the patient is lying on can be rapidly placed into the head-down position and that a suction catheter is at hand and switched on.

Should the patient regurgitate during induction of anaesthesia placing him in the head-down position and using suction will help clear his pharynx of gastric contents and reduce the likelihood of aspiration.

> The patient is then given 100% oxygen to breathe for a period of 3 minutes.

Pre-oxygenation is required to wash out nitrogen and ensure that the patient's functional reserve capacity (reserves of air in the lung) is full of oxygen. This allows the anaesthetist a little more time should intubation prove difficult.

> Pre-calculated doses of the rapidly acting induction agent *thiopental* (3–5 mg/kg) and of the depolarizing muscle relaxant *suxamethonium* (1 mg/kg) are then administered into the patient's drip.

The induction agent engenders sleep and the muscle relaxation allows intubation and initial ventilation.

> As the patient begins to lose consciousness the anaesthetic assistant applies 'cricoid pressure'.

This is a manoeuvre aimed at preventing regurgitation and aspiration of gastric contents by occluding the upper oesophagus with backward pressure on the cricoid cartilage.

> Once the patient is asleep and muscle relaxation has been signalled by muscle fasciculations the trachea is intubated and the cuff on the endotracheal tube inflated to ensure no leak around the vocal cords. Only then is the assistant instructed to remove the cricoid pressure.

A leak around the endotracheal tube is identified by air escaping round it on inflation. If air can get past so can vomit and secretions.

> Maintenance of anaesthesia requires a mechanical ventilator to deliver a mixture of oxygen and either oxygen-enriched air or nitrous oxide with the volatile anaesthetic *isoflurane* (1%). IV opioid analgesia can be administered in increments if required during the procedure and muscle relaxation is provided by one of the non-depolarizing drugs after the *suxamethonium* has been seen to wear off.

In this case all three parts of anaesthesia, sleep, muscle relaxation, and analgesia are required and given constant attention.

> At the end of surgery the volatile agent is turned off, 100% oxygen is administered, and *neostigmine* (and *glycopyrrolate*) as before are used to reverse muscle relaxation. The patient is placed in the lateral (recovery) position and his pharynx is suctioned to

remove any secretions that could be aspirated or cause laryngospasm. As the patient regains consciousness and his protective reflexes return the endotracheal tube is removed.

The patient continues to breathe oxygen via a face mask while transferring to the recovery area where he will undergo cardiorespiratory monitoring until he is ready to return to the surgical ward.

Clinical key points in anaesthesia

◆ Many different classes of drug are used to provide the classic triad of anaesthesia—sleep, analgesia, muscle relaxation

◆ Not every surgical procedure or anaesthetic requires all three components

◆ Anaesthetists require extensive knowledge of all the drugs they may use in order to tailor anaesthetics appropriately to the surgical procedure and any comorbidities the patient may have

◆ Anaesthesia and sedation should only be administered in areas with appropriate monitoring and staffing to conform with safety requirements

Background: anaesthesia

Anaesthesia can be thought of as a triad of:

◆ sleep

◆ analgesia

◆ muscle relaxation.

Depending on the nature of the surgery and the physical condition of the patient, it may not be necessary or desirable to provide all three components of anaesthesia during a specific procedure.

A patient with respiratory disease requiring inguinal hernia repair could have surgery performed under spinal anaesthesia, which would provide muscle relaxation, loss of sensation, and analgesia, but not sleep.

In contrast, a patient having a breast lump removed requires analgesia and could be either awake or asleep, but muscle relaxation is not necessary.

In some cases where the surgeon is entering a body cavity such as the abdomen or chest, all three components of anaesthesia are likely to be required.

Sleep

Inhalational anaesthetic agents can provide the triad of anaesthesia when given alone but at the expense of significant haemodynamic and ventilatory depression. Nowadays, it is common to use a combination of drugs to provide the different components of an anaesthetic allowing the anaesthetist to tailor the anaesthetic to the patient and the procedure, minimizing the dose of each component and thereby adverse effects.

IV anaesthetic agents, e.g. thiopental and propofol, are commonly used to induce anaesthesia (sleep) as they have a rapid action (the time taken to circulate from the injection site to the brain). Like most agents that produce anaesthesia, they cause cardiovascular and respiratory depression related to the dose. Propofol can be given by continuous infusion to maintain anaesthesia in an increasingly popular, but expensive, technique known as total IV anaesthesia (TIVA).

Maintenance of anaesthesia still usually occurs by inhalation of one of the volatile anaesthetic agents (gases), e.g. halothane, enflurane, isoflurane, sevoflurane, or desflurane. The anaesthetic gases are delivered to the patient from special vaporizers through a breathing circuit. The 'dose' of a vapour is expressed as a percentage of the inspired gas mixture and their potency as the MAC (minimum alveolar concentration required to prevent movement in 50% of patients receiving a surgical incision). The newer agents are nearly all effective in the 1–2% range.

As a result of a number of physiological changes (mainly in the lungs), anaesthetized patients require a higher concentration of oxygen to prevent hypoxia than non-anaesthetized individuals. It is common to use nitrous oxide (a weak anaesthetic agent) and at least 30% oxygen to 'carry' the anaesthetic gas to the patient. A mixture of oxygen-enriched air may also be used as the 'carrier gas'. Two of the inhalational agents, halothane and sevoflurane, are relatively pleasant to breathe and can be used to induce anaesthesia, e.g. in children in whom venous access may be difficult or in patients with airway problems. However, induction takes longer with inhalational techniques and the patient enters an excitement phase during which they may 'fight' the anaesthetic.

Analgesia

During most surgical procedures, analgesia is provided by one of the **opioid agents**. A number exist with differing durations of action, the commonest being *morphine* (long acting) and *fentanyl* (medium–short). These drugs can be given intravenously at induction and throughout the surgical procedure to block central pain receptors. They may be titrated in response to physical signs that the patient is in pain, e.g. tachycardia, hypertension, sweating.

All opioids produce the same side-effects no matter the route of administration. The most feared is respiratory depression, which is especially likely with the short-acting but very potent agents, e.g. *alfentanil* and *remifentanil*. Patients may also experience sedation, nausea and vomiting, and itchiness. The best way to minimize the risks of opioid analgesics is to administer them slowly in IV increments and to await a response before giving a further dose. All side-effects respond to IV *naloxone* (a specific opioid antagonist), which should also be given in increments in order to reverse the unwanted side-effect, but maintain analgesia.

Analgesia can also be provided by other agents either in combination with opioids or alone. The **NSAIDs** are very useful during body surface surgery and for dental and orthopaedic surgery. When used in combination with opioids they have an 'opioid sparing effect'. However, in certain groups of patients their use should be avoided, e.g. renal failure, asthma, and peptic ulceration, as these conditions can be exacerbated. Simple analgesics, such as *paracetamol* either alone or in combination with weak opioids may also be useful.

Local anaesthetic agents can be used to provide profound analgesia perioperatively. These agents block electrical impulses in all nerve fibres, thus preventing transmission of painful stimuli centrally, as well as causing autonomic and motor blockade. They are used as the main agents for central neural blockade (Fig. 2.1e).

Spinal anaesthesia

This involves the injection of a small amount of local anaesthetic into the subarachnoid space where it rapidly enters the nerve roots as they emerge from the spinal cord.

In order to avoid damage to the spinal cord, injection should be performed below the level of L2 vertebra (the spinal cord ends above this level in adults). As local anaesthetic is injected into the CSF, spread of the anaesthetic can be controlled by making the local anaesthetic solution heavier or lighter than CSF and by careful patient positioning (Fig. 2.1f). For example, a patient having spinal anaesthesia for haemorrhoidectomy would have the block performed in the sitting position with a 'heavy' solution of local anaesthetic—saddle block—to anaesthetize the perineum.

Local anaesthetics block all nerve types. Autonomic fibres, sensory nerves, and motor nerves are all anaesthetized with a spinal block. The onset of spinal blockade is rapid as local anaesthetic is able to penetrate the nerve roots very quickly from the subarachnoid space.

Hypotension can arise soon after spinal injection of local anaesthetic due to autonomic (sympathetic) blockade. This leads to vaso- and venodilatation resulting in venous pooling of blood (reduced preload) and reduced peripheral vascular resistance (reduced cardiac afterload). Treatment involves improving venous return by elevating the legs, using vasopressor drugs to vasoconstrict arteries, and careful use of IV fluids.

Opioid drugs may also be administered into the subarachnoid space, where they act directly on opioid receptors within the spinal cord and prolong the dura-

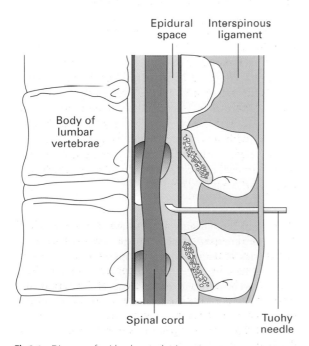

Fig 2.1e Diagram of epidural anaesthesia.

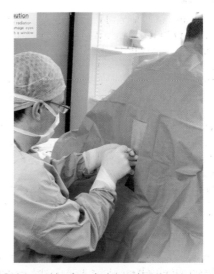

Fig 2.1f Patient position for spinal anaesthesia.

tion of both spinal and epidural anaesthesia and analgesia. However, respiratory depression is still a risk with this mode of administration. This may be late in onset (up to 24 hours after dosing) especially with the less lipid soluble opioids (morphine) as they persist in the CSF for longer.

Epidural anaesthesia

Injection of local anaesthetic into the epidural (extradural) space can be performed at any level of the spinal cord (cervical to sacral). It is most commonly performed in the thoracic and lumbar regions for abdominal, pelvic, and lower limb surgery. It is best to perform the epidural injection at the vertebral level of the dermatome in the middle of the surgical incision.

Catheters can be advanced into the epidural space to continue analgesia into the postoperative period, often for several days. The onset of epidural anaesthesia is slower than for spinal injection and the sensory and motor blocks are often less profound.

As with spinal block, epidurals cause autonomic blockade and can lead to hypotension. This is more evident in the volume-depleted patient as they are unable to compensate for fluid loss by vasoconstriction after central neural block.

As with spinal injections, opioid drugs can be added to the local anaesthetic to prolong the block. When used postoperatively for analgesia the use of opioid and local anaesthetic mixtures enables lower concentrations of both types of drug to be used. This helps to minimize motor weakness and opioid side-effects.

As well as central nerves, local anaesthetics can be used to block:

◆ peripheral nerves, e.g. digital nerve block for finger surgery

◆ larger nerves or groups of nerves, e.g. sciatic and femoral nerve block for foot surgery

◆ plexuses, e.g. the brachial plexus for arm surgery.

Used in this fashion an anaesthetic body part is produced with complete sensory loss and paralysis.

The commonest local anaesthetic agents in use are **lidocaine** (short duration of action) and **bupivacaine and ropivacaine** (long duration of action). Even if a specific nerve block is not possible for surgery, the surgeon can be encouraged to infiltrate the wound with local anaesthetic as this has been shown to improve pain control postoperatively.

Local anaesthetic toxicity

This can occur after inadvertent intravascular injection or if excessive dosage is used. Local anaesthetic toxicity presents as anxiety, light-headedness, and circumoral paraesthesia. If administration continues sedation and twitching may precede loss of consciousness, seizures, apnoea, and cardiac arrest due to ventricular fibrillation.

Prevention is better than treatment and careful injection with frequent aspiration should always be performed. If toxicity does develop, senior help should be sought, while the patient's airways are maintained, high flow oxygen administered, and, if necessary, treatment of seizures and cardiac arrest initiated.

Muscle relaxation

Certain types of surgery are facilitated if the anaesthetist can provide a reduction in skeletal muscle tone in the patient. Although in high dosage the inhalational agents can do this, it is safer to use specific **neuromuscular blocking drugs**. These drugs are also used to provide the profound muscle relaxation which enables endotracheal intubation to be carried out. The drugs block the action of acetylcholine at the neuromuscular junction so that action potentials are not translated into muscle contraction. Two types of muscle relaxants exist:

◆ **depolarizing agents**: those that first activate the acetylcholine receptor before blocking it, e.g. *suxamethonium*

◆ **non-depolarizing agents**: those that block the receptor without prior activation, e.g. *atracurium, vecuronium, rocuronium*.

Suxamethonium acts within a minute and lasts for about 3 minutes, its action being terminated by rapid metabolism. It is commonly used in emergency situations where the trachea must be intubated rapidly in order to protect the lungs from gastric acid aspiration. It is associated with two genetically determined complications: prolonged muscle relaxation and apnoea due to a metabolic enzyme deficiency and malignant hyperpyrexia. Although rare these complications are important as screening can detect other family members with the genetic abnormalities.

The non-depolarizing agents have a slower onset of action and are used to facilitate intubation where there is little risk of aspiration and to maintain muscle relaxation during surgery. At the end of surgery their action can be reversed by the use of an **acetylcholinesterase inhibitor** (*neostigmine*) given in combination with an **antimuscarinic agent** (*atropine, glycopyrrolate*) to prevent unwanted vagal (parasympathetic) effects such as excessive salivation and bradycardia.

Monitoring and equipment

Before administering an anaesthetic to a patient, the anaesthetist must ensure that all equipment that they require is to hand and working correctly. They must also ensure that appropriate monitoring equipment is available.

Guidelines exist to define acceptable levels of monitoring in the anaesthetized patient. As a minimum this must include cardiovascular monitoring using (Fig. 2.1g):

* ECG

* pulse oximetry (monitors peripheral oxygen saturation)

* non-invasive BP measurement, and

* respiratory monitoring using capnography (measurement of end-tidal carbon dioxide concentration and respiratory rate).

In addition, an oxygen analyser must be incorporated into the breathing circuit delivering the anaesthetic to ensure adequate oxygen concentrations are maintained.

For certain types of more complex surgery, e.g. aortic aneurysm repair, oesophagectomy, or where the patient is already very ill, more invasive monitoring may be required such as:

* intra-arterial BP measurement

* central venous pressure monitoring, or

* oesophageal Doppler monitoring of cardiac output.

A lot of equipment is required when conducting anaesthesia, which must be checked prior to use:

* if IV fluids are to be given during anaesthesia, then these must be prepared and an appropriate size of IV cannulae for drug and fluid administration selected

* all airway equipment to be used must be selected and checked before anaesthesia is induced, including laryngoscopes (the special light used to view the larynx at intubation), endotracheal tubes, and laryngeal masks

* any bacterial filters should be checked for patency and the breathing circuit should be inspected to ensure no leaks or blockages

* finally, the anaesthetic machine, which will be used to deliver oxygen and anaesthetic gases to the patient, should be thoroughly checked.

However, no mechanical or electrical monitor can replace the constant observation of the patient by the anaesthetist.

Sedation techniques

In acute medical practice, sedation is nearly always carried out using pharmacological methods (in non-acute situations the use of behavioural techniques or hypnosis may also be considered). It is important to remember that there is no clear line of demarcation between sedated and anaesthetized states. Careful use of drugs is essential, appropriate monitoring and resuscitation equipment must be to hand, and the responsible doctor must know how to use them correctly.

The agitated or restless patient

Doctors are often called to sedate the confused and restless patient. These patients are often elderly, and before sedation is used, it is vital to exclude specific causes for their disruptive behaviour. Hypoxia, pain, hypotension, infection, urinary retention, and the hallucinogenic effects of prescribed (and non-prescribed) medication can all lead to an agitated, confused patient. In these cases treating the cause will be more effective (and less dangerous) than giving sedation.

If sedation is required an oral dose of one of the antipsychotic drugs, e.g. *haloperidol*, may be given.

Diagnostic procedures

Sedation is widely used outwith the operating theatre for a variety of diagnostic procedures, e.g. endoscopy and bronchoscopy. The aim of sedation is to relax the anxious patient, but leave them able to co-operate during the planned procedure.

The drug in most common use is *midazolam* a short-acting benzodiazepine. It has anxiolytic and amnesic properties and has less 'hangover effect' than older agents. It has to be titrated carefully to avoid inadvertent overdosage.

The use of IV anaesthetic agents such as *propofol* in subhypnotic doses is not to be recommended for the non-anaesthetist. The drug has a rapid onset and offset, but changes in concentration can arise quickly, with a sedated patient rapidly becoming anaesthetized.

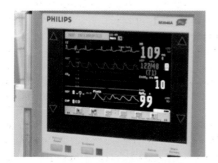

Fig 2.1g Monitoring screen showing pulse, BP, CVP, respiratory rate, and oxygen saturation.

In a very few cases the use of an opioid in combination with a benzodiazepine may be justified, but it is important to remember that not only is the effect greater but so are the side-effects and doses of both drugs should be reduced. The operator must be constantly aware of the risks of oversedation and loss of airway control.

Guidelines for the safe administration of intravenous sedation

◆ In all areas where IV sedation is administered, resuscitation and airway management equipment must be readily available and the medical and support staff versed in their use.

Fast facts—Anaesthesia and sedation

Safe anaesthesia depends on:

Preparation

◆ Patient assessment (i.e. cardiac, respiratory)

◆ Prophylaxis

◆ Premedication

Monitoring

◆ ECG

◆ Oximetry

◆ Capnography

◆ BP monitoring

◆ IV access

Anaesthesia consists of:

◆ Sleep (inhalational, IV)

◆ Muscle relaxation

◆ Analgesia (analgesics, local anaesthetic blocks)
Every case does not require all three, but every case requires analgesia.

Sedation

Safe sedation should be treated in the same way as anaesthesia with the same monitoring and supervision.

Recovery

All anaesthesia and sedation requires closely supervised recovery.

◆ IV access to the patient should be secured with a plastic cannula.

◆ Continuous monitoring of ECG and pulse oximetry with intermittent BP monitoring should be used.

◆ Oxygen saturation should not be allowed to fall below 92%, with oxygen being administered by face mask or nasal cannulae if necessary.

◆ Titrate the sedative drug slowly (midazolam 1 mg/minute) and await its effect. Conversing with the patient helps to gauge level of sedation—if the patient can no longer answer, they are oversedated and at risk.

Although modern sedatives are relatively short acting, subtle effects on CNS function can last for many hours. As such patients should be given the same advice on discharge as patients who have received a general anaesthetic. They should be accompanied home by a responsible adult and given written advice not to drive or operate machinery (including cookers, kettles) or take important decisions for 24 hours after the procedure.

Background: postoperative care

In the postoperative period there are again a number of issues that must be addressed to reduce the risk to the patient and make them as comfortable as possible. Many preoperative concerns continue into the postoperative period.

◆ recovery

◆ pain management

◆ postoperative nausea and vomiting management

◆ fluid management

◆ blood transfusion

◆ nutrition.

Recovery

Although most patients make an uneventful recovery from anaesthesia and surgery, a number will suffer early complications, some predictably, some not. Therefore, all patients recovering from anaesthesia must be nursed by trained staff, in an area properly equipped, such that any problems arising can be dealt with appropriately.

As a minimum, all immediately postoperative patients should be recovered:

◆ on a tipping trolley (although some patients can be managed on their bed)

◆ an oxygen supply and suction should be available

- minimum monitoring for every patient includes:

  - non-invasive BP; this is usually with an automatic BP monitor, timed to repeat the assessment every 15 minutes

  - ECG

  - pulse oximetry, to allow determination of oxygen **saturation**

  - in addition, within the recovery area there should be equipment for more advanced airways management, e.g. Guedel airways, endotracheal tubes, laryngoscopes, and cricothyroidotomy kits.

  - there must also be available a defibrillator and emergency cardiac drugs.

Before discharge from the recovery area all patients should be:

- conscious (perhaps still sleepy)

- able to maintain airways/breathing adequately

- warm

- pain free

- haemodynamically stable with minimal bleeding.

In the recovery area, the complications arising usually relate to the cardiovascular and respiratory systems, as well as pain and nausea.

Pain management

Pain is a complex sensation involving physical and psychological components. Acute (postoperative) pain is triggered by surgical incision and varies in intensity, from mild to severe. It is transitory in nature, lessening as the tissues heal.

A patient's perception of pain will vary, depending on many factors:

- site and type of incision (upper abdominal and thoracic incisions are most painful)

- reason for surgery

- previous experience

- personality type.

Thus there is likely to be great interindividual variation in experience of pain and requirements for analgesia after surgery.

> **ALWAYS REMEMBER PAIN IS WHAT THE PATIENT SAYS IT IS, NOT WHAT THE CLINICIANS THINK IT SHOULD BE**

Pain contributes to the physiological changes undergone by the body after tissue injury. Many of these changes that arise are part of the 'stress response to surgery' and are deleterious to the body leading to muscle mass breakdown, lethargy, thrombotic tendency, and susceptibility to infection. The presence of pain also has a number of adverse effects on specific organ functions:

- increased heart rate and BP leading to increased myocardial work (potential for myocardial ischaemia)

- rapid shallow breathing and inability to cough (potential for atelectasis, chest infection, and hypoxaemia)

- reduced bowel motility, which can be compounded by the use of opioid analgesics (leading to nausea and vomiting, ileus, and increased duration of fasting).

Therefore, good pain management is likely to have physiological, as well as psychological, benefits for the patient.

Treating postoperative pain

Commonly used techniques for the treatment of pain after surgery are drugs and local anaesthetic nerve blocks.

Preventing pain is easier than treating pain once it is established and steps are usually taken during anaesthesia to ensure that the patient wakes up pain free. This is done by administering analgesic drugs (opioids) as part of the anaesthetic technique often in combination with a nerve block.

A number of different classes of analgesic drug exists, and they often have a greater than expected effect (synergy) when used in combination. When prescribing analgesic agents the concept of an analgesia ladder can be used—start with mild drugs for mild pain and work up to the use of stronger agents for severe pain (Table 2.1e).

Traditionally, opioids have been given by intermittent intramuscular injection at the patient's request. This

TABLE 2.1e	Analgesic ladder
Minor surgery/mild pain	Simple analgesics, e.g. paracetamol 1 g × 4/day
Intermediate surgery/ moderate pain	Simple analgesic + NSAIDs, e.g. ibuprofen 200–600 mg × 4/day orally or diclofenac 50 mg × 3/day orally or suppository
Major surgery/severe pain	If possible give regular simple analgesic and NSAID plus opioid (morphine, diamorphine)

method of analgesia has been regarded as safe, but is acknowledged to lead to poor pain relief with troughs of inadequate analgesia and peaks where side-effects may be potentially dangerous, e.g. respiratory depression.

When presented with a patient in severe pain it is better to titrate opioid analgesia using small, frequent IV boluses until the patient is comfortable. Analgesia can then be continued, as a continuous IV infusion or using a patient-controlled analgesia (PCA) system.

The use of PCA allows the patient to titrate the dose of opioid they receive to their own needs within limits set by medical staff. A pump delivers a fixed dose of opioid when activated by the patient pressing a control button. After a successful bolus, the pump will not deliver any further boluses during a set period (usually 5 minutes).

Opioid drugs can also be administered as part of an epidural technique in combination with local anaesthetic agents.

Regardless of how they are administered, opioids have the same side-effects:

♦ sedation

♦ nausea and vomiting, and

♦ respiratory depression.

They should always be prescribed in conjunction with an antiemetic. If severe, oversedation or respiratory depression can be treated using the specific opioid antagonist, naloxone, titrated to effect.

Wherever possible the use of local anaesthetic agents should be encouraged in the treatment and prevention of postoperative pain. This may be in the form of:

♦ wound infiltration by the surgeon

♦ specific nerve blocks performed by the anaesthetist prior to surgery, or regional anaesthetic techniques, such as plexus blocks (brachial, lumbosacral)

♦ central nerve blocks (epidural, subarachnoid block).

Postoperative nausea and vomiting (PONV)

This is one of the commonest complications associated with anaesthesia and surgery, and may be extremely distressing for the patient. PONV has a complex aetiology with:

♦ patient factors (age, sex, history of motion sickness, or previous PONV)

♦ surgical factors (gynaecological procedures, eye surgery, ENT surgery), and

♦ postoperative factors (pain, use of opioids, movement).

A number of drugs are used in the treatment of PONV, most of which act centrally and as a result can be associated with a number of adverse effects:

♦ phenothiazines, e.g. prochlorperazine can cause sedation and extrapyramidal reactions (oculo-gyric crises)

♦ metoclopramide has a peripheral action, speeding gastric emptying as well as a central action. It can cause severe extrapyramidal reactions, especially in the young

♦ antihistamines, e.g. cyclizine, can be very sedating

♦ $5HT_3$ antagonists, e.g. ondansetron may act centrally and within the stomach mucosa. They can be associated with flushing and headache, but are generally well tolerated.

Often if PONV is severe, treatment with a combination of drugs from different classes is effective. In patients with a strong history of PONV, antiemetic drugs can be given prophylactically during anaesthesia.

Fast facts—Postoperative care (recovery, analgesia, postoperative nausea, and vomiting)

Recovery

♦ Immediate recovery from anaesthesia and surgery should take place in a dedicated area with specialist staff and equipment

—all patients who have received a general anaesthetic or sedation require oxygen until they are awake

—the main complications in the immediate recovery period relate to cardiorespiratory systems, pain, and nausea

Pain management

♦ Postoperative analgesia should be tailored for the individual patient

♦ Remember the concept of an analgesia ladder

♦ If a patient is in pain consider IV boluses of opioid to titrate them safely to comfort

Postoperative nausea and vomiting

♦ Postoperative nausea and vomiting is multifactorial and a combination of antiemetics is likely to be more successful than one drug alone

Fluid management

Scenario: fluid regimen following an uncomplicated laparotomy

> A fit 55-year-old man is scheduled to undergo a right hemicolectomy. The operation proceeds uneventfully with minimal blood loss.

The operation has been performed with no complications. As blood loss was negligible, the anaesthetist need only replace preoperative losses (preoperative fasting) and intraoperative losses from the gut surface and into the 'third space'.

> In theatre he receives 1500 ml of Hartmann's solution over 2 hours and has a urine output of 60 ml/hour. The anaesthetist has prescribed a further 500 ml of 5% dextrose over the next 4 hours and has then asked that the patient be reviewed, before further fluids are prescribed.

The operation has gone smoothly and the patient is previously fit. Ongoing third space losses into the gut are likely to be minimal. Therefore, when prescribing

TABLE 2.1f Fluid perscription for first 48 hrs post-operation

Date	Fluid	Volume	Time given
Day 1	Normal saline (0.9% NaCl)	500 ml	6 hours
Day 1	5% dextrose	500 ml	6 hours
Day 1	Normal saline (0.9% NaCl)	500 ml	6 hours
Day 1	5% dextrose	500 ml	6 hours
Day 1	Normal saline (0.9% NaCl)	500 ml	6 hours
Day 2	Normal saline (0.9% NaCl) + 10 ml KCl	500 ml	6 hours
Day 2	5% dextrose + 10 ml KCl	500 ml	6 hours
Day 2	Normal saline (0.9% NaCl) + 10 ml KCl	500 ml	6 hours
Day 2	5% dextrose + 10 ml KCl	500 ml	6 hours
Day 2	Normal saline (0.9% NaCl) + 10 ml KCl	500 ml	6 hours

500-ml bags are used to limit any potential for the patient receiving too large a bolus of fluid if there is a problem with the timing of the infusion.

fluid, take into account normal maintenance requirements for water (2–2.5 l) and electrolytes (1–2 mmol/kg of sodium) per 24 hours. Also take into account continuing losses (urine, vomit, diarrhoea, drain fluid), which are likely to be electrolyte rich.

> The patient is prescribed alternating 500 ml bags of 0.9% saline and 5% dextrose to run at 83 ml/hour.

On the second and subsequent postoperative day, potassium 10–20 mmol should be added to each bag of fluid (after the first 24 hours postoperation, potassium redistributes back into the intracellular compartment). IV fluid requirements will diminish as increasing amounts of fluid are taken orally.

Clinical key points in perioperative fluids

- In a normal 70 kg man urine output is 1500 ml/24 hours with a further 1000 ml of insensible loss
- Normal daily requirements are for 2000–2500 ml of water and 1–2 mmol/kg of both sodium and potassium
- Frequent assessment of the patient and all their observations and charts is required
- Owing to the renal effects of the metabolic response to trauma, water overload is much more likely to cause significant morbidity than hypovolaemia
- Fluid required = pre-existing deficit + normal maintenance + ongoing losses

Background: fluid management

Perioperative fluid management is an arithmetic exercise. The aim is to balance fluid and electrolyte input with output, in order to maintain stability. Replacing fluid loss is an inexact science depending heavily on frequent assessment of the patient, their blood chemistry, and observation charts.

Getting fluid balance wrong can be associated with increased perioperative morbidity. Too much fluid may be associated with oedema and altered lung compliance leading to reduced gas exchange and respiratory complications. Too little fluid can lead to renal dysfunction. Some knowledge of the volume and composition of fluid compartments within the body is required to help guide fluid therapy.

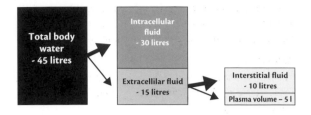

Total body water comprises 60% of lean body mass. Two-thirds of total body water or 40% of body weight comprises the intracellular fluid volume with the remaining two-thirds of total body water or 20% of body weight comprising the extracellular fluid volume. The extracellular fluid volume is further divided into interstitial fluid and plasma volume, which excludes red cell volume.

In a 70 kg man, the relative sizes of the various fluid compartments can easily be remembered by the 'rule of 1/3s'. Each compartment being distributed into 2/3–1/3 as shown.

Total blood volume is approximately 5 litres comprising plasma volume and red cell volume (2 litres).

The solute composition of plasma and interstitial fluid are very similar. Sodium is the principal *cation* (140 mmol/l) with chloride being the major *anion* (114 mmol/l).

Intracellular fluid differs from the extracellular fluid in having potassium as the major cation (150 mmol/l) with very little sodium (10 mmol/l). There is a high protein content intracellularly and the major anion is phosphate.

The cell membrane is freely permeable to water but only selectively permeable to different ions. Thus movement of water takes place between the intracellular fluid volume and the extracellular fluid volume to ensure equilibrium of the extracellular and intracellular osmolalities.

Water and electrolyte haemostasis

There are normally only minimal fluctuations in total body water from day to day. The main sources of water for the body are food and fluid ingestion, and water from metabolism. Fluid loss is usually defined as sensible or insensible. Insensible losses are from skin (sweat), lungs, and faeces. In health, sensible loss is the urine output. In disease or after surgery, other measured losses can occur from the gastrointestinal tract (nasogastric aspirate, vomit, diarrhoea), from drains, and as blood loss.

A normal individual will require about 2–2.5 litres of water a day to maintain stability.

In health, gastrointestinal excretions amount to about 6 litres/24 hours of which all but 100 ml is reab-

TABLE 2.1g In a healthy 70 kg man, in fluid balance, intake and output are as follows	
Volume	
Water intake	
Fluid intake	1500 ml
Food	600 ml
Water from metabolism	400 ml
Total	2500 ml
Water loss	
Sensible loss (urine)	1500 ml
Insensible loss (sweat, lungs, faeces)	1000 ml
Total	2500 ml

sorbed. In disease there is the potential for massive loss of electrolyte-rich fluid.

The healthy kidney has great concentrating capacity and can excrete the body's daily waste in as little as 0.5 ml/kg per hour. If urine output is less than this for any length of time, it may mean hypovolaemia has led to acute renal failure.

Patients also have to receive the correct type of fluid to maintain electrolyte homeostasis. In general:

- sodium requirement = 80 mmol per 24 hours (1–2 mmol/kg)

- potassium requirement = 60 mmol per 24 hours (1–2 mmol/kg).

There are two main groups of IV fluid (excluding blood): crystalloid and colloid.

Crystalloids

There are three commonly used IV crystalloid solutions for fluid replacement. They have differing electrolyte contents that affect their distribution in the total body water:

- 0.9% saline (normal saline): 154 mmol/l sodium and isotonic (same osmolality as extracellular fluid)

- Hartmann's solution: 140 mmol/l sodium, 5 mmol/l potassium, 110 mmol/l chloride (isotonic with extracellular fluid)

- 5% dextrose: sodium content is nil, essentially water but isotonic with extracellular fluid.

All sodium containing fluid remains in the extracellular fluid space, as it cannot gain access to intracellular fluid space due to the sodium/potassium pump. If the solution is isotonic, then no water moves across the cell membrane, i.e. 0.9% saline or Hartmann's solution expands only the extracellular fluid.

If 5% dextrose is infused, the glucose is rapidly metabolized and the water it is carried in distributes throughout the total body water (two-thirds to intracellular fluid, one-third to extracellular fluid).

Colloids

Colloid solutions contain large osmotically active particles which are too big to pass across capillary membranes and therefore they are largely retained within the plasma volume.

A number of solutions exist: dextrans, starches, gelatins and albumin, and fresh frozen plasma (FFP). They are more expensive than crystalloid, and some carry a risk of anaphylaxis and infection. They are used mainly as blood volume expanders. However, in disease states where capillary membranes can be leaky, the large particles can leak out into the interstitial fluid where they draw in more water, worsening oedema.

The metabolic stress response to trauma/surgery

The metabolic response to injury is roughly proportional to the severity of the trauma or surgical insult. In very minor surgery it is so small as to be of no real clinical relevance, but after major surgery it may be massive lasting for several days. The response to injury cannot be prevented, but its effects can be attenuated by appropriate fluid management, analgesia, and nutritional support.

Renal aspects of metabolic response to injury

Increased antidiuretic hormone secretion →
increased water retention
Increased aldosterone secretion → increased
sodium retention

These two changes result in a reduction in urine output and sometimes oliguria as well, meaning the kidneys are less able to deal with large water loads. Thus, giving excess hypotonic fluid can lead to water overload.

Perioperative fluid therapy

While most patients undergoing minor elective surgery will not require any form of postoperative IV fluid therapy, patients undergoing major elective surgery will require a period of IV fluid replacement.

Preoperative dehydration can be a significant problem particularly if patients have fasted for longer than 12 hours, received 'bowel prep', or have been vomiting.

Fluid management begins preoperatively by ensuring patients are well hydrated from the outset, and consideration should be given to commencing IV fluids in patients who have had a prolonged period of fasting, or had preoperative bowel prep.

Postoperatively, a fluid regimen should take into account intraoperative losses and their replacement, ongoing loss, and normal maintenance requirements.

Assessment

Repeated assessment of the patient is required when prescribing perioperative fluid regimens. This follows the usual format.

History

This should include a note of any losses before admission to hospital and/or intraoperative losses and replacement.

The type of surgery should be noted as bowel and intra-abdominal vascular surgery are associated with larger 'third space losses' (1–5 litres of plasma). This is where fluid moves from the plasma volume into the interstitial fluid after acute injury. Usually it resolves after 2–3 days and the fluid moves back to plasma volume.

Examination

Dry mouth is not uncommon in perioperative patients. Loss of skin elasticity is a late sign of hypovolaemia and cold. Vasoconstricted peripheries also suggest significant loss of volume.

Heart rate may be normal especially in previously fit patients and hypotension initially may only be apparent on moving from lying to standing.

Investigations

Fluid balance charts should be studied. These include not only urine output and fluid intake, but also other sources of fluid loss including nasogastric aspirate (or vomit), drain fluid, diarrhoea, and blood loss (Fig. 2.1h). It is important to remember that these types of fluid are electrolyte rich and these losses must also be replaced.

Also remember to take into account ongoing losses from skin and through breathing (insensible loss) and continuing third space loss after major surgery. Haematology and biochemistry should be checked

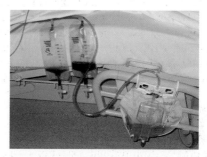

Fig 2.1h Drains and urine bag to monitor fluid loss.

regularly and can alert to inadequate or too vigorous fluid replacement.

Standard perioperative fluid regimens are therefore calculated as follows:

Fluid required = pre-existing deficit + maintenance + ongoing losses

Maintenance (for a 70 kg man) is based on 2–2.5 litres of water per 24 hours and 80–150 mmol/l of sodium.

This is normally provided as 1500 ml of dextrose 5% and 500–1000 ml of 0.9% saline. In the initial postoperative period, no replacement of potassium is required but after the first 24 hours, 10 mmol can be added to each 500 ml of fluid administered.

Pre-existing deficit should be estimated from history and examination. The type of fluid used for replacement will be dependent on the type of fluid lost.

♦ it is usual to replace blood loss of >20% blood volume with red cells

♦ crystalloid electrolyte infusion can be used for smaller losses, but it should be remembered that these will distribute throughout the whole extracellular fluid volume and thus three times the blood volume lost should be administered

---

Fast facts—Perioperative fluids

Fluids

If out = in = stable patient

♦ Fluid balance is an inexact science and frequent assessment of the patient, observations, and fluid charts is required

♦ Water without sodium expands the total body water (e.g. 5% dextrose)

♦ All infused sodium remains in the extracellular fluid (0.9% saline, Hartmann's solution)

Electrolytes

♦ Massive loss of electrolyte-rich fluid can occur from the gastrointestinal tract in disease

♦ Hyponatraemia postoperatively is usually due to over infusion of 5% dextrose

♦ Hypokalaemia may occur after the second postoperative day and fluid regimens should include 1–2 mmol/kg per 24 hours

---

♦ in the preoperative period, fluid deficits are often due to increased gastrointestinal loss of electrolyte-rich fluids and are replaced with crystalloid solutions

♦ it may be possible to replace pre-existing loss as a bolus over a short period of time while assessing response.

Ongoing losses are common after surgery. Loss from the gastrointestinal tract is common due to vomiting, nasogastric loss, or if there is a postoperative ileus, when fluid is lost to the gut lumen.

If these losses are considerable an appropriate sample should be sent for biochemical analysis so that appropriate replacement can occur. Third space losses continue for 48–72 hours after major surgery and are usually replaced as either 0.9% saline or Hartmann's solution.

Transfusion and blood products

Scenario 1: perioperative blood transfusion

A 79-year-old lady, with a history of congestive cardiac failure and ischaemic heart disease, is admitted with a history of altered bowel habit, tiredness, and increasing breathlessness on exertion. On examination she has a palpable mass in the right iliac fossa and a Hb of 7.5 g/dl, with a microcytic picture.

The history and examination are strongly suggestive of a right-sided colonic tumour. This has slowly been bleeding over many months and the patient now has a symptomatic anaemia (increasing breathlessness and tiredness). The microcytosis suggest an iron deficiency picture.

The patient's iron and ferritin levels are checked and the patient is transfused 4 units of red cell concentrate, with frusemide cover. Subsequent colonoscopy and CT scan reveal a caecal carcinoma with no metastases.

As the anaemia was symptomatic, the patient was transfused. In this situation the patient required red cells to improve oxygen-carrying capacity, but was not significantly hypovolaemic, and so the transfusion of blood (4 units of red cell concentrate, usually about 300 ml volume each) is covered by giving the patient oral frusemide 20 mg with alternate bags. This is to ensure that the patient does not become fluid overloaded, particularly as she has a history of congestive cardiac failure.

Following transfusion, the patient underwent a right hemicolectomy with an ileo-colic anastomosis, to remove the tumour. On the first postoperative day, her Hb was 8.7 g/dl, with a haematocrit of 0.3, and an albumin level of 29 g/l.

The low albumin and haematocrit all suggest a 'dilutional' cause for the low Hb, caused by crystalloid infusion during the operation and in the immediate postoperative period. At this level, and in view of the probable dilutional cause, the patient does not need a blood transfusion.

The patient made an uneventful recovery and was ready for discharge 8 days after her operation. She was mobile around the ward and was not breathless on exertion. Her Hb was 9.2 g/dl. She was commenced on oral iron sulphate therapy.

At this level (Hb 9.2 g/dl) the patient does not require transfusion, especially as she is not symptomatic. Her iron levels were depleted preoperatively and she was therefore commenced on oral iron therapy.

Current guidelines suggest that fit patients with no significant history do not need transfusion till the Hb reaches less than 7 g/dl. Patients with ischaemic heart disease require transfusion if the Hb is less than 8 g/dl. There is no real indication to transfuse any patient with a Hb greater than 10 g/dl.

Scenario 2: unanticipated intraoperative blood loss

A 35-year-old lady is to undergo right mastectomy and axillary clearance for breast cancer. She has undergone pre-assessment by a surgeon and anaesthetist and she is fit for surgery. Blood tests performed show her Hb is 11 g/dl preoperatively and blood has been sent for group, screen, and save.

Owing to the nature of surgery there is no indication to cross-match the patient, but because of the potential for blood loss from the axillary clearance a group and save is required.

During surgery the breast is found to be extremely vascular and bleeding is above average for the procedure. Surgical swabs are weighed during the procedure and are found to contain 600 ml of blood.

The blood content of swabs is assessed by simply weighing them (1 g = 1 ml).

As the surgeons begin to dissect the axillary contents there is some brisk blood loss from the axillary vein, which has been damaged. The patient becomes hypotensive and blood loss is estimated to have reached 1300 ml just as control over the bleeding vessel is obtained.

The patient has nearly 2 litres of recorded blood loss and will require blood for blood replacement.

The blood bank checks that the patient has had blood sent for a group, screen, and save. They are then able to tell the anaesthetist that as the patient has no unexpected red cell antibodies that they will perform a rapid ABO cross-match against donor blood and that blood will be available for the patient within 30 minutes.

The previous group and save allows a rapid supply of suitable blood.

Clinical key points for blood transfusion

- Patients with symptomatic anaemia should be transfused red cell concentrate. If the patient has a history of cardiac failure, consider giving covering oral frusemide to prevent pulmonary oedema

- Patients with an Hb of >10 g/dl do not need transfusion

- 'Fit' patients may not need to be transfused till the Hb is <7 g/dl

- Patients with ischaemic heart disease should be transfused if the Hb is <8 g/dl

- Patients undergoing major surgery should have at least a group and save preoperatively; patients undergoing complex surgery should be cross-matched preoperatively, so that blood is available

Background: transfusion and blood products

The safe practice of blood transfusion has been critical for the development and safe performance of many surgical procedures. However, transfusion of blood and blood products is not without risk due to the possibility of transfusion reactions and the spread of infection from donor to recipient. It is therefore important to

TABLE 2.1h	Blood groups		
Blood type	**% in UK**	**Red cell antigen**	**Antibody in plasma**
O	47	–	Anti-A, anti-B
A	42	A	Anti-B
B	8	B	Anti-A
AB	3	AB	–

give careful thought when considering the use of transfusion in clinical practice, to ensure the likely benefits outweigh the potential risks.

Blood groups

The ABO groups and the Rhesus system are the two most important blood groups in the clinical practice of transfusion medicine. The human red cell membrane contains a variety of antigens and individuals can have one of four major blood types depending on the antigens present.

Thus patients with blood group AB are 'universal recipients', as they have no antibodies to the major ABO antigens, while those with group O blood are 'universal donors' as their red cells have no A or B antigens. This, of course, does not take into account that other minor red cell antigens may be present and can cause a transfusion reaction.

Antibodies against the ABO red cell antigens occur naturally without prior exposure to 'foreign' red cells.

The Rhesus system is composed of many antigens, the most important of which is Rhesus D antigen. In the UK, approximately 85% of the population has the Rhesus D antigen and is labelled Rhesus positive. Antibodies to the Rhesus antigens do not occur naturally and require prior exposure to Rhesus-positive blood. In Rhesus-negative individuals (15% of the population) who have previously received a transfusion of Rhesus-positive blood, significant quantities of Rhesus antibodies exist and if a subsequent transfusion of Rhesus-positive blood is given, a serious haemolytic transfusion reaction can arise.

Blood grouping and cross-matching

The purpose of compatibility testing of blood is to prevent haemolytic transfusion reactions due to the presence of red cell antibodies of the ABO system and to other less common but clinically relevant blood group antigens.

The recipient's blood is ABO and rhesus typed by testing red cells with antisera containing anti-A, anti-B, and anti-D. This typing can be performed very quickly and

plays only a small part in the time it takes to complete compatibility tests.

An antibody screen is also performed on the patient's blood to detect any clinically significant red cell antibodies, which could give rise to a transfusion reaction. If there is a positive antibody screen, cross-matching with donor red cells may take more time as donor cells without the red cell antigen which reacts with the antibody in the recipient's blood must be identified.

If a cross-match is also requested the patient's serum is tested against the selected donor serum for ABO and other red cell antibodies (Coombs' cross-match). This test takes 30–45 minutes.

For many surgical procedures, the likelihood of requiring a blood transfusion is so low that it is unnecessary even to type the patient's blood. In some cases it is thought unlikely that transfusion will be required and so blood is not cross-matched but a group and antibody screen is performed and the serum saved so that blood can be issued quickly should the need arise (**group, screen, and save**). This prevents waste of a relatively scarce resource and also reduces lab costs.

If a blood transfusion is likely in view of the nature of the surgery or patient anaemia, then an elective blood **group, screen, and cross-match** is required.

Blood and blood products

Most blood banks now use almost all the whole blood donated as a raw material from which to make blood components. Very little blood (if any) is kept and issued as whole blood. This lowers the costs and makes components such as platelets, FFP, and cryoprecipitate more available. Red cell concentrate is the usual form in which blood is issued.

Red cell concentrates (RCC)

RCC consists of red cells in a little plasma, anticoagulant, and preservative solution. The volume is usually 250–350 ml with a shelf life of approximately 40 days. They contain little plasma and no viable platelets, and when used to replace red cell mass and blood volume during haemorrhage, are usually given with plasma expanders (haemacell, gelofusine) or large volumes of crystalloid.

In patients receiving massive transfusion (more than one blood volume) problems with coagulation can arise. This may be seen as oozing from the surgical field and from venepuncture sites. It is usually due to dilutional thrombocytopenia, as red cell concentrates given to replace blood loss contain no platelets (even in transfused whole blood platelets are non-functional being damaged by storage at 4°C). If confirmed by blood testing, platelet transfusion can be considered.

Platelet concentrates

Prepared from whole blood by the removal of 60 ml plasma and stored at room temperature for up to 5 days with about 70% retention of viability. They contain small numbers of red cells therefore it is preferable to use type-specific platelets where possible.

Disseminated intravascular coagulation is a serious derangement of both clotting and fibrinolysis. It can arise after massive transfusion, trauma, sepsis, or obstetric catastrophes. It causes generalized abnormal bleeding due to depletion of clotting factors, platelets and the antithrombotic effects of fibrin degradation products produced during fibrinolysis. Treatment is of the underlying condition, but after discussion with a haematologist it may be necessary to use platelets, FFP, and cryoprecipitate.

Fresh frozen plasma (FFP)

This is the liquid part of whole blood separated from the cells by centrifugation and contains all the plasma proteins. It usually has a volume of 250 ml per unit and can be stored frozen at −18°C for up to 1 year. It is often used to reverse deficiencies of clotting factors associated with warfarin.

Cryoprecipitate

Is produced by freezing single units of plasma. It is a concentrate of fibrinogen and factor VIII. It is used mainly in the treatment of disseminated intravascular coagulation.

Adverse transfusion reactions

Blood transfusion has significant risk, and should never be undertaken lightly.

Acute haemolytic transfusion reaction

This is rare but when it occurs, is severe and life threatening. It is usually due to ABO incompatibility and are nearly always the result of clerical errors with the patient being given the wrong blood. **Great care must be taken labelling blood samples and when checking blood products with patient name bands and case notes.**

If the patient is anaesthetized, the first signs of a reaction may be shock and abnormal bleeding with a degree of flushing. Other symptoms include back/chest pain, feelings of unease, headache, coughing, wheezing, and nausea.

Management involves stopping the transfusion and maintaining BP with crystalloid solutions, checking the patient details with the unit of blood, and informing the blood bank of a problem. A sample of blood should be taken and sent to the blood bank with the transfused unit, for further tests. If the reaction is severe, multiorgan failure and disseminated intravascular coagulation can develop: the treatment is supportive.

Delayed haemolytic transfusion reaction

This is very rare, occurring in patients who have been previously sensitized by transfusion or pregnancy, but in whom the level of red cell antibodies has declined to undetectable levels. After a second exposure to antigen, antibody production increases and after several days destruction of the transfused red cells begins. The reaction is often mild, but patients should be informed that they have irregular red cell antibodies, in case future transfusion is required.

Febrile reactions

This is among the commonest transfusion reactions but is mild and self-limiting. The patient experiences fever and chills and a haemolytic transfusion reaction should be ruled out. It is usually due to antibodies directed at donor leucocytes (or platelets) and the reaction can be prevented by using a white cell filter or leucocyte-depleted donations.

Allergic reactions

This is also very common and usually mild with the patient experiencing itching, flushing, and urticaria due to histamine release. It arises due to allergens in donor plasma reacting to antibodies on the recipient's mast cells and basophils. Antihistamines can be given to prevent recurrence.

Anaphylaxis

This is usually due to an idiosyncratic reaction to a substance in donor plasma. If not identified quickly and treatment begun, death may occur. Treatment is of anaphylactic shock with ABCs of resuscitation and the use of adrenaline (epinephrine) to maintain BP along with intravascular volume replacement.

Fluid overload

This may be common and underdiagnosed, especially in the very young or very old. Patients at risk should be identified before transfusion and blood given slowly with, if appropriate, a diuretic and careful monitoring to ensure pulmonary oedema does not arise.

Bacterial contamination

This is increasingly being recognized as an important cause of serious adverse reactions after transfusion. Severe septic shock can develop and requires supportive therapy and appropriate antibiotics. Great care when handling blood products is required from donation to delivery to the patient. Blood should be stored appropriately and not kept out of the fridge for any length of time before it is required. Platelet transfusions are often implicated, because these are stored at room temperature.

Indications for blood transfusion

In the acute situation where there is rapid ongoing blood loss, e.g. after trauma, intraoperatively, clinical assessment is used as a guide to the need for transfusion as measurements of Hb may not accurately reflect the degree of blood loss.

When deciding whether or not to transfuse, ongoing losses, haemodynamic instability, and the likelihood of postoperative bleeding all need to be considered. Most healthy individuals can compensate for losses of up to 40% blood. In these cases volume can be replaced with either crystalloid solutions or colloids (plasma expanders), such as gelofusine.

However, in those with cardiac and respiratory disease much smaller losses may give rise to tissue hypoxia, as the oxygen-carrying capacity of blood is reduced. In these individuals red cell transfusion may be considered after smaller volume blood loss, in order to increase oxygen-carrying capacity and to prevent the onset of tissue ischaemia.

Until recently, it was commonplace to order a blood transfusion if the Hb fell below 10 g/dl. Recent literature reviews and trials have suggested that this practice is unnecessary. More recent guidelines and consensus statements reflect the view that:

- Hb >10 g/dl: no transfusion required
- Hb <7 g/dl: transfusion is required.

In the range Hb 7–10 g/dl the decision for transfusion will be based on clinical assessment, e.g. symptoms of heart failure and organ ischaemia. In those patients with known or suspected heart disease, respiratory disease, the elderly, and those with postoperative complications, which lead to an increase in oxygen demand, transfusion may be indicated when Hb is <8 g/dl.

In summary the decision to transfuse a patient should not be taken lightly, but once taken the appropriate components should be given in the correct quan-

TABLE 2.1i	Possible blood ordering
Routine tariff	**Operation**
6 units of blood	Emergency aortic surgery
4 units of blood	Elective aortic surgery abdomino-perineal resection, total cystectomy
2 units of blood	Gastrectomy, splenectomy, open renal surgery
Group and save (G + S)	Remaining general, and arterial cases

Fast facts—Blood transfusion ('giving blood')

Two major systems of blood typing:

- ABO and Rhesus system:
  —48% of patients are group O ('universal donor')
  —3% of patients are group AB ('universal recipient')
  —85% of patients are Rhesus positive

Donated blood is split into:

- red cell concentrate
- platelets, and
- FFP (contains clotting factors)
- platelets and FFP are required if coagulopathy occurs with significant blood loss

Transfuse patient if:

- fit patient and Hb <7 g/dl
- patient with ischaemic heart disease and Hb <8 g/dl
- do not transfuse patient if Hb >10 g/dl

Reactions to transfused blood:

- febrile reaction—commonest, due to reaction with either white cells or platelets in the blood
- allergic reactions due to allergen in donated blood—treat with antihistamines
- severe problems (unusual)—include anaphylaxis and acute haemolytic reaction

---

tities. Undertransfusion is just as dangerous as an unwarranted transfusion.

Nutrition

Scenario: preoperative chronic malnutrition

A 62-year-old man is admitted for further investigations of painless jaundice and weight loss of >10% of initial body weight. Initial blood tests reveal a bilirubin of 200 mmol/l (elevated), albumin of 25 g/l (reduced), and a normal C-reactive protein.

The low albumin in this patient reflects a degree of chronic malnutrition, and the patient also has significant weight loss (>10% of normal body weight) and anorexia. The patient has a normal functioning gut and will be helped by additional oral nutritional supplementation, e.g. three sachets of 'Build-up' will provide about 9 g nitrogen/day.

The patient then undergoes investigations (ultrasound scan/endoscopic retrograde cholangiopancreatography/CT scan of chest and abdomen), which reveal a 2 cm mass in the head of the pancreas, with no obvious metastases. The investigations point to a localized tumour of the head of the pancreas.

A tumour of the head of the pancreas is the cause of painless jaundice in this patient. Treatment requires excision with a hope of cure or bypassing the obstructing lesion to allow bile drainage to achieve palliation.

The patient undergoes a pancreaticoduodenectomy (called a Whipple's procedure). At the time of the operation, a small feeding catheter is placed in the proximal jejunum and brought out through the abdominal wall.

This catheter is called a feeding jejunostomy and is used to feed the patient postoperatively—in this case the patient is unable to take much fluid orally (because of the surgery required to the stomach and duodenum) but still has a functioning small bowel, which can be used to feed the patient in the initial postoperative state. Usually about 1500 ml/day of polymeric elemental feed is given.

If the patient did not get a feeding jejunostomy at the time of the operation, then a period of postoperative parenteral (i.e. through a vein) nutrition is normally required. This parenteral feeding would be anticipated

Clinical key points for surgical nutrition

- Patients who have lost >10% of their normal body weight will require nutritional support
- BMI (body mass index) is a useful parameter to measure (weight in kg/height in m^2): a patient with a BMI of <20 is underweight and may have malnutrition
- There are three ways to provide nutritional support for patients:
  —*oral* (via the mouth: best way if possible)
  —*enteral* (via a tube in the stomach/jejunum: if unable to take food orally)
  —*parenteral* (via a venous catheter: if unable to take food by the oral or enteral route)
- Patients on TPN need close monitoring of blood electrolytes, LFT, and trace elements

to last less than 4 weeks and so would be given through a peripherally inserted central catheter (PICC) line. Usually 1500–2000 ml of total parenteral nutrition (TPN) are given in this way.

Background: surgical nutrition

Nutrition is an important aspect of surgery. Poor nutrition can lead to significant surgical problems, such as:

- impaired immunity
- delayed wound healing
- reduced muscle strength, leading to decreased respiratory movements and postoperative pneumonia.

Nutritional problems in surgical patients can occur preoperatively, postoperatively, and in certain surgical conditions.

Preoperative

- immobilized patients
- patients with a chronic inflammatory or infective illness
- patients with malignancy.

Patients with loss of 10% of their normal body weight will potentially have nutritional problems that need to be addressed.

Specific surgical conditions

Some conditions can make the patient significantly catabolic:

- pancreatitis
- severe trauma
- burns
- enterocutaneous fistula
- severe inflammatory bowel disease.

In addition, patients in intensive care with prolonged need for tracheal intubation (who are therefore unable to eat) will also require nutritional support.

Postoperative

- patients with prolonged ileus
- intra-abdominal sepsis
- colonic anastomotic dehiscence.

These problems will cause the patient to have a non-functioning gut and they will require nutritional support.

Patients undergoing major surgery (e.g. pancreatectomy, oesophagectomy) may require nutritional support, usually due to a prolonged ileus.

Assessment of nutritional status

There are various methods to assess nutritional status:

Weigh the patient

The easiest method is to weigh the patient and calculate the body mass index (BMI)

$$BMI = weight (kg)/height (m)^2$$

A BMI of 20–25 is ideal: a patient whose BMI is <20 is underweight and chronic malnutrition may be present.

Blood tests

Certain blood 'markers' can be checked that may be reduced if the patient is malnourished.

The commonest measured is serum albumin. However, the half life of albumin is 21 days; i.e. the patient must be malnourished for at least 3 weeks before the serum albumin drops due to a nutritional problem. Low albumin levels seen in the immediate postoperative period are in the main due to dilutional reasons caused by giving IV crystalloids (i.e. normal saline, 5% dextrose).

Other proteins, such as pre-albumin, and transferrin can be useful to measure, due to a shorter half life than albumin.

(Care must be taken in interpreting reduced plasma proteins as they can also be reduced if there is significant ongoing inflammation—in these instances it is useful to measure the C-reactive protein and if this is significantly raised, then measuring the plasma proteins as an index of malnutrition is unreliable.)

Anthropometric measurements

This involves indirectly measuring body fat stores by looking at, for example, the thickness of the skin-fold over the triceps (triceps skin-fold thickness): this method is not commonly used in surgical patients.

Nutrition requirements

Nutrition in normal circumstances consists of carbohydrate, fat, and protein (sometimes called macronutrients), vitamins and trace elements (sometimes called micronutrients), water, and electrolytes.

A patient's energy supply comes from carbohydrate, fat, and protein. A normal energy requirement is 25–35 kcal/kg per day (2100 kcal/day for a 70 kg man). Of this total energy intake, 50% should be supplied by carbohydrate, 20% by protein, and 30% by fat:

- 1 g of carbohydrate and protein will each give 4 kcal of energy
- 1 g of fat gives a lot more: roughly 9 kcal of energy.

Periods of fasting and starvation are common in surgical patients, as they can be fasted for investigations or operations.

In the first 24–36 hours of a fast, carbohydrates are used up first, as they are the most readily available store of energy: glycogen stores in the body (mostly in the liver and skeletal muscle) are broken down to glucose (a process called glycogenolysis).

After that initial period, fat stores are used (lipolysis) and protein is broken down to make glucose (gluconeogenesis).

The amount of protein required per day is usually expressed in terms of grams of nitrogen (as amino acids are broken down into nitrogen).

$$1 \text{ g } N_2 \text{ is equivalent to } 6.25 \text{ g protein}$$

A normal diet will consist of about 9 g N_2, but the body requirements can be markedly increased postoperatively, or when there is significant catabolism.

Methods of nutritional support

The method by which the patient is given nutrition is dependent on the state of the patient and the gastrointestinal tract. The following algorithm demonstrates how different routes might be used in different circumstances:

- **Oral.** If the patient is able to swallow and has a normal functioning gastrointestinal tract, the patient should be fed orally.

- **Enteral.** If the patient is unable to swallow sufficient nutrition, but has a normal gastrointestinal tract, then enteral feeding is used.

- **Parenteral.** If the patient has a non-functioning gastrointestinal tract (e.g. ileus or upper small bowel fistula), then a parenteral route is required.

Oral

If the patient is able to swallow and has a normal gastrointestinal tract, then additional nutritional supplements can be given to the patient, e.g. 'Build-up': three sachets per day can provide up to 9 g nitrogen a day.

Enteral

Methods of delivering enteral feeding include a fine bore tube via the nose into either the stomach (a nasogastric tube) or the jejunum (a nasojejunal tube).

If enteral feeding is required for a longer period (e.g. 4+ weeks), then a tube can be placed directly into the stomach (most commonly a PEG tube: percutaneous endoscopic gastrostomy) or a jejunostomy, which can be placed at the time of a major operation, which would be anticipated to require longer-term assisted feeding (such as pancreatectomy or oesophagectomy).

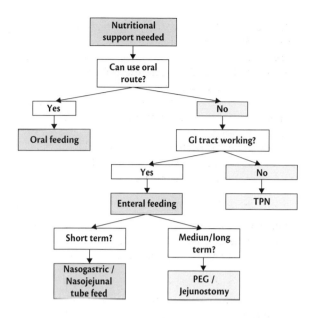

Enteral feeding can be provided as either:

- polymeric diets (with long chains of peptides), or
- elemental (when the peptides provided are shorter and easier to absorb: this can be necessary in certain surgical conditions, such as Crohn's disease).

The advantages of enteral feeding include improved gut immunity, decreased mucosal atrophy, it is cheaper than using the parenteral route and does not have the same spectrum of complications. Early enteral feeding can also be important in the postoperative patient, as it reduces the duration of postoperative ileus.

> **WHEN POSSIBLE USE THE GASTROINTESTINAL TRACT**

Parenteral (total parenteral nutrition)

Parenteral nutrition is the administration of nutrients via a vein. This is usually done by either a peripherally placed long line (called a **PICC** line: **P**eripherally **I**nserted **C**entral **C**atheter) or by a centrally placed catheter (usually by placing the catheter into the internal jugular or subclavian vein).

Giving feed by a short peripheral drip into the arm can only be used for a short period (24–48 hours), as the solution is hyperosmolar and can cause thrombo-

phlebitis. Remember that a feeding line should only be used for that purpose and drugs, and blood products should be given via a separate peripheral line.

A bag of TPN (usually given over 24 hours) generally consists of:

- 9–14 g N_2
- 2.5 litres fluid
- 500 ml 20% lipids
- electrolytes such as $Na/K/Ca/Mg/PO_4/Zn$
- trace elements
- water and fat soluble vitamins.

Remember that the TPN bag is essentially to provide the patient with food and vitamins. Some of the patients will, in addition, require a peripheral drip to give IV antibiotics or additional crystalloids, if they are dehydrated or have a significant fluid loss, such as a gastrointestinal fistula.

- **Monitoring a patient on TPN**. Patients receiving TPN must be monitored carefully to avoid electrolyte and fluid imbalance. In addition to weighing the patient every week, the patient must undergo regular blood monitoring:
  - daily bloods for U&Es/glucose/calcium/magnesium/phosphate
  - twice weekly LFTs/FBC/zinc
  - monthly copper, selenium (trace elements)
- **Complications**. Patients on TPN may develop complications, which may be related to either the line or the nutrients in the TPN bag.
  - Complications related to the line include problems such as *pneumothorax* or *haemothorax* in placing a central line or more significantly *line sepsis* (infections caused by having a central line) can be a problem in established lines. Consideration should be given to exchanging the central line over a guide wire for a new line every 7–14 days to reduce the chance of line sepsis.
  - Complications related to the actual TPN include deranged LFTs, electrolyte imbalance, and problems with control of the blood glucose. Hence the need to closely monitor electrolytes and glucose in patients on TPN.

Fast facts—Surgical nutrition ('feeding the surgical patient')

Normal requirements

- 25–35 kcal/kg/day of energy, plus vitamins, electrolytes, water, trace elements
- Energy is provided by 50% carbohydrate, 20% protein, 30% fat

Identify: patients at risk

- Preoperatively: >10% body weight loss. Patients with anorexia/cachexia/malignancy
- Certain conditions, e.g. gastrointestinal fistula, severely catabolic, burns patients, pancreatitis
- Postoperatively: prolonged ileus, gastrointestinal complications (e.g. anastomotic dehiscence)

Quantify

- Weigh the patient and compare with normal weight
- BMI (if <20 may have nutritional problems)
- Measure protein levels, e.g. albumin, pre-albumin, and transferrin

Management

- Nutritional support can be by the oral, enteral, or parenteral (venous) route
- Oral is the preferred route if patient able to swallow and gut functioning
- TPN required if gut not functioning
- Patients on TPN require close monitoring

Complications of total parenteral nutrition

- Line related: pneumothorax, haemothorax, line sepsis
- Feed related: deranged LFTs, electrolyte imbalance, hyperglycaemia

Postoperative problems

Chapter contents

ABC, Patient assessment and resuscitation 158

Scenario: postoperative collapse 158

Background: patient resuscitation 159

Assessment of the critically ill surgical patient 164

Scenario: postoperative recovery 164

Background: postoperative patient assessment 165

Postoperative complications: hypoxia 167

Scenario: hypoxia following an emergency laparotomy 167

Background: hypoxia 168

Postoperative complications: hypotension and cardiac ischaemia 173

Scenario 1: postoperative hypotension and ECG changes 173

Scenario 2: postoperative hypotension with a tachyarrhythmia 174

Background: postoperative hypotension 175

Postoperative complications: oliguria and electrolyte disturbance 179

Scenario: low urine output following an emergency laparotomy 179

Background: postoperative oliguria 181

Postoperative sepsis 184

Scenario 1: postoperative pyrexia and hypotension 184

Scenario 2: pyrexia, tachypnoea, and tachycardia 185

Background: postoperative sepsis 185

Deep vein thrombosis and pulmonary embolism 189

Scenario 1: postoperative painful swollen calf 189

Scenario 2 190

Background: deep vein thrombosis and pulmonary embolism 191

ABC, Patient assessment and resuscitation

Scenario: postoperative collapse

> The nursing staff call you urgently because a post-operative patient has 'collapsed'.

It is important for **medical staff to always listen and respond to the concerns of the nursing staff.** Surgical nurses have a wealth of experience that must never be dismissed. Delay in responding will rarely be in the patient's interests.

> The patient is tachypnoeic (24/min).

The patient appears to have an unobstructed airway and is breathing normally but rapidly. The first action must be to safeguard the patient's airways and breathing. In this case both are secure but **ill patients need oxygen** so high flow oxygen is given while resuscitation and assessment take place.

> He is barely conscious. The pulse is 110/min with a BP 85/40. The finger tip capillary refill time is very prolonged.

Tachycardia, hypotension, and coma indicate the patient has all the signs of shock (cause unknown as yet). The capillary refill time should be <2 seconds (the time taken to say 'capillary refill'). A prolonged refill time indicates poor peripheral perfusion, which reflects poor renal and brain perfusion.

> Examination of his urine output shows this to have been tailing off for about 3 hours and is now 20 ml/hour.

The **kidneys are the body's 'on-board' cardiac output monitor.** As the cardiac output drops kidney perfusion decreases and urine output falls. Higher brain function fails as cardiac output drops to low levels and the patient becomes increasingly disorientated, agitated, or comatose.

If cardiac output falls to very low levels, myocardial and cerebral ischaemia results and cardiac or respiratory arrest occurs.

> The patient is given 500 ml IV fluid (saline or gelofusine) over 15–30 min.

In hypovolaemia rapid fluid replacement is required. **The patient requires wide bore IV access.** The nature of the fluid is not important, but normal saline or gelofusine (a synthetic colloid) are preferred as they stay in the extracellular space (interstitial fluid/plasma volume).

The patient's pulse, BP, and urine output are monitored for improvement. The patient's Hb is checked and if it is 8 g/dl or less then blood should be given. This is particularly important in patients with a past history of myocardial infarction and presumed borderline myocardial ischaemia.

> The patient initially improves with reducing pulse, rising BP, and increasing urine output. However, the improvement stops and the BP once again falls. His Hb comes back as 6.1 g/dl, compared with a pre-operative value of 14 g/dl.

The further reduction in BP coupled with a very low Hb is a sign of probable bleeding. Resuscitation is required and will temporarily hold matters: stopping the bleeding is what is urgently needed. As it seems likely that the patient is bleeding, blood is required. The patient is given 2 units of blood over 1 hour.

> The patient is 6 hours post-left hemicolectomy. He is 69 years old with a past history of a myocardial infarction. The operation note shows nothing untoward.

It is vital that some knowledge of the operation is gained, either from the operative record or by consulting someone at the operation. An operative record consists of a surgical and anaesthetic record.

> The anaesthetic record shows the patient remained stable throughout the operation with no falls in BP or ECG changes. The patient received 2 litres of fluids during the operation and the blood loss record was 200 ml.

The anaesthetic notes will contain the intraoperative fluid chart. The notes indicate a straightforward operation.

> Examination shows the abdomen to be distended and tense.

The combination of shock (in this case probably hypovolaemic), an unexpectedly very low Hb, an abdominal operation, and a postoperatively tense distended

Clinical key points in shock management

- Always listen and respond to the concerns of the nursing staff

- Ill patients need oxygen. Give high flow O_2 through a Hudson mask with a reservoir bag

- Tachycardia, hypotension, and coma indicate that the patient is in shock

- The brain and kidneys are the body's 'on-board' cardiac output monitor. Increasing confusion or decreasing conscious level with falling urine output indicates organ dysfunction

- Establish IV access (wide bore cannula)

- In hypovolaemia rapid fluid replacement is required (500 ml bolus(es) of IV fluids)

- Monitor pulse rate, BP, and urinary output for signs of improvement. Early use of central venous pressure (CVP) monitoring should be considered, especially in the elderly

- Deal with the underlying cause

abdomen add up to intra-abdominal bleeding. **Deal with the underlying cause**—the patient will need to go back to theatre for an urgent laparotomy.

Background: patient resuscitation

It is important to have a well-practised method of assessment when faced with any emergency situation.

By following a simple plan, immediate life-threatening problems are identified and managed as they become apparent.

The approach takes causes of imminent death and deals with them in the speed in which they will kill:

Follow the letters of the alphabet, ABC

A Airway control with care of the cervical spine

B Breathing with the provision of adequate ventilation and oxygenation

C Circulation including haemorrhage control

D Disability of the central nervous system

E Exposure to make sure nothing has been missed

In other words—find out what is killing the patient at the moment and stop it by following a planned approach treating the potential causes in the right order.

Remember the need to **check and recheck** the patient and if problems are experienced always restart at Airway.

Remember ABC

This approach is appropriate no matter the circumstances—trauma, cardiac arrest, or postoperative complications.

Identify and quantify

A Airways (in trauma with care of the cervical spine)

An obstructed airway is the quickest way to death.

- **Is the airway clear?**

  - *Look at the patient*—are they able to speak? If the patient is unconscious, look in the airway.

    If the airway is compromised, it must be cleared of debris/vomit using fingers and suction, and the upper airway improved by the use of the **chin lift or jaw thrust method**. Only after these methods have been tried and the airway is still obstructed will other methods be used (see later). **Once an airway is opened and secured it must be maintained**.

    In the trauma situation the stability of the cervical spine is unknown; airway protection must be done initially without moving the neck. However, if it is not possible to open the airway without some movement of the cervical spine then the airway assumes the greater priority.

    In the patient with a surgical illness or postoperative problem the status of the cervical spine is highly likely to be known. Cervical spine instability may, however, still be an issue (i.e. rheumatoid arthritis) so **never assume the cervical spine is stable—ask.**

B Breathing (with additional oxygen)

Ill patients need oxygen—GIVE OXYGEN

Hypoxia is life threatening and the patient's ventilation is the next priority.

- **Is the breathing adequate?**

  - *Look at the patient*. Are they able to speak, are the accessory muscles of respiration being used, what is the respiratory rate? The respiratory rate is counted. The **normal respiratory rate should be between 12 and 18 breaths/min**. If the rate is <9 or >28 assisted ventilation may be necessary. If ventilation is absent or inadequate then manual ventilation with bag-and-mask is needed.

- *Examine the chest.* The position of the trachea should be established early on (deviation from the midline indicating a shift in the mediastinum possibly due to lung collapse or tension pneumothorax). Chest movement should be assessed, looking to ensure that it is equal on both sides.

C Circulation (with control of haemorrhage)

This part of the primary survey establishes whether there is an adequate cardiac output and an adequate blood volume to provide tissue perfusion.

Initially the pulse rate and capillary refill time (normal <2 seconds) are assessed. In the assessment of a shocked patient the presence of:

- a femoral pulse indicates a systolic pressure of >70 mmHg

- a radial pulse indicates a systolic pressure of >80 mmHg.

Signs of developing hypovolaemic shock such as sweating, confusion, and restlessness should be noted. Signs of external haemorrhage should be looked for rapidly and controlled by external pressure and the BP should be measured. Monitoring urine output is a vital part of the ongoing assessment of the hypotensive patient.

D Disability (of the central nervous system)

The objective here is to provide a rapid baseline for future comparison and in the initial primary survey it is perhaps best done using the AVPU system. This stands for:

A	alert
V	responds to verbal stimulus
P	responds to painful stimulus
U	unresponsive

E Exposure (to make sure nothing has been missed)

At this stage of the assessment it is important not to ignore **E** for exposure. It is important that the unexpected has not been missed. It is important to check to see that clothing, dressings, or the surface the patient is on may not be absorbing or masking any signs of severe external haemorrhage.

Resuscitation

Resuscitation should be proceeding as the primary survey identifies the problems but the two principal areas of concern are the management of **hypoxia** and the management of **hypovolaemia**.

If airway obstruction was identified this should have been relieved, and ventilatory support given as required. Patients who have suffered any significant medical, surgical, or traumatic event require oxygen. **Ill patients need oxygen.**

If there is any failure in the cardiovascular system this should have been corrected. At this stage, large-bore IV access should be obtained.

Secondary survey

The secondary survey is a full assessment of the patient.

During the secondary survey not only should the precise details of any surgery or illness be ascertained but also previous medical details of the patient should also be obtained. These should include details of:

- previous medical history

- drug history

- the nature of any recent operation and any intra-operative events.

The patient should be systematically and thoroughly examined. After a full clinical examination other forms of investigation should be used, e.g. pulse oximetry and ECG. Finally, if not already present, a urinary **catheter** may be passed.

Further investigations should now be considered, bloods taken as appropriate and possible radiological (e.g. CT) investigations carried out.

Monitoring and reporting

Having completed the primary and secondary surveys it is important to continually re-evaluate and monitor the patient's vital signs, their general *condition, and most importantly the response to any treatment.*

Management of airways

Management of the airway in any emergency situation is of paramount importance. To forget the airway or be drawn to other issues and not maintain the airway means that ventilation and tissue oxygenation will fail, carbon dioxide retention will occur, and the patient will probably die.

Hypoxia kills—and kills quickly

Manual methods

In the unconscious patient the most common cause of obstruction is the tongue. As the tongue is attached to the lower jaw, forward movement of the jaw will relieve the obstruction. This can be achieved by either the chin lift or the jaw thrust manoeuvre. **In a case of**

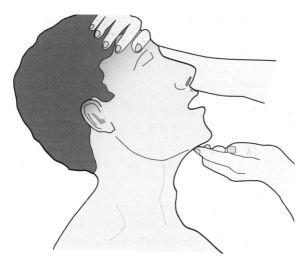

Fig 2.2a Chin lift.

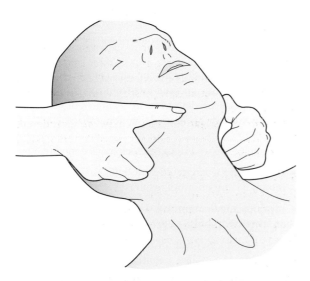

Fig 2.2b Jaw thrust.

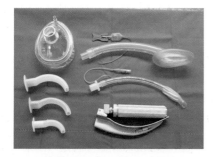

Fig 2.2c Masks and airways (clockwise: laryngeal mask, endotracheal tube, laryngoscope, Guedel airways, and face mask).

trauma these manoeuvres must be performed while maintaining in-line cervical spine stabilization.

- *Chin lift* (Fig. 2.2a). This simple manoeuvre lifts the tongue away from the posterior pharyngeal wall. In adults the jaw can be gripped firmly but in children great care must be taken because pressure on the soft tissues may occlude the airway further.

- *Jaw thrust* (Fig. 2.2b). By applying force behind the angle of the jaw on both sides the whole jaw can be lifted forward. This manoeuvre is of great importance in cases of trauma.

Mechanical devices (Fig. 2.2c)

Having opened the airway it is important to maintain that airway. It is here that mechanical methods can be helpful. These include:

- *Masks*. Masks should be clear so the mouth can be seen to ensure that vomiting will be noticed. The mask should form a complete seal on the patient's face.

- *Laerdal pocket mask*. This comes as a clear mask in a small case. The mask should be placed over the lower jaw and then lowered over the patient's mouth and nose. There is a one-way valve to prevent contamination of the rescuer.

- *Guedel airway*. The Guedel airway improves airway patency, but requires jaw support. It may cause oropharyngeal stimulation with coughing and vomiting unless the patient is deeply unconscious.

- *Laryngeal mask airway*. The mask is passed over the tongue and then pushed down in one movement into the hypopharynx. Correct positioning is accompanied by a slight bulging of the soft tissues in the front of the neck. The cuff is then inflated to form a seal (although this does not protect the trachea from gastric contents should the patient regurgitate).

- *Endotracheal tube*. Passing an endotracheal tube and inflating the cuff protects the airway. This is a skill that has to be practised regularly. If you have not passed an endotracheal tube before, do not attempt it, as failed attempts only add to the length of the patient's hypoxia. Most patients will be well oxygenated with a Guedel airway and high flow oxygen till senior help arrives.

Remember that in the emergency situation, it is **very rarely necessary to control the oxygen concentration**; in fact most times the **highest concentration possible is needed**. A closely fitting mask with a reservoir bag and high oxygen flow will produce inspired oxygen concentrations of about 90%.

Suction is also very important in maintaining a clear airway. Blood, vomit, and secretions may pool in the posterior pharynx and, although positioning of the patient may help, sucking these obstructions clear may be life saving. As this can interfere with breathing, suction should be performed in short bursts lasting no more than the time the operator can hold their breath.

Management of shock

Definition

Shock is a clinical state leading to **inadequate tissue oxygenation**, which causes impairment of cellular function.

Causes

Shock can arise from a variety of causes. The terminology usually reflects the underlying pathological change.

TABLE 2.2a The causes of shock

Hypovolaemic shock	due to reduced circulating blood volume
Cardiogenic shock	due to failure of the heart
Septic shock	due to circulating organisms or their toxins causing vasodilatation and myocardial dysfunction
Anaphylactic shock	due to an acute severe allergic reaction
Neurogenic shock	due to changes in the autonomic nervous system causing reduced pre-load due to pooling of blood

Hypovolaemic and cardiogenic shock are the commonest seen postoperatively.

Signs and symptoms

The signs of **hypovolaemic** shock are:

- hypotension (due to low circulating volume)
- tachycardia (due to trying to raise the cardiac output by increasing the heart rate)
- tachypnoea (increasing arterial oxygenation to compensate for lower delivery)
- peripheral vasoconstriction resulting in pallor and prolonged capillary refill time (shutdown of less vital circulatory beds)
- sweating (due to increased sympathetic tone)
- altered consciousness (due to underperfusion of the brain).

The human body, particularly younger patients, will compensate considerably before suddenly collapsing as all the systems fail due to increasing hypoxia and acidosis. The above signs, therefore, indicate the presence of established shock, and if not corrected will lead to death.

The aim is to **prevent these signs developing** and if they are present to aggressively resuscitate the patient.

If not corrected early, the pathological processes of multiple organ failure, diffuse intravascular coagulation, and acute respiratory distress syndrome can start and rapidly cascade.

Hypovolaemic shock

Hypovolaemic shock may be due either to haemorrhage, or significant fluid loss from the gastrointestinal tract (such as diarrhoea or a large output small bowel fistula); or an increase in generalized capillary permeability (sepsis).

The symptoms and signs of shock may be modified by:

- the patient's age (e.g. older patients may be unable to mount a compensatory response)
- previous medication (e.g. beta-blockade preventing an increase in pulse rate)
- pre-existing medical problems (e.g. hypertension resulting in a false negative normal BP, an implanted pacemaker preventing the normal response mechanisms).

TABLE 2.2b Clinical signs of hypovolaemic shock according to blood loss in an otherwise healthy patient

Volume—ml (% blood volume)	<750 (<15)	800–1500 (15–30)	1500–2000 (30–40)	>2000 (>40)
Pulse rate (/min)	<100	100–120	>120	>140
BP	Systolic Very low	Unchanged	Unchanged	Reduced
	Diastolic Very low	Unchanged	Raised (due to compensatory vasoconstriction)	Reduced
Capillary refill time	Normal	>2 seconds	>2 seconds	Absent
Respiratory rate	Normal	Normal	Tachypnoea	Tachypnoea

Management of hypovolaemic shock.

The objective of the management of hypovolaemic shock is to maintain tissue oxygenation and to restore it to near normal values. This entails applying the basic principles of resuscitation following the established ABC guidelines. **Patients with hypovolaemia should have a clear airway and have adequate ventilation with high flow oxygen.**

Circulatory control should begin by controlling any forms of external blood loss by direct pressure. Venous access should occur early with the largest cannula possible.

If the patient is hypotensive, IV fluids should be run wide open with a rapid re-evaluation after 500 ml of crystalloid. A cause should be identified.

Continual patient monitoring is essential, measuring pulse rate, BP, respiratory rate, capillary refill, urine output, and CVP.

For all hypotensive patients, if after 2 litres of crystalloid have been infused, the patient is still hypotensive, and if blood loss is the suspected cause, use warm blood transfusions. Other indications for blood transfusion would be obvious major blood loss (e.g. >700 ml immediately from a chest drain, multiple long bone or pelvic fractures, and finally heavily blood-soaked clothing and dressings.

Cardiogenic shock

This most commonly occurs after a myocardial infarction. Ischaemia leads to myocardial depression, pump failure, and therefore a reduced cardiac output.

Established cardiogenic shock has a very poor outcome. Treatment consists of oxygen, treatment of any cardiac arrhythmia, and possible use of inotropes to improve myocardial performance.

In patients with unexplained postoperative hypotension or tachyarrhythmia, consider myocardial infarct as the possible cause and check the patient's troponin-T (at least 6 hours after the onset of symptoms, to allow a rise in the troponin-T). **The commonest cause of an unexplained postoperative tachyarrhythmia is a myocardial infarct.**

Septic shock

Septic shock is caused by the release of bacterial toxins. There is a release of vasoactive inflammatory mediators such as kinins, which produce an increase in capillary permeability and a fall in peripheral resistance, although cardiac output may initially rise.

There may be fever associated with hypotension and the treatment includes oxygen, circulatory support and rapid admission to hospital where inotropes may be given. The pathogenesis of systemic inflammatory response syndrome (SIRS) is discussed later.

Anaphylactic shock

A profound allergic reaction can follow exposure to a foreign protein or drug. This is an acute medical emergency that requires aggressive management. Clinically, in addition to hypotension, caused by peripheral vasodilatation, the patient may have signs of bronchospasm and laryngeal oedema.

Oxygen and IV fluids are given in the first instance. **IV adrenaline (epinephrine) is given** to treat bronchospasm, vasodilatation, and to prevent further release of mediators of anaphylaxis. Later management includes the use of an antihistamine (e.g. chlorpheniramine) and steroids.

Fast facts—Resuscitation

Remember ABC

Airway with cervical spine control

Breathing with additional oxygen

Circulation with haemorrhage control

Disability: neurological evaluation

Exposure: to make sure nothing is missed

Airways

◆ **Hypoxia kills**

◆ Securing and maintaining an airway is the most important task

◆ Use simple methods first

◆ The manoeuvres used in airway management require repeated practice

Breathing

◆ **Ill patients need oxygen**

◆ Too rapid or too slow is almost as bad as not at all

◆ If the patient does not need ventilatory support (bagging) they will not tolerate it

Circulation

◆ **Hypovolaemia is the commonest cause of postoperative shock**

◆ Management of shock requires:

—the replacement of fluid losses

—adequate IV access for the task

—frequent assessment to ensure improvement

—control of haemorrhage (external and internal)

Neurogenic shock

Neurogenic shock may occur in head injuries or spinal cord damage. It is due to the interruption of the thoracolumbar sympathetic outflow, which causes a loss of sympathetic tone, resulting in arteriolar and venous dilatation. Sympathetic drive to the heart may also be lost, resulting in bradycardia and the normal response to blood loss. Beware as there may be associated hypovolaemic shock due to other injury.

Summary

In summary, to reduce the devastating effects of shock, think of the possibility, treat early, and resuscitate aggressively and appropriately. Then not only will the consequences of shock be prevented but also the problems of the acute respiratory distress syndrome (lung tissue damage) and multiple organ failure.

Assessment of the critically ill surgical patient

Scenario: postoperative recovery

> A 70-year-old man has had an inguinal hernia repair performed under spinal anaesthesia earlier in the day. The recovery nurse is concerned that his BP (currently 90/60 mmHg) is lower than preoperative values.

Low BP is a relatively common occurrence after anaesthesia and surgery. It may be due to the residual effects of anaesthetic drugs, but it may have more serious causes. If untreated, hypotension may progress to a level where organ perfusion and tissue oxygenation is inadequate—shock. **The first issue is to identify the ill patient; this can on most occasions be anticipated by what has gone before.**

> On examination the patient is receiving oxygen by face mask and appears to be pink and well oxygenated. He is alert and oriented and not complaining of any pain. His oxygen saturation is 98% and his respiratory rate is 16 breaths/min. His peripheries are warm and well perfused and there is no sign of any bleeding around his wound.

Initial management of the hypotensive patient involves checking the **A**irway (he is talking), **B**reathing (he is talking and his respiratory rate is 16/min), and **C**irculation. This may give a clue to the cause of the hypotension and also its severity. **All patients who are hypotensive must receive oxygen,** while further examination is made.

> The ECG shows his heart rhythm to be regular with no tachycardia or bradycardia.

Although acute changes are sometimes not seen on an immediate ECG, it is important to rule out a postoperative cardiac cause (check troponin-T levels at least 6 hours after the event if you are considering a myocardial infarct as the cause). **Differential diagnoses should be positively excluded.**

In many patients a minor degree of hypotension is well tolerated (no impact on cerebral, myocardial, or renal function) and apart from ensuring oxygen is being administered by facemask, no further treatment is required. If the degree of hypotension is more severe or the patient is elderly or has cardiac disease, treatment will be required.

> In this case the patient is well apart from a low BP with no signs of impending circulatory failure. Having ruled out the more sinister causes of hypotension, it is likely that in this case it is due to the residual effects of the anaesthetic he received.

Spinal and epidural anaesthesia cause a block of the sympathetic vasoconstrictor nerves, leading to vasodilatation and venous pooling of blood. The treatment of hypotension due to central neural blockade includes

---

Clinical key points in the assessment of the ill patient

- First identify the ill patient; this can usually be anticipated by what has gone before. The high-risk patient can be identified because of the nature of the surgery or past medical history

- A past history of myocardial infarction and chronic obstructive pulmonary disease places the patient at risk of both cardiac and respiratory complications following major surgery

- A postoperative patient should be getting better not worse

- Ill patients must receive oxygen

- Take a careful history, perform a thorough examination and investigate based on the likely diagnosis

- A positive diagnosis must be made based on the history and circumstances

administering oxygen and elevating the legs to improve venous return and occasionally using vasopressor drugs (usually ephedrine) in order to improve cardiac output and to produce vasoconstriction.

Background: postoperative patient assessment

The initial recognition, investigation, and treatment of a critically ill surgical patient must be performed rapidly and accurately.

The following provides a framework to aid in recognition that something is wrong with these patients. It is also a guide to their early investigation and management.

There are three stages to the management of the critically ill surgical patient; **the IQM principle**:

* identify
* quantify
* manage.

Identify

Early identification is of paramount importance. The identification of a deteriorating patient can be very difficult. Careful preoperative assessment, knowledge of the patient, documentation of any events (e.g. operation note, anaesthetic record, and any assessment) along with a recorded routine assessment of the postoperative patient, together help to create a safe environment for patient care.

Two factors can help in early identification:

1. The first is the concept of a '**patient at risk**'. This is another way of saying that certain preoperative, operative, and postoperative issues put the patient at high risk of complications.

   The 'at-risk' patient must be actively managed with frequent documented assessments searching for postoperative problems, rather than waiting for them to become clinically apparent.

   (a) *General medical condition*—medical conditions that can predispose the patient to complications, e.g.

   * chronic respiratory disease—prone to postoperative respiratory sepsis
   * ischaemic heart disease—prone to peri/postoperative myocardial ischaemia/infarction
   * diabetes—prone to peri/postoperative hypo/hyperglycaemia and infection.

   (b) *Surgical pathology*. Whether the patient is an emergency or elective case is also important to the risk profile. Emergency patients will have had less preoperative work-up, and are usually sicker. Patients who have undergone emergency surgery will automatically be 'at risk'.

   Knowledge of the nature of an operation is important. For example, gastrointestinal anastomoses may leak (usually after 5–7 days), producing localized and then generalized sepsis. Routine repeated abdominal examination may reveal a situation which is either not improving or deteriorating, indicating all is not well. Early radiological examination (contrast studies) could then outline an anastomotic 'leak', which should be dealt with before generalized sepsis and patient deterioration has occurred.

   (c) *Intraoperative surgical difficulties*. Concerns about intraoperative events should place the patient in a higher 'at-risk' group. Gut viability and intraoperative bleeding would be issues that would result in a 'closer' eye being kept on the patient.

   (d) *Recent postoperative events*. Patients who have experienced a postoperative event (e.g. angina, myocardial infarction, respiratory tract infection, or operation site complication), are clearly at risk of a repeat event.

2. The second factor is the use of aids as identification of deteriorating patients can be difficult.

   (a) 'Early warning scores' bring together physiological criteria recorded by the nursing staff. Table 2.2c shows one such chart. As can be seen

TABLE 2.2c Early Warning Scoring System (EWSS) physiological score. The patient is scored from all five groups: a total score of 3 or greater triggers referral for more senior input

Score	3	2	1	0	1	2	3
Heart rate		<41	41–50	51–100	101–100	111–130	>130
Systolic BP	<71	71–80	81–100	101–200		>200	
Respiratory rate		<9		9–14	15–20	21–29	>29
Temperature		<35.1		35.1–38.4		>38.4	
Response to stimulus				Awake	Verbal	Pain	Unresponsive

different combinations of recordings can trigger concern. Allied to this should be a protocol that maps the process when the 'trigger point' is crossed.

(b) Following an operation, patients receiving appropriate care should get better. A postoperative patient who does not show a noticeable improvement in their general condition may be developing complications. This may be that:

- the wrong diagnosis/treatment had been given
- the treatment has been inadequate
- a complication/new event is acting against the expected improvement.

After treatment and with appropriate care, the signs of illness should diminish and parameters improve:

- heart rate returning to normal
- good urine output
- tachypnoea and/or oxygen saturation should improve
- pyrexia should settle
- white cell counts should come down.

Any deviation from the expected patient pathway should provoke a search for the cause of this failure to improve.

Quantify
Patient history

It is essential to review the patient as a whole and not just the recent operation site. The history of the presenting illness often gives valuable clues as to why the patient is now ill.

- Surgical pathology
  - pancreatitis
  - sepsis
  - anastomotic leak
  - peritonitis
  - advanced malignancy
- Surgical difficulties
  - inoperable neoplasm
  - difficult anastomosis
- Recent postoperative events
  - pneumonia
  - myocardial infarction.

The patient must be considered as a whole and their pre-existing state of health, their drug therapy, their nutritional state, and their age be reviewed.

- Underlying health
  - diabetes
  - pulmonary disease
  - ischaemic heart disease
- Drug history
  - steroids, NSAIDs, angiotensin-converting enzyme inhibitors
- Poor nutrition
  - enteral feed
  - total parenteral nutrition
- Age and general well-being
  - very old
  - obese/cachectic.

Clinical examination

Valuable clinical information can be gained from the end of the bed, just by observing and listening to the patient. As with any examination of a compromised patient, following the ABCs helps ensure a thorough assessment of the patient.

1. Is the **Airway** clear?
   - check for evidence of aspiration or foreign bodies such as dentures
   - has the patient had recent neck surgery or insertion of necklines?
   - is the patient able to cough and clear his secretions alone or with the aid of physiotherapy?

2. Is the **Breathing** adequate?
   - observe the respiratory rate/pattern, both sides of the chest expanding symmetrically
   - is there evidence of a pneumothorax?
   - is the patient cyanosed?

3. Is the **Circulation** adequate?
   - what is the heart rate and rhythm?
   - what is the patient's BP in relation to their normal/preoperative level?
   - what is the peripheral perfusion like; is the patient shocked?
   - is the urine output adequate?

4. Can the patient's **Diagnosis** provide any clues?

Further investigations are required as indicated: e.g. those for the investigation of myocardial damage, sepsis, renal failure, etc.

Management

The initial management and resuscitation should be commenced along with assessment of the patient:

- administer oxygen if the patient is not already receiving it. If the patient remains cyanosed increase the inspired concentration (CO_2 retention is rarely a problem). Check SpO_2 (oxygen saturation), arterial blood gases, and do a CXR
- administer fluids if required. Place a urinary catheter and measure hourly urine output. Give a fluid challenge of e.g. 200 ml 0.9% saline, and assess response by changes in heart rate, BP, CVP, and urine output. Repeat this as necessary
- if cardiac failure is suspected, consider giving a diuretic, e.g. frusemide
- take blood for assessment of FBC, U&Es, and cardiac enzymes if indicated
- send appropriate cultures if sepsis is suspected and commence best guess antibiotics.

ICU or HDU transfer (this requires senior input) may be indicated by:

- respiratory failure requiring ventilation, either inadequate oxygenation (PO_2 <6 kPa with an FiO_2 1.0 on a non-rebreathing mask) or rising $PaCO_2$ (>8 kPa, pH <7.3)
- the need for advanced cardiovascular monitoring, e.g. pulmonary artery flotation catheter, oesophageal Doppler monitoring, and inotropic support
- fluid and electrolyte abnormalities requiring close observation
- the need for renal replacement therapy (dialysis)
- a need for 1 to 1 nursing.

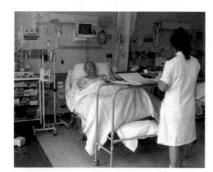

Fig 2.2d HDU care (oxygen, monitoring and 1-to-2 nurse to patient ratio).

Fast facts—Assessment of the critically ill surgical patient

'Prevention is better than cure'

The 'at-risk' patient

- Past medical history
- Surgical pathology
- Intraoperative events
- Recent events
- **Manage along lines of IQM principle**

Identification

- Treated ill patients should get better
- Routine medical reviews
- Early warning scoring systems

Quantify

- Airway
- Breathing
- Circulation
- Diagnosis

Management

- Ill patients need oxygen
- Fluid requirements
- Ask for help
- Frequent review
- Consider need for HDU/ITU care

The mainstay of care of the critically ill patient is clinical examination and observation of the patient (Fig. 2.2d). However, several techniques and the use of more complex monitoring procedures can be used to aid diagnosis and guide the management of these patients.

Postoperative complications: hypoxia

Scenario: hypoxia following an emergency laparotomy

You are asked to review a 69-year-old man who is 3 days post-emergency laparotomy for an obstructing carcinoma of the descending colon. He has become unwell with a fall in his oxygen saturation and confusion.

A postoperative patient should be getting better not worse, therefore some event *has* taken place. This task is to identify the event, quantify it and manage it.

> A review of the patient reveals that there are no airway issues causing this change as he is talking normally, though confused as to time and place. His oxygen saturation is 89%, though was 94% in the preceding 2 days. His respiratory rate is 20/minute.

The oxygen saturation has reduced postoperatively. This can be accounted for in a number of ways: postoperative chest infection, heart failure with or without a myocardial infarction or pulmonary embolus. Intra-abdominal sepsis and sedative drugs may also cause this deterioration. A careful examination and investigation is required, rather than simply assume a chest infection.

> A review of the patient's notes shows he has a past history of both myocardial infarction and chronic pulmonary airways disease.

This past history places him at risk of cardiac and respiratory complications following major surgery.

> The operation note shows that he underwent a left hemicolectomy with primary re-anastomosis of the bowel ends following on-table bowel lavage.

It is therefore possible that this anastomosis has leaked and the resultant sepsis is accounting for his condition.

> Examination of the patient shows a slight drop in the BP with a rise in the pulse. Chest examination reveals coarse crepitations at the left base. Abdominal examination is unremarkable with no evidence of peritonism.

The examination suggests that the problem is likely to be a chest infection, in line with his past respiratory history. However, potential diagnoses require to be positively ruled out rather than assuming the likeliest candidate is responsible.

> CXR confirms a left basal collapse. ECG is unchanged from his preoperative one.

This appears to support the working diagnosis and is enough to start antibiotics and chest physiotherapy. Occasionally **rhythm changes such as atrial fibrilla-**

Clinical key points in postoperative hypoxia

- Tachypnoea is an early sign of respiratory compromise
- The first indication of hypoxia may be a fall in oxygen saturation on routine pulse oximetry
- All ill patients require oxygen, give high flow O_2 therapy while taking a history and performing the examination
- Increasing confusion and reducing consciousness are late signs of hypoxia
- Examine the cardiorespiratory systems looking for signs of heart failure and pulmonary infection
- CXR and ECG will help to diagnose heart failure and pulmonary infection
- If hypoxia exists in the presence of a normal CXR, rule out pulmonary embolism (PE) by ventilation (V)/perfusion (Q) scan or chest CT
- Treat chest infection with antibiotics (with sputum culture) and chest physiotherapy, heart failure with diuretics, and PE by anticoagulation

tion (AF) can be caused by sepsis or a new myocardial infarction so care must be taken in not jumping to conclusions.

In this case, senior input is required as to whether a contrast examination of the large bowel anastomosis is required, to exclude a leak.

> Frequent assessments show the patient is improving and therefore the diagnosis appears correct.

Failure to improve would indicate that either the diagnosis is wrong or incomplete, or the therapy inadequate.

Background: hypoxia

Disorders of the respiratory system are a common cause of postoperative morbidity and mortality.

The importance of oxygen and the effects of hypoxia

The need for oxygen is fundamental to life. Cell death rapidly occurs should there be a complete lack of oxygen (anoxia). **Hypoxaemia** (a reduction in the oxygen content in the blood) leads to insufficient oxygen being delivered to the tissues, forcing them into anaerobic metabolism. The acid by-products of this are less easily excreted than carbon dioxide and metabolic acidosis can occur. Cellular and organ dysfunction may then arise if tissue **hypoxia** (inadequate supply of oxygen) is ongoing.

All organs are affected by hypoxia but the clinical features will be related to the degree and duration of inadequate oxygen supply.

- In the brain, hypoxia can be a cause of confusion and agitation and if very severe proceeds to loss of consciousness. **Hypoxia is the commonest factor associated with postoperative confusion in the elderly.**

- The heart responds to hypoxia by increasing heart rate, which in turn increases myocardial oxygen demand. If this demand cannot be met, myocardial ischaemia or infarction may occur.

- Impairment of renal and hepatic function leads to accumulation of toxins, which cause further cardiac and brain dysfunction. Hypoxia is a contributory factor in postoperative acute renal failure.

Oxygen delivery

To understand hypoxia, oxygen delivery to the tissues should be understood.

The partial pressure of oxygen in the atmosphere is 21 kPa. By the time it reaches the alveoli this has fallen to 13 kPa (as a result of humidification, and mixing with alveolar CO_2). This is the **oxygen cascade**.

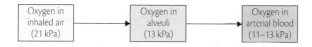

Oxygen passes from the alveoli into the pulmonary capillary blood along a concentration gradient. Most is combined with Hb, which is almost fully saturated at normal arterial oxygen tensions (98%) and very little is dissolved in plasma (unless breathing 100% oxygen).

Oxygenated blood then passes back to the left side of the heart and then on to the systemic circulation and the tissue capillaries where oxygen again passes along a concentration gradient into the tissues.

Deoxygenated blood returns to the alveoli via the venous system and the pulmonary arteries.

In summary, delivery of oxygen to the tissues depends on the following factors:

- clear airways
- adequate ventilation
- adequate concentration of oxygen in inspired air
- no diffusion barrier to oxygen at alveolar–capillary interface
- matching between ventilation and perfusion of the lung

- appropriate cardiac output from both the left and right sides of the heart to ensure oxygen uptake in the lungs and distribution to the tissues
- adequate and normally functioning Hb to carry oxygen in the blood.

Anything that impacts on the above factors may alter oxygen delivery. In times of stress to the body, e.g. after surgery or during exercise, oxygen demand will increase.

Delivery may be increased by an increasing inspired oxygen concentration and by increasing cardiac output (increasing heart rate and contractility, ensuring appropriate ventricular filling). Anaemia (low Hb) will reduce the ability of the blood to carry oxygen.

The assessment of the suitability of a patient to withstand surgery and anaesthesia is closely related to their ability to increase oxygen delivery to vital tissues during, and after, the stress of surgery. Optimizing all the above factors will maximize the patients' reserves.

Identification and quantification of hypoxia

Patient factors increase the risk of hypoxia and respiratory complications:

- *smoking* (smokers have a relatively high level of carboxyhaemoglobin. Carbon monoxide has a 240 times greater affinity for Hb than oxygen. It therefore prevents Hb binding oxygen and only slowly dissociates. Oxygen administration speeds up this process and abstinence, even for 24 hours, will reverse most of this.)
- *chronic pulmonary disease*
- *age and obesity* (decreased functional residual capacity; the volume of lung after the end of normal exhalation, from which actual oxygen uptake occurs)
- *perioperative opiates and sedatives* (hypoventilation)
- *abdominal/thoracic surgery* (particularly emergency surgery, due to diaphragmatic splitting by raised intra-abdominal pressure and poor respiratory effort due to inadequate analgesia)
- *orthopaedic surgery* (as a result of fat emboli from the marrow during manipulation of bones).

Identifying those at high risk of lung complications and actively trying to optimize respiratory function preoperatively are the keys to reducing hypoxic and respiratory events. A number of strategies may be used:

- preoperative optimization of lung function with chest physiotherapy, bronchodilators, and cessation of smoking
- effective analgesia (epidural analgesia, use of local anaesthetic techniques)

- careful postoperative fluid management (prevention of a large positive fluid balance)
- early postoperative chest physiotherapy
- monitored oxygen therapy (pulse oximetry to ensure good oxygenation).

History and examination are the first steps in the management of patients with respiratory complications. Hypoxia itself causes non-specific symptoms, but should always be suspected as a cause (and result) of postoperative complications.

Examination

- *Inspection*—cyanosis is a late and unreliable sign of hypoxaemia. Significant hypoxia can exist before cyanosis is apparent. However, other signs may indicate hypoxaemia: **an altered mental state**, obvious respiratory distress, tachypnoea, or a very slow respiratory rate and the use of accessory muscles of respiration.

- *Palpation*—tracheal deviation is an important sign (see below).

Crepitus suggests subcutaneous emphysema (air), which, although rarely a major problem in itself, indicates the need for investigation for the source if not already obvious. It can occur in association with pneumothorax, ruptured oesophagus, and mediastinal injury. Chest expansion should be assessed, as asymmetry indicates problems on the side that moves less.

- *Percussion*—dullness suggests consolidation or fluid. Hyper-resonance may indicate the presence of a pneumothorax. It is important to assess any associated distress and tracheal deviation that may indicate a tension pneumothorax. If suspected then immediate release of the pressure with a needle is indicated.

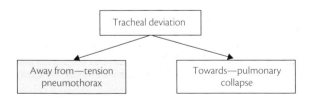

- *Auscultation*—noisy breathing may mean airways obstruction. Auscultation may also help with the diagnosis of atelectasis or lung collapse, pulmonary oedema, pneumothorax, bronchospasm, or pleural effusion.

Investigations

1. *Pulse oximetry*. This is a non-invasive technique that uses infrared/red light to determine the percentage saturation of arterial blood (Hb) with oxygen. A small probe can be placed on the finger or ear lobe to give a continuous display of oxygen saturation. Normally for arterial blood this should be above 97%.

   However, due to the way oxygen is carried by Hb, a substantial decrease in oxygen tension (PaO_2) can occur before saturation begins to fall (Fig. 2.2e). An oxygen saturation of 90% generally equates to an arterial PaO_2 of only 8 kPa (normal **arterial** PaO_2 is 13 kPa).

   Pulse oximetry may be unreliable in the presence of abnormal Hb, e.g. carboxyhaemoglobin formed from carbon monoxide where the oximeter will overestimate oxygen saturation (smokers have high CO contents), and with peripheral shutdown in hypovolaemic shock.

   What level of oxygen saturation is safe? There is no hard and fast rule but one suggestion is that postoperative hypoxaemia be regarded as a PaO_2 of less than 8 kPa or SaO_2 less than 90% with a 'safe' lower limit of 93%.

2. *Arterial blood gas analysis*. The measurement of the **partial pressure of oxygen (PaO_2)** and **oxygen saturation (SaO_2)** in a fresh sample of arterial blood

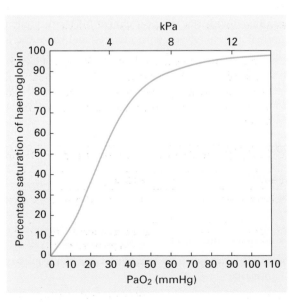

Fig 2.2e Oxygen dissociation curve.

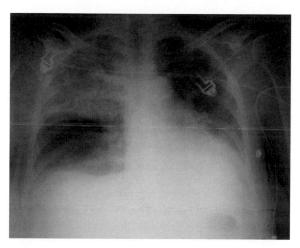

Fig 2.2f Chest X-ray of right middle and lower lobe pneumonia.

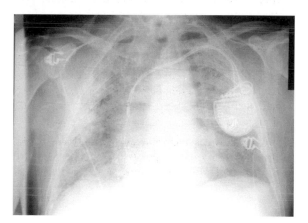

Fig 2.2g Chest X-ray of acute pulmonary oedema (note pacemaker).

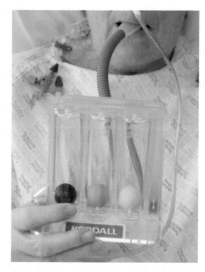

Fig 2.2h Incentive spirometry (inspiration makes the balls rise).

3. *CXR.* In the postoperative setting a CXR can provide useful information (Fig. 2.2f, 2.2g). The state of the lung fields and any evidence of fluid, collapse, or air may help to decide the likely cause and appropriate treatment of problems.

4. *Respiratory function tests.* In postoperative patients only 'bedside' tests are appropriate. Of these, spirometry is probably the simplest. It is useful to monitor the response to bronchodilators and physiotherapy and the two are combined with an incentive spirometer where the patient can see increasing numbers of coloured balls rising with respiratory effort (Fig. 2.2h). The patient inspires ('sucks') to raise the balls as the aim is to inflate the lungs not deflate them.

Summary

The clinical detection of postoperative hypoxaemia can be difficult. However, pulse oximetry provides a simple, non-invasive way of detection in the vast major-

remains the gold standard by which hypoxaemia is determined. It also measures $PaCO_2$ (adequacy of ventilation—$PaCO_2$ rises as ventilation falls) and acid/base status (pH, base excess, and bicarbonate level).

TABLE 2.2d The likely causes of hypoxia and the CXR findings

Cause	CXR findings	Cause of hypoxia
Pulmonary oedema	Diffuse, bilateral, symmetrical changes	Diffusion barrier to oxygen due to fluid in alveolar tissue
Bronchopneumonia	Localized unilateral changes, or localized bilateral asymmetrical changes	Shunting of blood through areas not being ventilated
Pulmonary embolus	Normal, no gross changes	Increased dead space with ventilation of non-perfused lung
Adult respiratory distress syndrome	Widespread localized bilateral asymmetrical changes	Shunting of blood through areas not being ventilated

ity of patients. It also provides the best means of monitoring progress and the level and duration of treatment.

The commonest causes of a low SaO_2 in the early postoperative period are:

- hypoventilation
- alveolar–capillary perfusion barrier
- ventilation/perfusion (V/Q) mismatching.

Hypoventilation results in hypercapnia and hypoxaemia, which can be overcome by increasing the concentration of inspired oxygen. A number of causes exist in the postoperative period:

- airways obstruction
- reduced ventilatory drive—depressant effects of anaesthetics, cerebrovascular accident
- peripheral factors—residual neuromuscular blockade, pain, tight dressings, obesity.

Alveolar–capillary perfusion barrier
Pulmonary oedema
The fall in SaO_2 is due to:

- the tissue between the alveoli and the capillaries being oedematous ('water-logged'); therefore, oxygen diffuses less efficiently
- the lungs with this fluid load become stiff and difficult to inflate and more susceptible to infection.

This is much more likely to occur in elderly patients. The usual causes are patients being fluid over-loaded and/or postoperative myocardial ischaemia/ infarction.

V/Q mismatch is the commonest cause of hypoxia.

Atelectesis/pulmonary sepsis
In the early postoperative period, alterations in lung mechanics causing small airway closure and reductions in cardiac output related to anaesthesia, lead to mismatching of ventilation (V) and perfusion (Q) within the lung, resulting in hypoxaemia. These changes may persist for 3–4 days after operation, depending on the magnitude and site of surgery (thoracic and upper abdominal procedures are worst). Air is then trapped in these small airways, which have closed and as it is absorbed the alveoli collapse (atelectasis). Secretions from these lung units cannot be expectorated and may become infected, worsening hypoxia through collapse and consolidation of the alveoli.

The use of regional anaesthetic techniques may help to minimize the effect of altered lung physiology in the perioperative period.

Pulmonary embolism
The first signal of a pulmonary embolism may be a sudden fall in the SaO_2, which may rapidly recover. In the absence of CXR changes of cardiac failure or pnemonia a pulmonary embolism must be excluded.

Management
Treatment of the hypoxic patient is aimed at improving oxygen delivery. Careful preoperative assessment helps to identify those at risk and allows time to optimize those factors involved in oxygen delivery, e.g. correction of anaemia, treatment of existing respiratory disease.

If hypoxia develops the priority is to improve oxygenation by working through ABCs.

Ensure a clear **Airway** as the upper airway can obstruct in sedated patients due to loss of tone. Secretions may also accumulate and cause obstruction while the patient is too sleepy to cough and clear them. It is best to recover patients in the lateral position using simple manoeuvres—**chin lift, jaw thrust, and head tilt**—to maintain a clear airway. If the patient is unable to talk and obviously sedated, an oropharyngeal airway can be used. If there is loss of consciousness endotracheal intubation may be necessary, but should be performed by a skilled operator.

Next the adequacy of **Breathing** should be checked. Hypoventilation due to the residual effects of muscle relaxants or opioids may require pharmacological treatment. Bronchospasm is also not uncommon perioperatively.

Oxygen therapy is given to treat hypoxia and is most effective when the underlying cause is hypoventilation.

Once an adequate airway is achieved, then oxygen should be administered. If there is adequate spontaneous ventilation, then a simple variable performance device, e.g. Hudson type face mask (5 litres/min oxygen initially) or nasal catheter (2 litres/min oxygen initially) should be used. The flow of oxygen should be adjusted according to the measured oxygen saturation by pulse oximetry or arterial blood gas analysis (aim for e.g. 95%, PaO_2 >9 kPa).

If high oxygen flows are required (10–15 litres/min) then a Hudson reservoir mask should be used. Failure to achieve adequate oxygenation with this suggests the need for aggressive treatment of the cause, or more invasive management of oxygen therapy. This may be with continuous positive airway pressure via a tight-fitting face mask or endotracheal intubation, or intermittent positive pressure ventilation via an endotracheal tube.

The dangers of giving oxygen to patients who rely on hypoxic drive have been overstated and **controlled low-dose oxygen has virtually no part in postoperative oxygen therapy**. Giving 30–50% oxygen is usually sufficient to restore oxygen saturation to a satisfactory level. This can be achieved using a nasal cannula with an oxygen flow of 2–3 litres/ min or 4–5 litres/min via a face mask.

In some cases where there is a large shunt (under-ventilated but perfused lung), oxygen alone does not improve oxygenation. It may be necessary to intubate the patient's trachea and use a mechanical ventilator to reventilate the collapsed alveoli, possibly in conjunction with bronchoscopy to identify and aspirate a mucus plug in a bronchi.

The **circulation** should next be assessed remembering that if cardiac output is low (or normal but inadequate for the body's demands) hypoxia can result. If there is hypovolaemia due to blood loss, oxygen-carrying capacity will also be reduced as a result of anaemia. This will contribute to tissue hypoxia. A FBC should be taken and any anaemia treated. If there are signs of fluid overload then diuretics may be considered.

Patients with inadequate respiration

If there is inadequate spontaneous ventilation then attempt to ventilate immediately with a tight-fitting face mask and self-inflating bag. Call for anaesthetic help. Endotracheal intubation may be required.

Manoeuvres to improve respiration

Patients should ideally be allowed/encouraged to sit up. This tends to restore functional residual capacity and gives the diaphragm and chest wall an added mechanical advantage.

Analgesia should be optimized to facilitate breathing, expectoration, and physiotherapy. Other methods include physiotherapy, direct suction via an endotracheal tube, or cricothyroidotomy. If the patient has aspirated, antibiotics should also be considered.

Naloxone is a specific opioid antagonist and can be used to treat opioid-induced respiratory depression. It may also reverse analgesia unless titrated very carefully.

If there is mechanical interference with respiration due to fluid, blood, or air in the pleural space then aspiration should be considered. A suspected tension pneumothorax should be decompressed by immediate needle thoracentesis without waiting for an X-ray.

Fast facts—Postoperative hypoxia (a lack of oxygen)

Aim to anticipate and prevent hypoxia in every postoperative patient.

Causes

- Pulmonary atelectesis
- Pulmonary oedema
- Pulmonary infection
- Pulmonary embolus
- Pneumothorax

Clinical features

- Anxiety
- Confusion
- Tachypnoea

Manage along lines of IQM principle

Investigations

- Pulse oximetry
- CXR
- Arterial blood gases

Management

Appropriate assessment guides logical management of hypoxic patient

---

Formal chest drainage will then be required whether the diagnosis was correct or not.

If bronchospasm is a feature, this should be managed initially by nebulized bronchodilators, e.g. salbutamol 2.5–5 mg/4 hourly.

Postoperative complications: hypotension and cardiac ischaemia

Scenario 1: postoperative hypotension and ECG changes

A 75-year-old man becomes hypotensive 2 days following an above-knee amputation for chronic arterial disease.

Hypotension on the second postoperative day (in the absence of obvious haemorrhage) **is classically due to myocardial infarction**. In this case, the patient has a history of peripheral vascular disease. These patients are also likely to have coronary artery disease.

> The patient is given 100% oxygen while he is reviewed. He has until now had an uneventful postoperative course. He has a past history of myocardial infarction.

Ill patients need oxygen.

A full history and examination should be performed to look for clues as to the cause of his low BP. Hypovolaemia, arrhythmias, sepsis, and ventricular failure should all be excluded. His past history clearly places him at risk of a postoperative myocardial ischaemic event.

> The patient gives no history of chest pain, but does appear to be tachypnoeic with a respiratory rate of 24 breaths/min.

Postoperative myocardial infarction can be difficult to diagnose. Only 25% of patients will present with 'crushing central chest pain'. Tachypnoea can be an early sign of developing left ventricular failure, which is associated with myocardial infarction. Myocardial ischaemia reduces ventricular performance. Any angina should be treated and precipitating factors corrected once identified in order to prevent a worsening cycle of ischaemia and left ventricular dysfunction.

> On examination, the patient is cold and clammy, BP is 95/50 with a pulse of 105/min. His chest has scattered fine crepitations.

Hypotension associated with poorly perfused peripheries and increased heart rate may be due to hypovolaemia or left ventricular failure. Perioperative fluid balance charts should be checked to look for imbalance between input and output. The surgical wound site should be inspected for haemorrhage. A small fluid challenge may be administered if there is doubt about the diagnosis (200 ml).

In this case examination of the chest is suggestive of heart failure with developing pulmonary oedema. Jugular venous pulse may also be elevated.

> An ECG shows a rate of 125/min and the acute changes of a myocardial infarction, which when compared with the preoperative ECG are new.

Comparing new and old ECGs is the easiest way to decide whether a cardiac event has occurred. **The diagnosis of myocardial infarction is usually supported by a rise in the troponin-T enzyme.** Bloods should also be sent for FBC to exclude anaemia and electrolyte abnormalities.

> CXR shows elements of heart failure but not localized pulmonary collapse or consolidation.

The results of clinical examination and investigation both confirm that the patient is developing heart failure as the result of a postoperative myocardial infarction. A further differential diagnosis could be pulmonary embolus (PE). This is unlikely in view of the ECG and CXR changes. Where there has been a PE the CXR is often normal, although the ECG may show evidence of right ventricular strain (classically S_1–Q_3–T_3).

Scenario 2: postoperative hypotension with a tachyarrhythmia

> A 72-year-old lady is first postoperative day following urgent laparoscopic cholecystectomy. Routine observations have shown a fall in her BP with a rise in her pulse. Her oxygen saturation is 93%.

As before the patient should receive 100% oxygen while a full history, examination, and investigations are performed.

> She has no pain but feels breathless and dizzy when sitting up. Her pulse is 110/min irregularly irregular (probable atrial fibrillation (AF)). Her BP was 100/60 mmHg with a preoperative level of 130/85 mmHg. Chest auscultation reveals diffuse fine crepitations. ECG confirms fast AF with a ventricular rate of 110–120/min.

The initial impression is that the patient has developed AF, resulting in reduced cardiac output due to loss of atrial contraction. This reduces ventricular filling and so the volume ejected by the heart during systole falls. Hypotension and heart failure can then arise.

Perioperatively, many causes of arrhythmia can exist (hypoxia, hypercapnia, electrolyte disturbance, acid–base imbalance, myocardial ischaemia, sepsis, drugs). Treatment of the cause may correct the rhythm disturbance. In some cases specific anti-arrhythmic therapy will be required.

Clinical key points in hypotension and myocardial ischaemia

- All ill patients require oxygen, give high flow O_2 therapy while taking a history and performing the examination

- If there is a past history of cardiovascular (cardiac and peripheral vascular) problems, then the risk of cardiac complications after major surgery is high

- Check the BP on both arms, note any abnormal cardiac rhythms (arrhythmias can cause hypotension and myocardial ischaemia)

- Examine the chest for signs of cardiac failure

- Myocardial infarction does not present with chest pain in the majority of postoperative patients

- Investigation should include cardiac enzymes including troponin-T, FBC (for anaemia), ECG, and CXR (looking for heart failure)

- Check the patient continues to receive their normal cardiac medications before and after surgery, by another route than oral if necessary

---

Blood tests for U&Es and FBC are all normal. A troponin-T level is requested to exclude myocardial infarction as a cause and a CXR confirms evidence of mild pulmonary oedema. The preoperative ECG shows she was in controlled AF prior to surgery. On questioning the patient usually takes digoxin but had vomited up the tablets for a couple of days prior to admission (when ill with cholecystitis) and has not been prescribed this medication while in hospital.

Many things happen to the patient when they are admitted as an emergency and important issues can be forgotten by both patient and staff. **Check the patient's current medication.**

Uncontrolled AF in the postoperative period requires urgent treatment. The combination of increased heart rate and low cardiac output can precipitate myocardial ischaemia, which may further worsen the situation.

If the patient is cardiovascularly unstable, d.c. cardioversion may be required. However, in this case, hypotension is mild and time can be taken for drugs to act.

The patient is prescribed digoxin and a diuretic with good results.

Background: postoperative hypotension

Hypotension

Low systemic arterial pressure (<90 mmHg or >30% reduction from preoperative value) is not an uncommon postoperative finding. As the blood flow to many organs is pressure dependent, hypotension can, if serious, lead to organ dysfunction. **Hypotension causing inadequate organ perfusion and tissue oxygenation is defined as 'shock'.**

Causes of immediate perioperative hypotension

Many of the drugs used in anaesthesia can cause a fall in BP (IV and inhalational anaesthetics, opioids). They can result in both systemic vasodilatation and direct myocardial depressant effects. Early in the postoperative period **residual anaesthetic drug effects** can be a cause of hypotension. This may be especially likely in patients receiving other cardiac drugs (e.g. beta blockers, angiotensin-converting enzyme inhibitors), who are in no pain.

Patients who have received spinal or epidural anaesthesia may also have a low BP after surgery, as a result of autonomic blockade. In these cases, the heart rate is usually normal or low and the patient's hands and feet are warm and well perfused.

In many patients these findings are well tolerated and apart from ensuring that oxygen is being administered by face mask, no further treatment is required. If the degree of hypotension is causing concern, the patient is elderly or suffers from concurrent cardiac or respiratory disease, treatment will be necessary. Oxygen must always be given, venous return can be improved by elevating the legs, and if necessary a small volume of IV fluid (200 ml) can be infused.

If hypotension occurs in association with flushing, appearance of a rash (urticaria), and with bronchospasm, the patient may be having an allergic reaction. **Anaphylactic type reactions** can occur even with no prior exposure to a drug. Treatment as ever follows the ABCs:

- oxygen is administered; all drugs and blood transfusions are stopped.

- IV fluid is given as crystalloid or colloid, and adrenaline (epinephrine) is given in small increments intravenously (or intramuscularly) until BP improves.

- senior assistance should be sought early.

Postoperative hypotension

Systemic arterial pressure is normally closely controlled to ensure tissue perfusion. It can be calculated as follows:

Mean arterial pressure (MAP) = cardiac output (CO) × systemic vascular resistance (SVR)

As cardiac output is affected by heart rate and stroke volume, it can be seen that **hypotension can result from reduction in:**

- heart rate
- ventricular filling (stroke volume falls—less in less out)
- ventricular contractility (pump power)
- peripheral resistance.

Heart rate

Bradycardia

A heart rate of 45–50/min may be well tolerated and even normal. However, in the elderly it may result in hypotension. A low heart rate is therefore treated on its effects.

A **low heart rate** may be due to myocardial ischaemia, sinus bradycardia because of sympathetic block (e.g. beta-blockers, high spinal/epidural anaesthesia), or parasympathetic stimulation (e.g. vasovagal attack).

Treatment is initially with atropine, which counteracts the effect of the vagus nerve, allowing more unopposed sympathetic action, thereby raising the heart rate. If there is no response, then other causes must be sought, such as complete heart block.

Tachyarrhythmias

These are common perioperatively and are mostly benign requiring no treatment. Specific causes are:

- anaesthetic drugs, e.g. halothane
- hypoxia/hypercapnia
- pain
- electrolyte and acid–base disturbance.

Fast heart rates are often associated with hypotension as a result of the shorter time available for ventricular filling. This is more so when there is loss of atrial contraction as in AF.

Patients with ischaemic heart disease are particularly at risk from a prolonged tachycardia, as it increases cardiac work, which requires more oxygen to be delivered. Coronary heart disease may limit this and the myocardium becomes even more ischaemic, worsening still further myocardial performance.

Ventricular filling: hypovolaemia

This can result from inadequate replacement of pre-operative and/or intraoperative losses, or to ongoing losses after surgery. The fluid lost may be from the intravascular compartment (haemorrhage), or the extra-cellular and intracellular compartments (intestinal obstruction, peritonitis, vomiting, and diarrhoea).

Continued bleeding is usually obvious from inspection of the wound site or any drains, but it may be concealed particularly in the abdomen or chest, even if drains are present. Usually, postoperative haemorrhage is due to inadequate surgical haemostasis but coagulopathy must be considered especially if there has been a large transfusion, sepsis, pre-existing clotting abnormality, or if anticoagulants have been given.

Classically, hypotension due to hypovolaemia is accompanied by tachycardia and peripheral vasoconstriction. This is the body's attempt to protect the vital organs (brain, heart, and kidneys) from inadequate blood flow. The patient is cold and clammy, with poor capillary refill in the hands and feet. Urine output is likely to be low and jugular venous pressure (or CVP) will be low or normal.

In some patients, heart rate may not be elevated due to the effect of drugs they may be receiving (beta-blockers, anticholinesterases used to reverse muscle relaxation). Patients who are extremely hypothermic can have profound vasoconstriction and as they re-warm, hypovolaemia can be unmasked.

Hypovolaemia causes a reduction in cardiac stroke volume by reducing venous return and cardiac preload. Two other conditions cause a reduction in preload and cause profound hypotension:

- **Tension pneumothorax** (impedes venous return due to raised intrathoracic pressure) and
- **PE** (obstructs right ventricular outflow with signs of right ventricular failure) both compromise cardiac output.

Pneumothorax should be considered in all patients where a central venous line has been inserted or where thoracic surgery has been performed. Heart rate and jugular venous pulse will be elevated and examination of the chest will show the characteristic findings of hyper-resonance, tracheal shift away from the affected side, and absent breath sounds.

After a large pulmonary embolus, there is breathlessness and hypotension with tachycardia, elevated jugular venous pulse, and cyanosis.

Contractility: low cardiac output

In the postoperative period, left ventricular failure is most commonly due to myocardial ischaemia/infarction or to excessive use of IV fluids.

There is poor peripheral perfusion as once again the body tries to maintain blood flow to vital organs. Heart rate is elevated and jugular venous pressure or CVP will be elevated or normal. These compensatory mechanisms, however, further increase myocardial work and oxygen demand and so further deterioration in ventricular function follows.

It can be difficult to distinguish between hypotension due to hypovolaemia and that due to cardiac failure. If there is doubt a small fluid challenge can be administered with caution. In the very elderly, or those with a history of myocardial ischaemia, consideration should be given to the early insertion of a CVP monitoring line.

Peripheral vascular resistance: sepsis

This may be a common finding especially after emergency surgery. Initially, hypotension exists as part of a hyperdynamic picture with a warm, vasodilated, tachycardic patient with bounding peripheral pulses, and a raised cardiac output. The hypotension results from loss of fluid through damaged, leaky capillaries into the interstitial fluid space.

As the septic process continues and organ function further deteriorates, the picture changes to that of low cardiac output, with tachycardia, vasoconstriction, and the cold, clammy picture of cardiac failure.

Identification and quantification of hypotension

As always history, examination, and investigation are the tools used to make a diagnosis and guide therapy. Always **give oxygen while assessing the patient**.

BP measurement must be carried out regularly in the postoperative period. Early on this should be at least hourly until the residual effects of anaesthesia have worn off. Then for a variable period of time depending on the seriousness of the surgery and the presence of intercurrent cardiac disease, measurements should be made at least every 4 hours.

History

This allows an assessment of cerebral function to be made. The patient should be questioned about any features that could have led to hypotension, e.g. chest pain, irregular heart beat, bleeding, vomiting, etc. All fluid charts and other observation charts should be consulted as should the drug kardex. Postoperative BP should always be compared with preoperative values.

Examination

BP should be checked again and a full examination of the patient performed with close attention to the heart, lungs, and surgical wound. Also any evidence of reduced peripheral perfusion should be sought (cold hands, feet) and if there is delayed (>2 seconds) capillary refill.

Investigations

Some simple investigations can be performed that can guide the diagnosis and treatment:

- confirm **BP** and continue to monitor BP

- monitor heart rate and rhythm with **continuous ECG**

- a 12-lead ECG should be obtained, and blood taken for FBC (possibly coagulation screen), U&Es, and cross-matching if there is evidence of continued blood loss

- a blood sample should also be taken to exclude myocardial infarction (troponin-T)

- pulse oximetry should be used to ensure that even if hypotensive, the patient is well oxygenated

- if not already in place, a urinary catheter should be passed to help monitor the response to treatment

- a CXR should also be obtained and looked at to exclude a pneumothorax, heart failure, and pulmonary sepsis/collapse.

Fast facts—Postoperative hypotension (common postoperative problem)

BP (BP) = cardiac output* (CO) × systemic vascular resistance (SVR)

*CO = heart rate (HR) × stroke volume (SV) i.e. changes in:

- heart rate, i.e. AF

- stroke volume, i.e. hypovolaemia, myocardial ischaemia

- vascular resistance: i.e. sepsis

can all affect BP

Manage along lines of IQM principle.

Identify and quantify

- History, examination and investigation (FBC, ECG, CXR, U&Es, CVP, oximetry)

Manage

- Give oxygen

- Treat as hypovolaemia till proved otherwise (i.e. give fluid challenge)

- If poor response to fluid challenge and CVP normal, consider inotropic drugs (get senior help)

- Constantly reassess

Management

As stated above initial management of the hypotensive patient begins with the ABCs of resuscitation.

Oxygen should be administered in the first instance while adequacy of breathing and the circulation are assessed. Venous return can be improved by elevating the legs if feasible (usually by raising the foot of the bed).

Hypovolaemia where there is hypotension in association with tachycardia and poor peripheral perfusion requires IV administration of appropriate fluid. This should be infused with care especially in the elderly. Early consideration of the use of CVP monitoring to guide therapy should be made.

Low cardiac output if due to reduced myocardial contractility requires correction of the cause if possible (e.g. drugs, electrolytes, arrhythmias, hypoxia, hypercapnia). Specific treatment of fluid overload with diuretics may be necessary and inotropic agents to support the heart may be required. Such therapy is guided by the use of CVP monitoring (or by pulmonary artery pressure monitoring or oesophageal Doppler monitoring of cardiac output).

Treatment of suspected sepsis relies on early recognition and intervention with antibiotics and further surgery if necessary to remove the source of infection. As it is likely that large volumes of IV fluid will be required as well as inotropes, invasive monitoring will be required and senior help should be called early.

As always it is important to reassess the patient frequently in order to ensure improvement is sustained.

Myocardial ischaemia/infarction

Myocardial ischaemia is most likely to occur in patients with pre-existing coronary artery disease. In the postoperative period a number of situations arise that may precipitate ischaemia:

- *hypotension*—numerous causes (see above)

- *hypertension*—this is a common finding in the postoperative period especially if the patient is in pain, is hypoxic or hypercapnic. Increased peripheral resistance increases myocardial work and oxygen demand. If this increase in oxygen demand cannot be met, ischaemia results

- *tachycardia*—causes are similar to those for hypertension. Again myocardial oxygen demand is increased and if supply cannot also be increased, ischaemia will occur

- *hypoxia*—this causes both hypertension and tachycardia in the presence of reduced oxygen supply.

It is important to intervene early if angina should occur. Any causative factors should be treated, oxygen and anti-anginal therapy given, and a 12-lead ECG should be performed. Ideally, continuous monitoring of ECG and pulse oximetry should take place in those known to be at risk throughout the immediate postoperative period.

Myocardial infarction

Perioperative myocardial infarction carries a high mortality (>50%). It commonly occurs on the second to third postoperative days, but may happen at any time during or after surgery.

In those patients without a history of ischaemic heart disease, the incidence of perioperative myocardial infarction is less than 1%. The risks are significantly higher in those with a past history of angina or a previous myocardial infarction. As mentioned in preoperative assessment, a short time interval between myocardial infarction and surgery increases the incidence of reinfarction.

Other factors that can be identified preoperatively which increase the likelihood of myocardial infarction include: evidence of heart failure, arrhythmias, aortic stenosis, and poorly controlled hypertension.

Certain types of surgery are associated with an increased incidence of myocardial infarction. Vascular surgery in particular carries perioperative risks of infarction of 5–20% for some high-risk procedures (e.g. carotid endarterectomy, aortic surgery).

Intraoperative factors may also influence infarction rates. Hypotension, hypertension, and tachycardia are all risk factors, as is hypoxia. In particular these can occur around the time of endotracheal intubation and extubation. The anaesthetist can modify the response to these manipulations to try to limit myocardial ischaemia.

There is some evidence that the use of regional anaesthetic techniques may reduce the likelihood of perioperative myocardial ischaemia/infarction.

Risk reduction

Identification of at-risk individuals and delay of surgery after myocardial infarction.

- Best medical therapy of risk factors for infarction, including: angina, hypertension, arrhythmias, cardiac failure, hypercholesterolaemia. In particular there is evidence that perioperative use of beta-blockers and 'statins', in certain high-risk groups, may greatly reduce the incidence of perioperative myocardial infarction.

- Anaesthetic techniques: should be tailored to the procedure and the patient's medical status. Regional

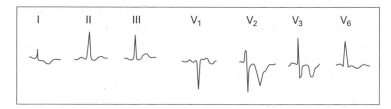

Fig 2.2i ECG showing myocardial infarction.

anaesthetic techniques may confer a benefit. All patients at risk of myocardial infarction should receive postoperative oxygen therapy. It may be necessary to continue this for up to 3 days after surgery (longer if complications arise).

◆ Postoperative recovery: careful monitoring of the

Fast facts—Myocardial ischaemia/infarction

◆ Those with a past history of coronary artery disease are at highest risk

◆ Postoperative monitoring of at-risk individuals is crucial to early detection of problems

◆ Perioperative myocardial infarction has a mortality of greater than 50%

◆ Common precipitating factors are:

—hypo/hypertension

—hypoxia

—tachycardia

◆ Precipitating factors should be treated rapidly to avoid escalation

◆ Classical symptoms of myocardial infarction are present in only a minority of patients postoperatively

◆ Consider the likelihood of myocardial infarction in patients with:

—confusion

—hypotension

—breathlessness/tachypnoea, or

—arrhythmias

◆ **Manage along lines of IQM principle**

◆ Ensure that patients receive their usual cardiac drugs in the perioperative period (by another route if necessary)

---

cardiovascular and respiratory systems should occur, with as a minimum, continuous ECG, pulse oximetry, and regular non-invasive BP measurement. Prompt treatment of any factors that can precipitate infarction will be necessary.

Diagnosis

Myocardial infarction in the postoperative period may be difficult to diagnose. The classical history of 'crushing' central chest pain is present in less than 25% of patients. Myocardial infarction should be considered as a possible cause of hypotension, arrhythmia, and breathlessness.

As always, the diagnosis will be made from history, examination, and investigations. A 12-lead ECG may show evidence of elevated ST segments, rhythm abnormalities, or conduction defects. These may differ from the preoperative ECG if one has been taken. Blood should be taken for measurement of FBC (anaemia as a cause of decreased oxygen supply), U&Es, and cardiac enzymes. The troponin-T will be elevated if infarction has occurred.

Treatment

After ensuring the ABCs of resuscitation have been followed, it is important to discuss the patient with senior cardiology colleagues for their further specialized management. Adequate analgesia, if required, should always be administered in the meantime.

Postoperative complications: oliguria and electrolyte disturbance

Scenario: low urine output following an emergency laparotomy

A 65-year-old man presents with a 3-day history of vomiting and constipation on a background of altered bowel habit for 2–3 months. The diagnosis of bowel obstruction is made and the decision taken that the patient requires urgent laparotomy.

Before going for surgery a full assessment of the patient's fluid and electrolyte status must be undertaken.

- a full history is taken from the patient including severity and amount of vomiting, feelings of thirst, and amount of urine being passed
- examination should look for evidence of fluid depletion such as dry mouth, hypotension, and tachycardia
- investigation must include FBC (may be evidence of haemoconcentration) and U&Es.

Where there is significant fluid depletion, urea may be elevated. As fluid lost from the gastrointestinal tract is rich in electrolytes, there can be significant depletion of sodium, potassium, and chloride. These deficits should at least be partially corrected prior to surgery.

> The patient feels 'dry' and blood tests confirm dehydration (urea >10 mmol/l) and hypokalaemia (K+ <2.4 mmol/l). The patient has been catheterized and urine output is only 25–30 ml/hour. A nasogastric tube has also been passed and aspirates of 100 ml/hour are being obtained.

This man has significant pre-existing fluid and electrolyte deficits as well as continuing losses, which must be taken into account before surgery. He is initially prescribed rapid infusion (500 ml/hour) of 0.9% saline with 10 mmol of potassium per hour. Infusion pumps should always be used to administer infusions containing large quantities of potassium, to safeguard against accidental rapid infusion and potential cardiac arrythmias. He should be regularly reviewed.

> After 2 hours (1000 ml of saline) he is feeling less thirsty but he continues to have 100 ml/hour of nasogastric aspirate and urine output remains low at 30–40 ml/hour.

Given the 3-day history of vomiting, the patient could easily have a fluid deficit of several litres. Continued replacement with electrolyte-containing fluid is required.

> A further 2 litres of 0.9% saline and 1 litre of 5% dextrose is prescribed with each 500 ml bag containing 10 mmol of potassium. The fluid is to be given at a rate of 250 ml/hour for the first 4 hours, then the rate is to be reviewed.

The patient must be reviewed regularly to ensure continued improvement. If he continued to be oliguric despite fluid replacement then discussion with senior staff regarding placement of a central venous catheter and involvement of the renal physicians would be required.

> At his next review the patient is feeling better. His urine output has improved to 50–70 ml/hour and it looks less concentrated. He still has nasogastric aspirate of 50–100 ml/hour. U&Es have been re-checked and the results show the urea has fallen to 7 mmol/l and the potassium has increased to 3.2 mmol/l. The surgeons are now keen to take the patient to theatre for a laparotomy.

In theatre, the anaesthetist continues to replace normal maintenance and ongoing losses. This is usually done using Hartmann's solution, which is isotonic with extracellular fluid.

The patient has diverticulitis and undergoes a Hartmann's procedure. The operation takes 2 hours and blood loss is minimal. While in theatre he receives 2500 ml of Hartmann's solution. Urine output remains at about 70 ml/hour. The anaesthetist prescribes 500 ml of 0.9% saline over 4 hours (125 ml/h) and then asks that the patient is reviewed before further prescription is made.

TABLE 2.2e   A method of calculating fluid balance (per 24 hours)

	Volume (ml)
Insensible losses	
Respiratory	400
Skin/sweat	500
Faeces	100
Urine	1500
Total	**2500**
Abnormal losses	
Drains	Measure
Stomas/fistulae	Measure
Vomit/nasogastric aspirate	Measure
Other losses (diarrhoea)	Measure
Total	**May be litres**
Input	
Food	800
Metabolism	400
Water	1300

> The patient initially does well. However, on his second postoperative day he is noted to have a falling urine output and continued large nasogastric aspirates. His stoma has had only minimal output. A full assessment of the patient is required. Fluid balance charts must be inspected to ensure that all losses (nasogastric, urine, stoma, and insensible losses) are being measured.

Patients with pyrexia have greater insensible losses and 'third space' losses (into the gut, wounds) must also be estimated.

Considerable losses of electrolyte-rich fluid can occur from gastrointestinal secretions, which are sequestered into the gut lumen during obstruction. In this case the diagnosis is a postoperative ileus.

The patient is prescribed increased IV fluid in the meantime. As well as normal maintenance of 2–2.5 litres/24 hours, he needs extra electrolyte-rich fluid at the rate of his nasogastric aspirate with an extra 20–30 ml/hour for other gastrointestinal and 'third space' loss.

In most cases postoperative ileus will settle within 2–3 days.

In patients who are fasting, fluid normally obtained from food and drink must be given by the IV route. As well as water there is a requirement for electrolytes (sodium, potassium, chloride). Appropriate crystalloid fluids should be used for fluid replacement—usually 0.9% saline or Hartmann's solution with 5% dextrose (acts as water only).

Clinical key points in oliguria

- The early identification and treatment of patients with oliguria may prevent the development of acute renal failure

- History, examination, and investigation are the key to successful management

- Always rule out urinary obstruction (including blocked catheters) as a cause of oliguria

- The commonest cause of oliguria in the postoperative period is hypovolaemia

- A urinary catheter should be placed to monitor urinary output in response to treatment

- In patients with a history of cardiac disease or the elderly a central venous catheter may be required to monitor CVP response to fluid challenge

Fluid required = pre-existing deficit + normal maintenance + ongoing losses

Background: postoperative oliguria

Postoperative oliguria may be defined as:

- **a urinary output of less than 20 ml/hour (in adults).**

Early identification of patients with low urine output, and appropriate intervention may prevent the development of renal failure. However, especially in the elderly, over-enthusiastic intervention without appropriate monitoring may precipitate heart failure.

Again it is important to be aware of those patients '*at risk*' of developing problems with renal function in the perioperative period:

- major elective surgery (especially aortic surgery, hepatic surgery, pancreatic surgery)

- emergency surgery especially if there is preoperative sepsis/shock

- patients with low cardiac output states (arrhythmias, heart failure)

- patients with potential hypovolaemia (blood loss, massive gastrointestinal losses)

- patients receiving certain drugs with the potential to cause renal problems (aminoglycosides, NSAIDs, angiotensin-converting enzyme inhibitors, diuretics).

Ideally most of these 'high-risk' patients will have been identified preoperatively and will have had a CVP line inserted to guide fluid therapy. The patient should be well hydrated pre- and postoperatively. Giving 'at-risk' patients any nephrotoxic drugs or even worse, more than one (i.e. gentamicin and ibuprofen) is clearly inadvisable.

Aetiology

The causes of oliguria can usefully be thought of as:

1. *Pre-renal*. This is the commonest cause of postoperative oliguria and is due to relative underperfusion of the kidney as a result of hypovolaemia.

2. *Renal*. The result of intrinsic damage to the kidney leading to acute tubular necrosis (ATN). May be due to renal ischaemia (underperfusion of the kidney due to hypovolaemia or sepsis) or to nephrotoxicity (e.g. gentamicin, NSAIDs). ATN is the second most common cause of oliguria postoperatively.

3. *Postrenal*. Caused by obstruction to renal outflow (**blocked catheter**, more rarely due to compression of ureters by intra-abdominal mass, large prostate gland).

The management of the oliguric patient will depend on identification of the problem (or those at risk) and frequent assessment of the patient and the effect of any interventions.

Identify/quantify

History

Ask the patient how they feel, e.g. they may feel thirsty or dry. Ask the nurse in charge for any relevant information. Look at drug charts to ensure no potentially nephrotoxic drugs (gentamicin, NSAIDs) have been given. Finally look at the fluid balance charts and add up the input and the (total) output.

Examination

A thorough assessment of the patient is required. Look for dry mucous membranes, check the BP and heart rate. Hypotension and tachycardia may suggest hypovolaemia or sepsis.

Listen to the heart (triple rhythm) and lungs (crepitations) for any evidence of fluid overload. Increased respiratory rate and arrhythmias may be suggestive of sepsis.

Check any monitoring the patient has, e.g. pulse oximetry. The patient should be catheterized if this has not already been performed and patency of the urinary catheter should be checked (by flushing).

If the patient has a central venous line this should be checked, the pressure measured, and any trend up or down noted.

Investigations

Check the Hb, U&Es (serum potassium, urea, and creatinine may all be elevated in renal failure).

Arterial blood gases should be taken, as a metabolic acidosis can develop in renal failure and hypoxia can itself lead to renal compromise.

It may also be useful to send urine to the laboratory for measurement of urinary osmolality and urinary sodium. This helps to distinguish between pre-renal causes of oliguria (high urinary osmolality, low urinary sodium) and ATN (low urinary osmolality and high urinary sodium), where the kidney is unable to preserve sodium and concentrate the urine.

Management

In the majority of cases postoperative oliguria is a result of hypovolaemia. Repeated assessment to guide fluid challenges is the basis of management.

If oliguria persists despite adequate fluid loading acute renal failure must be considered. Senior clinical help should be sought early in the management of patients with problems of fluid balance in the postoperative period, including advice from renal physicians.

A urine output of 0.5 ml/kg per hour (at least 30 ml urine output per hour) should be the aim of therapy. A urinary catheter, if not already present, should be passed and urine output monitored hourly.

The following is a suggested plan of management of the oliguric patient:

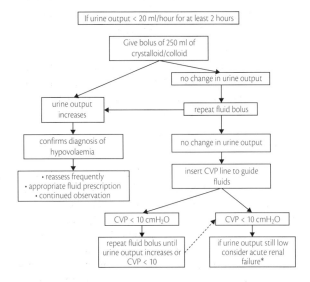

Acute tubular necrosis

Acute renal failure in the form of ATN may occur if there is persistent oliguria (20 ml/hour for 24 hours).

- In the oliguric phase there is:
  - retention of water
  - retention of sodium.
- Together these may cause left ventricular failure and pulmonary oedema:
  - retention of potassium (K^+).
- This may lead to cardiac arrhythmia and even cardiac arrest.
  - retention of H^+.
- This may precipitate a metabolic acidosis.
- Fluid and electrolyte balance must be maintained:
  - water is restricted to 400 ml/day
  - urine and gut sodium loss are measured and replaced

*Involvement by renal physicians is required for appropriate management.

- potassium intake is restricted and serum potassium is closely monitored and any abnormal rise aggressively treated with dextrose and insulin or calcium resonium

- metabolic acidosis may occur and may require sodium bicarbonate

- renal dialysis is the definitive treatment.

♦ ATN usually resolves within 1–3 weeks. If the oliguria persists then a renal biopsy is necessary to investigate the possibility of renal necrosis.

♦ As ATN recovers, there is a diuretic phase, which may last for 3–4 weeks. This is associated with sodium and potassium loss together with large volumes of water. This again mandates careful monitoring of fluid balance and U&Es.

Common postoperative electrolyte abnormalities

Hyponatraemia

This is a relatively frequent finding in the postoperative patient and is usually iatrogenic. It can occur when fluid regimens replace electrolyte-rich fluid losses (gastrointestinal tract, third space) mainly with 5% dextrose, instead of more 'physiological' sodium-containing solutions, such as Hartmann's solution.

In most postoperative patients, the metabolic response to surgery includes antidiuretic hormone secretion (producing water retention) exacerbating the imbalance.

Symptomatic hyponatraemia is unusual until serum sodium falls below 125 mmol/l when lethargy, nausea, and altered consciousness can occur. Life-threatening fits and coma can arise with plasma sodium concentration of <115 mmol/l.

Treatment consists of careful assessment of fluid balance and appropriate prescription of electrolyte containing fluids. Acute symptomatic hyponatraemia is a medical emergency and will require treatment with hypertonic saline under the auspices of senior medical staff and with appropriate monitoring.

Hypokalaemia

Hypokalaemia in the perioperative period is usually due to reduced intake and increased loss. The kidneys are less efficient at retaining potassium than sodium. During the first 24 hours after surgery, there is a shift of potassium from the intracellular to the extracellular fluid volume. After this time, potassium re-enters cells and replacement will be required (1–2 mmol/kg per 24 hours). This requirement will be increased in those

---

Fast facts—Oliguria and electrolyte disturbance

Oliguria

♦ Postoperative oliguria is defined as a urine output of <20 ml/hour

♦ Oliguria if untreated may develop into acute renal failure

Patients at risk

♦ Major elective and emergency surgery

♦ Pre-existing hypovolaemia

♦ Low cardiac output states

♦ Those receiving potentially nephrotoxic drugs

♦ **Manage along lines of IQM principle**

Identify

♦ Pre-renal (underfilling/hypoperfusion)

♦ Renal (prolonged hypoperfusion/nephrotoxic) drugs

♦ Postrenal causes (outflow obstruction/blocked catheter)

Manage

♦ Fluid challenge

♦ Invasive techniques (CVP monitoring) used to guide further therapy

♦ Acute renal failure requires help from renal physicians:

—fluid restriction

—inotropic support

—dialysis

Electrolyte disturbance

♦ Postoperative hyponatraemia is often dilutional due to replacement of electrolyte-rich losses with water (dextrose 5%)

♦ Potassium replacement

—not required in the first 24 hours

—after which 1–2 mmol/kg per 24 hours

♦ Hyperkalaemia of >6.5 mmol/l requires urgent correction: insulin with 50% dextrose

with ongoing losses from the gastrointestinal tract or to the 'third space'.

Symptoms due to hypokalaemia include loss of appetite, nausea, and cardiac conduction abnormalities with a risk of cardiac arrest.

Treatment is with potassium supplementation either intravenously (at a rate no faster than 40 mmol per hour), or orally.

Hyperkalaemia

This is occasionally seen postoperatively, often as a complication of chronic or acute renal failure. Characteristic ECG changes occur with tall, peaked T waves, widened QRS complexes, and eventually asystole.

Treatment is required urgently with serum potassium levels of >6.5 mmol/l. Potassium is driven intracellularly by giving a bolus of insulin, with 50% dextrose to prevent hypoglycaemia while giving calcium gluconate IV antagonizes the effect of low potassium on the heart. These are temporary measures and total body potassium must be reduced by using ion exchange resins (calcium resonium) or by dialysis.

Postoperative sepsis

Scenario 1: postoperative pyrexia and hypotension

> A previously healthy 35-year-old man underwent appendicectomy for a gangrenous appendix 5 days ago. The nursing staff are concerned that he has been pyrexial and hypotensive and since catheterization has a low urine output.

In all cases of hypotension management begins with checking the ABC. The findings will direct subsequent examination and investigation. **As in all cases of hypotension, give oxygen.**

> On examination the patient is found to be slightly confused. His temperature is 39°C, heart rate is 110/min and BP is 90/40 mmHg. His peripheries are warm and pulses are bounding.

This picture suggests that the patient is toxic (confused, pyrexial). His cardiovascular signs are in keeping with someone who is septic (hyperdynamic circulation). His low urine output is a worrying feature and may be due to hypovolaemia or the effect of the septic process on the kidneys.

> Although initially not catheterized over the last 8 hours he has passed only 80 ml of urine. His charts show that he has been receiving 100 ml/hour of crystalloid since returning from theatre and that he is in a positive fluid balance of 1200 ml.

In sepsis, there is marked vasodilatation and blood vessels become leaky so that fluid moves into the interstitial spaces causing intravascular hypovolaemia. Fluid requirements may therefore be very high. It will be important in a case like this to monitor fluid balance carefully for although the circulation is initially hyperdynamic, factors released from cells during the septic process cause myocardial depression, and cardiac failure can ensue.

The patient should receive high flow oxygen by face mask. An examination of his chest and abdomen should be made to detect any signs of an infective process.

Blood should be taken for haematology (high white count in sepsis) and for U&Es to check the renal function (high urea and creatinine). Blood cultures should also be taken and if there is any sputum that should be sent for culture also.

Best guess antibiotic therapy can then be commenced and altered after the results of investigation if necessary. The patient should be catheterized in order to monitor response to a fluid challenge (rapid infusion of a crystalloid bolus). If this fails to improve BP and urine output a further bolus may be given but caution is required. Insertion of a central venous catheter may be necessary in order to prevent the development of pulmonary oedema. Discuss with senior medical staff to ensure appropriate management.

> The results of blood tests show that the patient has a high white count (18 × 10⁹/l) and a high urea (9.5 mmol/l). On examination his abdomen is extremely tender in the region of his wound. His urine output improves slightly following a 500 ml bolus of normal saline, but he remains hypotensive. After discussion with senior medical staff it is felt he may have a pelvic abscess and an abdominal CT scan confirms this. A percutaneous drain is inserted into the abscess radiologically to drain the pus collection.

Scenario 2: pyrexia, tachypnoea, and tachycardia

A 73-year-old patient is 5 days postoperative following an oversew of a perforated duodenal ulcer. He has made a slow recovery with a prolonged postoperative ileus, is on IV fluids, and has a urinary catheter *in situ*. He complains of right shoulder tip pain and on examination has a temperature of 38°C, respiratory rate of 20/min, tachycardia of 110/min, and decreased air entry in the right basal lung field.

The rising temperature and respiratory rate suggest infection. The potential sites of infection are (in order) respiratory, abdominal (subphrenic), and urinary.

Pain in the shoulder tip should alert you to the possibility of a subphrenic abscess, as the diaphragm is supplied by the phrenic nerve, which can be irritated by the abscess. The phrenic nerve 'refers' the pain to the shoulder as it shares the same root value as the dermatomes of the shoulder (C3, C4, C5). **High flow oxygen should be given**. Bloods should be checked (FBC, U&Es, LFTS, glucose), blood, sputum, and urine sent for culture and sensitivity, and an erect CXR ordered.

Clinical key points in postoperative sepsis

- Early identification of the possibility of sepsis is important

- All patients with hypotension should have high flow oxygen

- On detection of sepsis, search for a source of infection (respiratory, abdominal, urine, blood)

- Treat the complications of sepsis (organ dysfunction or shock) promptly with correct fluid management, oxygen, and appropriate antibiotics

- Pain in the shoulder tip is suggestive of a subphrenic abscess in a septic patient

- CT scan of the abdomen is a useful investigation to exclude an intra-abdominal abscess

- Deal with the source of the infection (e.g. percutaneous drains)

The WCC is elevated at $20 \times 10^9/l$, and CXR shows a raised right hemidiaphragm with right basal atelectasis. The patient was commenced on IV co-amoxiclav and metronidazole and an oral contrast CT scan requested.

These results would be compatible with an infection either from the lungs or from the abdomen (subphrenic abscess). A broad-spectrum antibiotic regimen is started to cover a wide range of anaerobic and aerobic organisms, as the clinical picture is of sepsis (although there is as yet no proven organism). **The CT scan will help determine whether there is a subphrenic collection** (abscess) and also if there is any ongoing leak from the oversewn perforated duodenal ulcer.

Two hours later his urine output falls to 15 ml/hour. He is given a fluid bolus challenge of 200 ml gelofusine but over the next hour his urine output remains at 8 ml/hour. In view of this a central venous catheter is inserted and the CVP is measured at 6 cmH$_2$O. He is given a further bolus of 1 litre of gelofusine over 4 hours and his urine output increases to 30 ml/hour. Bacteriology phone to confirm the presence of *E. coli* in the blood culture.

The presence of infection (*E. coli*) confirms the clinical suspicion of sepsis (SIRS plus proven infection). As this has been associated with an organ dysfunction (renal dysfunction with decreased urine output), this is severe sepsis.

The CT scan shows a large right subphrenic abscess with no ongoing leak from the duodenum. The abscess was drained percutaneously by the radiologist and a drain left in the right subphrenic abscess. The pus sent from the subphrenic abscess also grew *E. coli*. Following drainage of the abscess, the patient made a satisfactory recovery.

Background: postoperative sepsis

Despite apparent improvements in the care of the critically ill patient, the mortality from severe sepsis remains high (40% of patients with septic shock die). Severe sepsis and septic shock in the postoperative patient remain a clinical challenge, with the source of infection coming from various sites—the most common sources being:

- surgical wounds
- chest
- intra-abdominal collection
- central venous lines
- urine.

The earliest manifestation of sepsis is a systemic response to the infection, called the systemic inflammatory response syndrome (SIRS).

Systemic inflammatory response syndrome

SIRS is a systemic response to a number of clinical problems that induce an inflammatory response, including pancreatitis, peritonitis, ischaemia, and severe trauma. The mediators of this response include:

- cytokines (e.g. tumour necrosis factor, interleukins 1, 6, and 8)
- complement
- leukotrienes and proteases.

These mediators interact with various cellular systems (e.g. macrophages, neutrophils, platelets, lymphocytes) to produce a complex inflammatory response. This response produces changes in the body, manifest by various clinical parameters, allowing assessment as to whether a patient has SIRS. These parameters include:

- *respiratory rate* (≥20 breaths/min)
- *temperature* (≥38°C)
- *pulse* (≥90 b.p.m.)
- *white cell count* (≥12 or ≤4).

The presence of two or more of the above parameters defines the presence of SIRS. Once SIRS is established, several systemic changes occur, including:

- loss of microvascular integrity and increased vascular permeability
- systemic vasodilatation
- depression of myocardial contractility
- poor oxygen delivery and increased tissue oxygen debt
- increased microvascular clotting.

If the SIRS response is related to a proven infection (e.g. urinary or respiratory), then this is termed sepsis, i.e. **SEPSIS is SIRS in the presence of a proven infection**. If this sepsis is severe then in conjunction with the above systemic changes, certain vital end organs can be affected by relative underperfusion, leading to dysfunction of the organ. These organs include:

- brain (confusion and altered mental state)
- kidneys (reduced urine output)
- lungs (hypoxaemia and pulmonary consolidation, pulmonary oedema)
- liver (jaundice and deranged clotting)
- gastrointestinal tract (stress ulceration).

Once several organs are affected by the process, this is termed multiorgan dysfunction, which carries an extremely high mortality (98% mortality if three organs are affected). The following standard terminology is recommended:

- *sepsis*: SIRS resulting from proven infection
- *severe sepsis*: associated with organ dysfunction, hypoperfusion, or hypotension. Examples of perfusion abnormalities include: oliguria, metabolic acidosis, or altered mental state
- *septic shock*: severe sepsis with hypotension (i.e. systolic BP <90 mmHg) with no other cause for hypotension, despite adequate fluid loading.

TABLE 2.2f The mortality rates for the above 'grades' of SIRS

	SIRS	Sepsis	Severe sepsis	Septic shock
Mortality rate (%)	7	15	20	40

The poor outlook that occurs once septic shock and multiorgan dysfunction syndrome develop, makes it very important to identify sepsis early, before the problem cascades. This should be done by a process of early identification, quantification, and management, as in previous sections.

Identification

Maintain a high index of suspicion in the postoperative patient, and look out for patients who may be exhibiting early signs of sepsis, i.e. SIRS. Be aware of any patient with two or more of the following signs, who by definition have SIRS:

- fever or hypothermia (the latter due to heat loss secondary to peripheral vasodilation)
- leucocytosis or leucopenia
- tachycardia
- tachypnoea.

In addition to the above, it is important to check for signs of dysfunction of the more important organs, such as the brain, kidneys, lungs, and the heart. Check each of these organs, looking for signs such as altered mental state, oliguria, hypoxaemia, and hypotension, respectively. Having identified a potential problem, the next step is to quantify the problem.

Quantification

History and examination

Ask the patient about any respiratory or urinary symptoms. Examine the patient's chest, abdomen, urine, and peripheral or central lines (e.g. thrombophlebitis) for any obvious source of infection. Examine the calves for any evidence of a deep vein thrombosis (DVT), as this may also present as a postoperative pyrexia.

Action

1. Check for any site of infection—this will include looking at:

   ◆ blood (cultures samples should be taken from peripheral blood and from central lines if present)

   ◆ urine, chest, and wound (send urine, wound, and sputum for Gram stain and culture).

   If the patient is already on antibiotics, send a stool sample to exclude *C. difficile* (the cause of pseudomembranous colitis).

2. Take blood samples for:

   ◆ FBC (including platelet count) and clotting studies; thrombocytopenia, coagulopathy, raised or decreased white cell all suggest sepsis

   ◆ check the C-reactive protein (inflammatory markers)

   ◆ U&Es, blood sugar

   ◆ LFTs

   ◆ blood gases (may show hypoxaemia—due to poor organ perfusion, acidosis).

   There may be evidence of renal impairment, hyperglycaemia, low albumin, impaired liver function (clotting abnormalities with a raised prothrombin time), or hypoxaemia.

3. Erect CXR. Remember that the CXR may be normal in patients with early adult respiratory distress syndrome even though they may be tachypnoeic and hypoxaemic—the radiological signs of adult respiratory distress syndrome follow on after the clinical signs. The X-ray is taken erect to look for air under the diaphragm (pneumoperitoneum).

4. Once cultured, commence best guess antibiotics, while awaiting sensitivities. Co-amoxiclav with metronidazole is a good best-guess combination. If necessary you may need to consider an aminoglycoside such as gentamicin—starting with a loading dose unless there is significant renal impairment. It is important to check the gentamicin levels 6–14 hours postdose, and to check on a gentamicin nomogram (such as the Hartford nomogram) to determine the time interval between doses of gentamicin. *(These nomograms should be available on the ward or from the bacteriology department, with whom it is important to liaise.)*

5. The patient may require further imaging studies (such as CT scan of the abdomen in the patient scenario), to identify possible causes of infection such as subphrenic abscess or pelvic abscess, which can occur in patients following abdominal surgery.

Having identified and quantified the problem, a management plan for sepsis is needed.

Management

The management of septic patients can be divided into supportive measures and specific measures. The supportive measures are designed to preserve organ function while specific measures deal with the underlying cause.

Supportive measures—it is important to support the vital organs in patients with severe sepsis, including the lungs, kidneys, and cardiovascular system.

Respiratory support: oxygenation

It is critical to ensure adequate oxygenation and ventilation. The hypoxaemia that is common in the early stages of sepsis can usually be overcome by using high flow face mask oxygen therapy. The response can be judged by pulse oximetry and arterial blood gas analysis. If the response to high flow oxygen is inadequate, continuous positive airway pressure provided by face mask at a pressure of usually 5–10 cmH$_2$O may help. If respiratory failure is severe, then endotracheal intubation and ventilatory support in the ICU will be required.

◆ **i.e. high flow oxygen → continuous positive airway pressure if required → intermittent positive pressure ventilation if required.**

Renal support: adequate urine output

A urine output of at least 0.5–1 ml/kg/hour should be maintained, and if not already present the patient should be catheterized to accurately assess the urine output. If the kidney is underperfused, ATN may occur (see section on fluid balance on p. 145, and note the differences between pre-renal and renal failure).

Tachycardia, hypotension, and oliguria should be treated by administering a fluid bolus in the first instance—usually with a bolus of 250 ml of crystalloid (e.g. normal saline or Hartmann's solution). If there is no response to two to three boluses of crystalloid, then a CVP line should be inserted, by either an internal jugular or subclavian route. If the CVP is low (<5 cmH$_2$O) in association with tachycardia, hypotension, and oliguria more fluid is required. Further boluses of fluid are given and the effect on the above parameters is observed.

If an adequate CVP is reached (e.g. 10–12 cmH$_2$O) and the patient remains hypotensive, then inotropes, such as dopamine or noradrenaline, should be considered. This will have to be done in either a HDU (High Dependency Unit) or ITU (Intensive Care Unit) setting. It is common to guide inotrope therapy either with a pulmonary artery catheter or oesophageal Doppler to measure cardiac output and systemic vascular resistance.

If severe oliguria persists despite adequate fluid loading and good peripheral perfusion, 20 mg IV frusemide may be given. It is important that frusemide is withheld until there is adequate fluid loading (as frusemide can be nephrotoxic).

Cardiovascular support

Basic cardiovascular monitoring of heart rate, BP, and hourly urine output should be commenced. It is important to establish the cardiac rhythm, as any change from sinus rhythm may indicate sepsis. One of the commonest problems seen in these patients is the development of AF. If the ventricular rate response to AF is high ('fast AF') and the BP compromised, then the patient may be given amiodarone 200 mg slow IV bolus. Should the AF persist, the patient should be commenced on IV digoxin.

More invasive monitoring of the patient's cardiovascular system would include inserting a central venous line (via the internal jugular vein or subclavian) and an arterial line (a small venous cannula inserted into the radial artery). The arterial line can be connected via a transducer to obtain direct intra-arterial measurement of the BP and also gives access for repeated blood gas analysis. Monitoring of cardiac output is by pulmonary artery flotation catheter or oesophageal Doppler.

Other systems that need support

1. *Coagulopathy.* Disseminated intravascular coagulation may occur in sepsis. Management consists of removal of the source of the sepsis along with treatment with fresh frozen plasma, platelets, cryopre-

cipitate, DeFIX (activated Factor IX) and other factors as directed by coagulation tests. Vitamin K may be required in patients with a prolonged INR.

2. *Gastrointestinal bleeding.* Stress ulceration may occur in uncontrolled sepsis. IV H$_2$ blockers such as ranitidine or oral cytoprotective drugs such as sucralfate are effective.

3. *Nutrition* (see section on Nutrition on p. 152). Severe sepsis produces an increase in energy expenditure and is associated with a hypercatabolic state, which can lead to breakdown of protein and a negative nitrogen balance. The negative nitrogen balance can be minimized by nutritional support, preferably by the enteral route (via a small bore nasogastric or nasojejunal 'clinifeed' tube), but total parenteral nutrition given via a central venous line may be required. Total parenteral nutrition is indicated in cases of gastrointestinal tract obstruction, mesenteric ischaemia, and short bowel syndrome. Enteral nutrition is the preferred route and has been shown to reduce mortality in trauma and surgical patients.

Specific measures

Once the sepsis has been identified and quantified, the other aspect of management of sepsis is in the control of the source of the sepsis.

If the source of the sepsis is the chest, then in addition to antibiotics, chest physiotherapy is useful to clear infected sputum from the lungs. Occasionally the thickened secretions need to be cleared by bronchial toilet, and if severe a bronchoscopy may be indicated to clear the main bronchial tree.

If the source of the sepsis is within the abdomen, then prompt management of intra-abdominal prob-

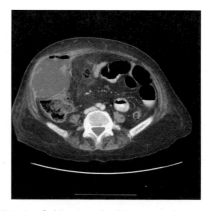

Fig 2.2j CT scan of a large pericolic abscess secondary to caecal cancer.

Fast facts—Postoperative sepsis (infection after an operation)

- **SIRS**—earliest stage, presence of two or more of the following:
  - —fever
  - —tachycardia
  - —tachypnoea
  - —raised WCC
- **Sepsis**—SIRS with proven infection
- **Severe sepsis**—sepsis with organ dysfunction
- **Septic shock**—sepsis with hypoperfusion
- **Multiorgan dysfunction syndrome**—sepsis with multiorgan dysfunction
- **Organs to be aware of**
  - —brain
  - —lungs
  - —heart
  - —kidneys
- **Manage along lines of IQM**

Investigations

- High index of suspicion in any patient with SIRS

Quantify

- Examine vital organs and their function
- Check FBC, U&Es, glucose, arterial blood gases, clotting studies
- Culture—blood, urine, wound swabs
- Consider CXR/CT scan of the abdomen

Management

- High flow oxygen (ill patients need oxygen)
- Start best-guess antibiotics (e.g. co-amoxiclav and metronidazole) till cultures available
- Monitor urine output, BP, pulse, ± CVP, oxygen saturation
- Inotropes if normal CVP and hypotensive
- Treat cause of sepsis
  - —antibiotics and physiotherapy for respiratory source
  - —drainage of abdominal abscess
- Renal replacement therapy if ATN develops

lems should be undertaken—a CT scan is a useful investigation to look for intra-abdominal abscesses (seen as a collection of fluid, occasionally with gas in the fluid, due to the presence of gas forming organisms) (Fig. 2.2j)—these collections can be drained either by percutaneous insertion of drains radiologically or by a repeat laparotomy.

Other potential problems may be due to the type of operation that the patient has had, e.g. if the patient has had an anastomosis performed (such as in anterior resection of the rectum), then this anastomosis may dehisce ('fall apart'), in which case the patient will develop signs of peritonism and sepsis. The anastomosis can be checked by performing a single contrast enema, which may show a leak of contrast at the anastomosis. If a leak is confirmed, then the patient needs an urgent laparotomy, to take down the anastomosis and form a temporary colostomy (in the case of a colorectal anastomosis).

Remember that any delay in the treatment of postoperative sepsis may result in the downward spiral of sepsis, leading to severe sepsis, multiorgan failure, and death. Always be on the lookout for early sign of SIRS, and consider these patients to have sepsis till proven otherwise.

Deep vein thrombosis and pulmonary embolism

Scenario 1: postoperative painful swollen calf

Seven days following a colectomy for colonic cancer a 56-year-old lady complains of a painful, swollen calf. There is no history of trauma.

The complaint of a **painful swollen calf** in the postoperative period indicates the possibility of a postoperative DVT. This patient has risk factors which would predispose the patient to a DVT—trauma/operation, underlying malignancy, and bed rest. History of local trauma or tripping may indicate a muscle haematoma due to direct injury or muscle tear.

On examination the patient has a low-grade pyrexia and the calf is hot, swollen, and tender. Measurement of the calves shows a 6 cm difference in circumference.

The triad (heat, swelling, and pain) is typical of a DVT. The heat and pain are due to inflammation, and the swelling due to oedema and venous obstruction. The swelling can be objectively assessed by measuring the circumference of the calf at a defined distance from the tibial tuberosity.

These findings can be viewed as a 'late' sign and are caused by the intraluminal thrombus promoting vein wall inflammation. This implies a degree of fixation of the thrombus to the vein wall, which may reduce the likelihood of embolization.

Diagnosing DVT clinically can be difficult. Only 50% of patients with a clinically apparent DVT, actually have one. Furthermore, when a DVT is present, 50% are 'silent' (i.e. no clinical signs).

> A duplex ultrasound is obtained and shows a thrombus (Fig. 2.2k).

Duplex scan is the first investigation of choice. Duplex scanning is a combination of colour Doppler ultrasound and B-mode ultrasound (see Vascular investigation on p. 102, p. 116).

> The patient is treated with low molecular weight heparin and oral anticoagulation (warfarin) is started.

Patients with DVT are treated by anticoagulation, initially by injection (low molecular weight heparin) to allow the oral medication (warfarin) to achieve therapeutic levels. Oral anticoagulation continues for 3 months.

Anticoagulation reduces the risk of thrombosis propagation into more proximal veins, PE, and the incidence of chronic venous insufficiency. The latter is also assisted by wearing support stockings to aid venous return and function.

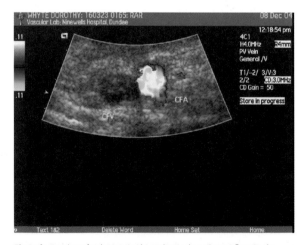

Fig 2.2k Duplex of a deep vein thrombosis showing no flow in the femoral vein (grey) with blood flow in the femoral artery flow (colour).

Scenario 2

> Six days following an aortic aneurysm repair a patient becomes hypotensive and hypoxic.

This patient is severely ill and their life is at risk. Follow ABC with a particular emphasis on giving oxygen. The first task is resuscitation, then diagnosis; the latter requires positive exclusion of a number of potential diagnoses. The key ones are dealt with in the accompanying chapters.

> On examination the patient's BP is 85/40, with an oxygen saturation of 89%. The patient is confused but otherwise the examination is unremarkable. The legs are normal.

This history and findings can represent a massive PE. The investigation of choice depends on the presenting symptoms. **Haemodynamic upset indicates that the thrombus is interfering with the outflow from the right side of the heart.**

> A contrast-enhanced CT of the chest is obtained. This shows a blood clot in the main branches of the pulmonary artery (Fig. 2.2l).

A **contrast-enhanced chest CT is** rapid and gives a prompt diagnosis in a life-threatening situation and allows appropriate therapy to start. A large PE can block the major branches of the pulmonary artery, reducing the outflow of the right side of the heart, leading to hypotension and signs of right heart failure.

These large emboli can be seen easily on a CT scan. More often the emboli are smaller, and beyond the

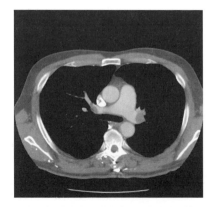

Fig 2.2l CT scan of pulmonary embolus with darker thrombus within the lighter contrast-enhanced pulmonary arteries.

major branches of the pulmonary arterial outflow. These emboli tend not to cause hypotension, but clinically can infarct segments of the lung. This may result in pleuritic chest pain (catching chest pain with inspiration), haemoptysis, and hypoxia. These smaller emboli can be difficult to see on a CT scan and in these patients a **VQ (isotope ventilation/perfusion) scan** is appropriate.

Unexplained oxygen desaturation, with either non-specific or no symptoms, may also indicate a PE. A high index of suspicion is required at all times in the postoperative period.

> High-dose low molecular weight heparin (200 u/kg per day) is prescribed on reasonable suspicion. Warfarin is commenced once the diagnosis is confirmed.

As with DVT, anticoagulation is the treatment. The main difference between DVT and PE treatment is

---

Clinical key points in the diagnosis of deep vein thrombosis and pulmonary embolism

- Ask about any pain and swelling of the calf. This may indicate a DVT

- The risk of a DVT is higher following pelvic or leg surgery or in cases of malignancy

- Examination of the legs should look for swelling, difference in size and tissue tension comparing the legs

- Investigation should also include pulse oximetry as a PE will reduce the O_2 saturation

- A duplex ultrasound scan is performed to examine the deep veins of the leg for venous thrombosis

- The management of DVT/PE is anticoagulation, initially with subcutaneous injections of low molecular weight heparin and in the longer-term warfarin

- In the case of suspected PE which does not cause haemodynamic compromise, a VQ radioisotope scan is indicated

- In the case of suspected massive PE causing haemodynamic upset (fall in BP) a contrast-enhanced CT of the chest should be performed

- An inferior vena caval filter is indicated if anticoagulation is contraindicated or where recurrent PE occurs despite adequate anticoagulation

---

that the anticoagulation is continued for 6 months for the latter.

Proven adequate anticoagulation is usually sufficient to prevent further thrombo-embolic episodes. However, despite proven adequate anticoagulation, if further episodes of embolism occur or if anticoagulation is contraindicated (usually due to bleeding), then an **inferior vena caval filter** is indicated. This is placed via the femoral vein under radiological control to the infra-renal inferior vena cava. This acts as a barrier to catch emboli and protect the pulmonary circulation.

Background: deep vein thrombosis and pulmonary embolism

DVT is a cause for referral to hospital and a common postoperative event. Migration of the thrombus to the lungs (PE) can be fatal.

A number of factors predispose to DVT and PE. These include:

- a past history of venous thrombo-embolism

- a history of recent trauma, surgery (especially major joint replacement, peripheral vascular reconstruction, and surgery for cancer—after surgery, there is increased activation of the coagulation system for at least 10 days)

- immobility

- pregnancy

- malignant disease.

Up to half of DVTs are silent. Lower limb DVT is responsible for more than 90% of pulmonary emboli, but is clinically apparent at the time of the pulmonary emboli in only 10% of patients.

Fresh thrombus is soft, friable, and may for most of its length be free floating. It is only when the inflammatory change associated with early organization of thrombus occurs that the clinical symptoms develop. It is this process that attaches the thrombus to the vein wall. Asymptomatic pulmonary emboli occur in about 50% of clinically diagnosed proximal DVTs and 30% of isolated calf vein thrombosis.

Classically, venous thrombosis is due to interplay between three factors (Virchow's triad):

1. reduced blood flow through the vein

2. vein wall damage, and

3. hypercoagulable blood.

The first and last are the most important. DVT occurring with no obvious predisposing factors can be the result of a primary hypercoagulable state (*thrombo-philia*). The body has a number of mechanisms to prevent unwanted coagulation. Disorder of these can result in a hypercoagulable state.

Identify
Clinical features

1. *Deep vein thrombosis.* While DVT can often be asymptomatic, the main symptoms of lower limb DVT are calf pain and swelling. Signs include pitting oedema, tenderness, erythema, increased temperature, and dilated collateral superficial veins. Extensive iliofemoral DVT may rarely be complicated by the development of phlegmasia alba dolens ('painful white leg'), phlegmasia cerulea dolens ('painful blue leg') or progress to venous gangrene.

   Phlegmasia alba dolens (painful white leg) is characterized by a swollen, painful, pale limb. The pallor is due to the acute oedema. It may progress to phlegmasia cerulea dolens (painful blue leg); this usually occurs in patients with an advanced malignancy. Twelve to 40% develop pulmonary emboli and half will progress to venous gangrene with an overall mortality of 20%.

2. *Pulmonary emboli.* Pulmonary emboli may present with acute onset dyspnoea, pleuritic chest pain, and haemoptysis. However, it is not uncommon for pulmonary emboli to cause very little in the way of symptoms or signs. Postoperative pulmonary emboli may present as confusion, tachypnoea, or even a patient not progressing in an expected manner.

   Clinical signs may include low-grade pyrexia, cyanosis, tachycardia, hypotension, and a raised jugular venous pulse.

   Massive pulmonary emboli may present as sudden cardiovascular collapse and cardiac arrest. Initially, it can be very difficult to differentiate between a pulmonary embolism and a myocardial infarction.

Quantify
Investigation of lower limb deep vein thrombosis

It is important not only to make a correct diagnosis of deep venous thrombosis and pulmonary emboli, but also to define the site/extent of the problem. If the condition is suspected then the patient is protected from any potential deterioration by anticoagulation.

Venous duplex ultrasonography has become the investigation of choice for potential DVT. B-mode ultrasound shows a black and white picture of the vein, when the thrombus within the lumen can be seen. The thrombus

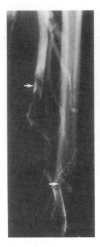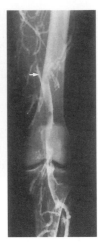

Fig 2.2m Selected venograms showing 'intraluminal filling defects' which, in the vascular system, are diagnostic of acute thrombosis as outlined by radiographic contrast material (arrows). These are examples of extensive deep venous thrombosis involving the infrapopliteal veins of the calf, the popliteal vein, and the deep venous system of the thigh. The 'propagating tail' of the thrombus is identified in the mid-thigh.

also prevents the ultrasound probe compressing the vein. Colour flow Doppler shows flow in the vein, and with DVT there is interference of flow through the vein.

An ascending venogram is invasive and is a second line investigation in cases where duplex ultrasonography is inadequate or unavailable. It visualizes from the tibial veins to inferior vena cava. Thrombosis is seen as a filling defect within the deep veins (Fig. 2.2m). Complications of phlebography are contrast reactions, DVT, and pulmonary embolus.

Investigation of pulmonary embolus

Low oxygen saturation is probably the commonest initial finding raising the possibility of a pulmonary embolus. Pulmonary embolus may not be clinically apparent and as a result in high-risk specialities (e.g. vascular surgery) oxygen saturation measurement is included in the routine nursing observation.

Arterial blood gas analysis can show a degree of hypoxia and hypocapnoea (a reduction in pCO_2), due to tachypnoea.

Plain CXR is rarely diagnostic of PE, but is of use in order to exclude other pathology (such as pulmonary collapse secondary to bronchial plugs).

Non-specific changes such as evidence of right heart strain and/or ischaemia with or without T-wave inversion should be sought. The classic pattern S1–Q3–T3

TABLE 2.2g

	Ventilation deficit	Circulation deficit
Moderate PE	No	Yes
Pneumonia	Yes	No
PE	No	Yes
Normal	No	No

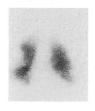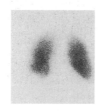

Fig 2.2n Perfusion–ventilation scintigrams using $^{99}Tc^m$-macroaggregated albumin and $^{81}Kr^m$ gas, respectively. The labelled macroaggregates stick in the pulmonary capillary bed. The pair of scintigrams show an unmatched perfusion defect typical of a pulmonary embolus in the right mid-zone.

(S-wave in lead I, Q and T-waves in lead III) is occasionally seen. The main purpose of an ECG is to rule out a myocardial infarction.

CT may also allow rapid diagnosis of pulmonary emboli in cases of haemodynamic upset. Its accuracy is almost equal to the more invasive pulmonary arteriography. As it identifies clots within the first few divisions of the pulmonary artery it is not recommended when the emboli are thought to lie more peripherally.

Pulmonary radioisotope ventilation perfusion scan (VQ scan) is a radioisotope scan. Two isotopes are used: technetium-labelled microspheres are injected and are distributed by the circulation. The second part is the inhalation of radioactive gas or aerosol.

VQ scans are notorious for being unhelpful in a significant number of cases (Fig. 2.2n). A recent CXR is required as areas of collapse and consolidation may produce a similar appearance. It is therefore most helpful in the presence of a normal CXR.

Pulmonary arteriography is the 'gold standard' for the diagnosis of pulmonary emboli. If available (uncommonly) and there is profound cardiovascular collapse or hypotension this is the first-line investigation. Emboli cause intraluminal filling defects and loss of branches of the pulmonary arterial tree. It also allows the delivery of targeted thrombolysis.

Management
Treatment
The aim of the treatment of DVT is threefold:

- reduction of the risk of PE
- prevention of the propagation of the thrombosis, and
- aiding the resolution of the thrombus to minimize any post-thrombotic syndrome.

The usual treatment of DVT is anticoagulation, limb elevation, and compression stockings. Anticoagulant therapy reduces further thrombosis, enabling the body to dissolve the clot.

Wearing below-knee compression stockings has been shown to halve the incidence of 'postphlebitic limb' after iliofemoral thrombosis.

Low molecular weight heparin is given for a minimum of 6 days and until warfarin has produced an INR of >2.0 for 2 consecutive days.

Warfarin is continued for a minimum of 3 months with an INR of 2.0–4.5. This reduces the risk of recurrent DVT or PE from 80% to 5%.

The mortality rate in patients with symptomatic PE is 30% without treatment and 2% with treatment. In a patient with suspected PE oxygen should be administered and the patient treated with low molecular weight heparin prior to investigation.

If PE is confirmed and the patient is stable, anticoagulation should be continued and oral anticoagulants (i.e. warfarin) commenced. Both methods of anticoagulation should be used till the oral anticoagulation is in the therapeutic range. Oral anticoagulation is required for 6–12 months.

Anticoagulation
Three forms of anticoagulation are available:

- unfractionated heparin
- low molecular weight heparin, and
- warfarin.

Unfractionated heparin was the first line of treatment, but has now been superseded by low molecular weight heparin. The principal mode of action is by increasing the binding of coagulation factors.

IV administration is effective immediately and has a half-life of 90 minutes. Subcutaneous administration is as effective and safe as IV unfractionated heparin, peaks at 4–6 hours, and lasts for about 12 hours.

The bleeding risk with IV unfractionated heparin is about 10% after 5–10 days of treatment. The anticoagulant effect is reversed by administering IV protamine.

Heparin-induced thrombocytopenia may develop some days after starting heparin, due to heparin-associated antiplatelet antibodies. Therefore the platelet count should be monitored in patients requiring heparin for more than 5 days.

Low molecular weight heparin binds with factor Xa. The treatment does not require monitoring, except in renal failure (low molecular weight heparin is excreted by the kidneys).

Low molecular weight heparin and warfarin are started together and low molecular weight heparin is stopped when the INR is therapeutic. Bleeding complications are fewer with low molecular weight heparin compared with unfractionated heparin, although the platelet count should be monitored (the incidence of heparin-induced thrombocytopenia is about 1%).

Warfarin reduces the activity of the vitamin K-dependent coagulation factors. Warfarin has a half-life of 36–40 hours. A reduced dose may be required in patients with liver failure, and in patients receiving parenteral nutrition and antibiotics.

As thrombin has a half-life of 36 hours warfarin is therefore ineffective for about 48 hours. Warfarin initially leads to a temporary hypercoagulable state for approximately 24–72 hours. The target INR should be 2.0–4.0.

Lifetime warfarin should be considered for patients with a second venous thromboembolus, those with thrombophilia (increased tendency to clot), and patients with a first venous thromboembolus and malignancy, until the latter has been eradicated. The risk of major bleeding with therapeutic warfarin therapy is approximately 0.5–1% per month rising with age.

Inferior vena caval filtration

An inferior vena caval filter is designed to simply catch the clot on the way from the lower body to the lungs.

Inferior vena caval filters are placed percutaneously under local anaesthesia via the common femoral, internal jugular, or antecubital vein. The filter is normally positioned in the infrarenal vena cava but it can be sited above the renal veins if necessary.

Absolute indications for insertion of an inferior vena caval filter are recurrent pulmonary embolus despite proven effective anticoagulation or where anticoagulation is contraindicated due to an increased risk of bleeding.

Fast facts—Deep vein thrombosis/pulmonary embolism (blood clot within deep veins)

Epidemiology

- DVT is common in postoperative patients (10–20%); PE is a cause of sudden postoperative death (1–2%)

Predisposing factors

- ↑ age
- Malignancy
- Trauma
- Sepsis

Clinical features

DVT

- Asymptomatic
- Hot, tender, swollen calf

PE

- Confusion
- Pleuritic chest pain, haemoptysis
- Circulatory collapse

Manage along lines of IQM principle

Investigations

DVT

- Duplex scanning

PE

- Contrast-enhanced chest CT in patients with haemodynamic upset
- VQ radio-isotope scan
- ECG: S1–Q3–T3

Management

DVT

- Anticoagulation for 3 months

PE

- Anticoagulation for 6 months
- Inferior vena caval filter with recurrent PE despite anticoagulation or when anticoagulation is contraindicated

TABLE 2.2h Useful normal values

Biochemistry	
Sodium	135–147 mmol/l
Potassium	3.5–5 mmol/l
Urea	4–12 mmol/l
Creatinine	80–190 mmol/l
Albumin	36–50 g/l
Alkaline phosphatase	65–150 U/l
Bilirubin	0–17 mmol/l
Corrected calcium	2.1–2.55 mmol/l
Glucose	3.3–5.8 mmol/l
Thyroid-stimulating hormone	0.4–4 mU/l
Troponin	<0.1 mg/l
C-reactive protein	<5 mg/l
Haematology	
Hb	13–18 g/dl
White cell count (WCC)	4–11
Platelets	150–400

Index

ABC resuscitation 158–60
  airways management 160–2
  monitoring and reporting 160
  secondary survey 160
  shock management 162–4
abdominal angina 20, 27
abdominal aortic aneurysm 111–12
  popliteal artery aneurysm 112
  sudden abdominal pain and collapse
    110–11
abdominal distension
  small bowel obstruction 23
  and vomiting 18–19
abdominal pain
  acute right lower 17–18
  and constipation 34–6
  cramping 32–3
  Crohn's disease 25
  and jaundice 64–6
  recurrent 19–20
  repeated right upper 61
  severe left lower 33–4
  severe upper central 53–5
  sudden, and collapse 110–11
  upper, with vomiting 61–3
  and weight loss 20–1
abdominoperoneal resection 39
ABO groups 150
ABPI 102
abscess
  breast 82, 84
  pelvic 187
  perianal 47, 48–9
  pilonidal 49–50
  subphrenic 185, 187
achalasia 5–6
acute gastritis 14
acute haemolytic transfusion reaction
  151
acute limb ischaemia 99, 100, 105–7
acute pancreatitis 53–7, 58
acute right lower abdominal pain 17–18
acute tubular necrosis (ATN) 181, 182–3,
  187

adenocarcinoma
  colorectal tumours 36
  oesophagus 6, 7
  stomach 10, 15
adenomas
  gastric cancer 15
  hepatocellular 70
adenomatous polyps, colonic 36, 37
adhesiolysis 24
adhesions
  large bowel obstruction 44–5, 46
  small bowel obstruction 23
adult respiratory distress syndrome
  187
  aspiration of gastric contents 128
advance directives 133
airways management 159, 160–2
  equipment
    during anaesthesia 134
    postoperative 161–2
alcohol
  acute pancreatitis 54–5
  chronic pancreatitis 57, 58
  cirrhosis 69
allergic reactions to transfusion 151
alveolar–capillary perfusion barrier 172
amaurosis fugax 100, 109
ampulla of Vater, carcinoma of the
  59–61
amputation 103, 104–5
anaemia 148
anaesthesia and sedation 138, 142
  adverse transfusion reactions 151
  agitated or restless patients 141
  analgesia 138–40
  and anticoagulation prophylaxis 130
  diagnostic procedures 141–2
  general anaesthesia for a varicose
    vein operation 133–5
  history taking 125
  for a laparoscopic cholecystectomy
    136–7
  monitoring and equipment 141
  muscle relaxation 140

myocardial ischaemia/infarction risk
  178–9
postoperative care 142–4
postoperative pain prevention 143
rapid sequence induction for an
  emergency laparotomy 137–8
regional 135, 140
  myocardial ischaemia/infarction
    risk 178
  toxicity 140
risk of aspiration of gastric contents
  128–9
safe administration of intravenous
  sedation 142
sedation techniques 141
sleep 138
spinal anaesthesia for an inguinal
  hernia repair 135–6
anal cancer 39
anal fissure 46–7, 50–1
analgesia 138–40
  for a laparoscopic cholecystectomy
    136–7
  patient-controlled (PCA) 144
  postoperative pain prevention 143–4
anaphylactic shock 162, 163
  and blood transfusion 151
  hypotension 175
anaplastic carcinoma, thyroid 94
anastomosis 46
angina
  abdominal 20, 27
  preoperative assessment 125
angiodysplasia 42–3
angiography 103
angioplasty 103
antibiotic prophylaxis 130–1
anticoagulation prophylaxis against
  DVT/pulmonary embolism
  postoperative 190, 191, 193–4
  preoperative 130
antral ulcer 13
aortic aneurysm 98
aortomesenteric bypass 28

appendicitis 17, 18, 21–3
    appendicectomy 18, 22, 23
    preoperative care 124–5
arterial blood gas analysis 170–1
arterial occlusive disease *see* chronic
    arterial occlusive disease
arteritis ulcers 118
ascites 70
aspiration of gastric contents, risk of
    128–9
assessment of the critically ill surgical
    patient 164–5
    IQM principle 165–7
asthma, preoperative assessment 126–7
atelectasis 172
atherosclerosis 97
atrial fibrillation (AF)
    hypotension 174, 175, 176
    sepsis 188
at-risk patients, postoperative care 165,
    181
autoimmune chronic gastritis 14
autoimmune thyroiditis (Hashimoto's
    thyroiditis) 94

bacterial contamination of blood
    products 151–2
barium swallow 2
    achalasia 5
    diffuse oesophageal spasm 6
    oesophageal cancer 7
Barrett's metaplasia 3, 7
bile duct clearance 57
biliary colic 61, 62, 63
biliary disease 69
biliary system 63
    gallstone disease 63–4
    malabsorptive syndromes 29, 30
    repeated right upper abdominal pain
        61
    upper abdominal pain and vomiting
        61–3
bilirubin 65, 66
    obstructive jaundice 67–8
bleeding on defecation
    painful 46–7
    painless 47
blood grouping and cross-matching 150
blood groups 150
blood loss, unanticipated intraoperative
    149
blood per anum 31–2
blood products 149–51
blood transfusion 149–50
    adverse reactions 151–2
    indications for 152
    perioperative 148–9
body mass index (BMI) 154
body water, total 146
bradycardia 176
branchial cyst 90

breast 83–4
breast abscess 82, 84
breast cancer 83, 84–6
breast cyst 82
breast lumps 81–2
    abscess 84
    carcinoma 83, 84–6
    cyst 82
    discrete 82
    fibrocystic changes/fibroadenoma 84
    hot, painful 82–3
    multiple 82
    non-tender ill-defined 83
breast mouse 82
bronchospasm 172
Buerger's sign 102

caecal cancer 20, 23, 24
caecal rupture 35
caecal volvulus 43
calf, postoperative painful swollen
    189–90
cancer
    anal 39
    breast 83, 84–6
    caecal 20, 23, 24
    colorectal 31–3, 36–9
    gastric 10, 11, 12, 14–16
    gastro-oesophageal 11
    liver 70–2
    oesophageal 2, 3, 6–8
    pancreas and ampulla of Vater 59–61
    testicular 74
    thyroid 91, 94, 95
cardiac arrhythmias, preoperative
    assessment 126
cardiac failure, history of, and blood
    transfusion 148, 149
cardiogenic shock 162, 163
cardiotomy 6
cardiovascular disease 125–6
carotid artery disease 100, 109–10
carotid endarterectomy 100, 109
    consent issues 132
cerebrovascular accident (CVA) 109
cervical spine status, and airways
    management 159
Charcot's triad 64, 65
chest infection, prevention of 131
chest X-ray (CXR), hypoxia investigation
    171
Child–Pugh classification of cirrhosis 69,
    70
chin lift method 159, 160–1
cholangiocarcinoma 67, 71–2
cholangitis 64, 65
    obstructive jaundice 68
cholecystectomy
    acute pancreatitis 57
    anaesthesia for a laparoscopic
        procedure 136–7

biliary colic 61, 63
cholangitis 66
cholecystitis 62
gallstone disease 63, 64
preoperative care in diabetic patient
    123–4
cholecystitis 6l, 62, 63
cholecyst-jejunostomy 60
cholecystostomy 64
choledochojejunostomy 60
choledocholithiasis 64, 67
cholelithiasis *see* gallstones
cholestatic jaundice 67
chronic arterial insufficiency 118
chronic arterial occlusive disease 100–1
    acute limb ischaemia 99, 100, 105–7
    amputation 104–5
    carotid artery disease 100, 109–10
    diabetic foot 107–8
    foot pain at night 98–9
    leg pain with walking 97–8
    peripheral 98, 101–5
    sudden painful numb foot 99
    sudden weakness of right hand
        99–100
chronic gastritis 14, 15
chronic leg ulceration 113–14, 117–19
chronic malnutrition, preoperative
    152–3
chronic pancreatitis 57–9
chronic respiratory disease 165
chronic venous disease *see* venous
    disorders
chronic venous insufficiency 113, 114,
    117–18
cirrhosis 68–70
CLO (Campylobacter Like Organism) test
    12
clopidogrel 128
coeliac artery 27
coeliac plexus block 59
collapse, and sudden abdominal pain
    110–11
colloids, fluid management 147
colon 36
    polyps 36
    volvulus 43–4
colorectal cancer 31–3, 36–9
colorectal conditions
    abdominal pain and constipation 34–6
    anal carcinoma 39
    angiodysplasia 42–3
    blood per anum 31–2
    diverticular disease 33, 34, 41–2, 43
    intestinal obstruction 44–6
    recurrent diarrhoea and cramping
        abdominal pain 32–3
    severe left lower abdominal pain 33–4
    tumours 36–9
    ulcerative colitis 32–3, 39–41
colour duplex scanning 102, 103

compartment syndrome 106
compression stockings 129, 193
compression therapy, chronic recurrent
    leg ulcer 114
confusion, postoperative 169
congestive splenomegaly 70
consent issues 132–3
constipation 34–6
    diverticular disease 42, 43
    large bowel obstruction 44
contraceptive measures 128
contractility, and hypotension 176–7
Coombs' cross-match 150
corkscrew oesophagus 6
coronary artery disease 100, 176
corticosteroids 128
Courvoisier's sign 59, 67
cricoid pressure 137
Crohn's disease 20, 25–7
    malabsorptive syndromes 29
cross-matching of blood 150
cryoprecipitate 151
crystalloids, fluid management 146–7
cyclical mastalgia 81
cystic hygroma 90

deep vein thrombosis (DVT) 190–2, 194
    identification 192
    investigation 192–3
    management 193–5
    postoperative painful swollen calf
        189–90
    preoperative prophylaxis 122, 129–30
defecation
    and painful bleeding 46–7
    and painless bleeding 47
delayed haemolytic transfusion reaction
    151
dermoid cyst 89
diabetes
    anaesthesia 136
    chronic leg ulceration 118
    chronic pancreatitis 58, 59
    perioperative care 123–4, 127, 128
    postoperative care 165
    preoperative assessment 127
    preoperative care for cholecystectomy
        123–4
diabetic foot 107–8
diarrhoea, recurrent 32–3
diffuse oesophageal spasm 6
disseminated intravascular coagulation
    151
diverticular disease 33, 34, 41–2, 43
diverticulitis 33, 41, 42
drug-induced acute gastritis 14
Duke's classification, colorectal cancer
    38, 39
duodenal conditions
    acute upper abdominal pain 8–9
    haematemesis 11

ulcer 8, 9, 11, 12–13
    vomiting and weight loss 10–11
duodenum 12
dyspepsia 2
dysphagia 1, 2
    gastro-oesophageal reflux 5
    motility disorders 4–5
    oesophageal cancer 7

Early Warning Scoring System (EWSS)
    165–6
ECG changes
    myocardial infarction 179
    and postoperative hypotension 173–4
elastic compression stockings 129, 193
electrolyte disturbance, postoperative
    183
    following an emergency laparotomy
        180
    hyperkalaemia 184
    hypokalaemia 183–4
    hyponatraemia 183
electrolyte haemostasis 146
embolectomy 28, 106
emboli
    acute limb ischaemia 106
    carotid artery disease 109
    pulmonary see pulmonary embolism
emergency procedures
    laparotomy
        postoperative hypoxia 167–8
        postoperative oliguria 179–81
        rapid sequence induction 137–8
    postoperative care 165
empyema of gall bladder 63
encephalopathy, hepatic 70
endarterectomy, femoral 103
endarteritis 118
endoscopic retrograde
        cholangiopancreatography (ERCP)
    acute pancreatitis 55, 58
    choledocholithiasis 64
    obstructive jaundice 67–8
    pancreatic cancer 60
endotracheal tube 161
enteral nutritional support 154–5
epididymal cyst 74
epidural anaesthesia 140
epigastric hernia 78–9
extracellular fluid 146

facial nerve palsy 90
faecal peritonitis 33, 42
familial polyposis 36, 37
fasciotomy 106
febrile reactions to transfusion 151
feeding jejunostomy 153, 154
femoral endarterectomy 103
femoral hernia 18, 19, 75–6, 77, 78
    small bowel obstruction 23
femoro-popliteal bypass 103–4

fibroadenoma of breast 82, 84
fibrocystic change in breast 84
fibrosis 128
fistulae
    Crohn's disease 25, 26
    diverticular disease 33, 41, 42
fistula-in-ano 47, 49
fluid balance
    calculation 180
    charts 147, 181, 182
fluid management 145–6
    assessment 147–8
    colloids 147
    crystalloids 146–7
    following an uncomplicated
        laparotomy 145
    metabolic stress response to
        trauma/surgery 147
    perioperative fluid therapy 147
    sepsis 184
    water and electrolyte haemostasis
        146
fluid overload
    oliguria 182
    in transfusion 151
follicular carcinoma 94
foot
    diabetic 107–8
    night-time pain 98–9
    sudden painful numbness 99
fresh frozen plasma (FFP) 151
fundoplication 4

gall bladder
    empyema of 63
    mucocele of the 63
gallstone ileus 64
gallstones 61, 63–4, 65–6
    acute pancreatitis 54, 55, 57
    cholecystitis 61, 62, 63
    obstructive jaundice 67
gangrene 192
    diabetic foot 108
gastrectomy 15
    malabsorptive syndromes 29
gastric cancer 10, 11, 12, 14–16
gastric contents, risk of aspiration of
    128–9
gastric polyps 15
gastric resection 15
gastric ulcer 8, 11, 12, 13
gastritis 11, 14, 15
gastroenterostomy
    gastric cancer 15
    gastric outlet obstruction 10, 11
    pancreatic cancer 60
gastrointestinal stromal tumours (GIST)
    15
gastro-oesophageal cancer 11
gastro-oesophageal portal hypertension
    70

gastro-oesophageal reflux 1, 2, 3–4, 5
    preoperative assessment 127
gastro-oesophageal reflux disease 3–4
gastro-oesophageal sphincter 3
gastro-oesophageal varices 11
general anaesthesia 133–5
Gilbert's syndrome 67
Glasgow scoring system, acute
        pancreatitis 57
gluconeogenesis 154
glycogenolysis 154
goitre 94, 95
    multinodular 92, 94, 95, 96
Graves' disease 93, 94, 95, 96
groin hernia 75–9
    epigastric 78–9
    femoral 78
    incisional 79
    inguinal 77–8
    recurrent swelling 75
    umbilical 78
    vomiting and tender swelling 75–6
groin swelling, painless 73–4
Guedel airway 161

haematemesis 11
haematoma, perianal 50, 51
haemochromatosis 69
haemolytic transfusion reaction 151
haemorrhoidectomy 47, 48
haemorrhoids 47, 48
haemostasis, water and electrolyte 146
haemothorax 155
hand, sudden weakness of the right
        99–100
Hartmann's procedure 34, 35, 36
Hashimoto's thyroiditis (autoimmune
        thyroiditis) 94
headache, postdural puncture 136
heartburn 1–2
heart failure 125–6
heart murmurs 126
Helicobacter pylori
    gastric cancer 15, 16
    peptic ulcers 12–13
hemicolectomy 25
    Crohn's disease 26
    small bowel obstruction 24
heparin-induced thrombocytopenia 194
hepatectomy, partial 71
hepatic encephalopathy 70
hepatic jaundice 67
hepatitis 69
    protection against hepatitis B 131–2
hepatobiliary system, malabsorptive
        syndromes 29, 30
    see also liver
hepatocellular adenoma 70
hepatocellular carcinoma (HCC) 71
hepatoma 7
hepatomegaly 2

hepato-renal syndrome 68
hepatosplenomegaly 89
hernia 18, 19, 20, 76–7, 78
    epigastric 78–9
    femoral 18, 19, 75–6, 77, 78
        small bowel obstruction 23
    groin *see* groin hernia
    incisional 23, 79
    inguinal 18, 19, 20, 75–6, 77–8
        small bowel obstruction 23
        spinal anaesthesia 135–6
    inguinoscrotal 73, 74, 77
    irreducible 75, 76
    large bowel obstruction 45, 46
    para-umbilical 78
    preoperative repair in elderly man
        122–3
    reducible 75, 76
    sliding 3, 4, 78
    small bowel obstruction 23, 34
    umbilical 78
hiatus hernia 2, 3–4
high-dependency units (HDUs), transfer
        to 167
HIV, protection against 131–2
hoarseness 87–8, 91
hormone replacement therapy (HRT) 128
hydrocoele 73, 74
hyperkalaemia 184
hypertension
    postoperative 178
        sepsis 184
    preoperative assessment 126
hypertensive peristaltic oesophagus 6
hyperthyroidism (thyrotoxicosis) 93–4,
        95–6
hypokalaemia 183–4
hyponatraemia 183
hypoplasia 120
hypotension
    postoperative 164–5, 175–6, 177
        contractility 176–7
        and ECG changes 173–4
        heart rate 176
        hypovolaemia 176
        identification and quantification
            177–8
        myocardial ischaemia/infarction
            178–9
        sepsis 177
        with a tachyarrhythmia 174–5
    preoperative, causes 175
hypoventilation 172
hypovolaemia 158, 160
    hypotension 176, 177, 178
    hypoxia 173
    oliguria 181, 182
hypovolaemic shock 158–9, 160, 162–3
hypoxaemia 168, 170
    investigations 170, 171–2
    sepsis 187

hypoxia, postoperative 159, 160, 168, 173
    effects 168–9
    following an emergency laparotomy
        167–8
    identification and quantification
        169–72
    importance of oxygen 168
    management 172–3
    manoeuvres to improve respiration
        173
    myocardial ischaemia 169, 178
    oxygen delivery 169

ileostomy 40
incentive spirometry 171
incisional hernia 23, 79
inferior mesenteric artery 27
inferior vena caval filtration 191, 194
inflammatory bowel disease 32–3
inguinal hernia 18, 19, 20, 75–6, 77–8
    small bowel obstruction 23
    spinal anaesthesia 135–6
inguinoscrotal hernia 73, 74, 77
inotrope therapy 188
insulin, perioperative care 123–4, 128
intensive care units (ICUs), transfers to
        167
intermittent claudication 97, 98, 101, 103
interstitial fluid 146
intracellular fluid 146
IQM (identify, quantify, manage)
        principle, postoperative patient
        assessment 164–7
irritability, hyperthyroidism 93–4
ischaemia, acute limb 99, 100, 105–7
ischaemic heart disease
    blood transfusion 149
    hypotension 176, 178
    postoperative care 165
ischaemic rest pain 98, 101
ischaemic ulcers 98, 99

jaundice 66
    and abdominal pain 64–6
    classification 67
    diagnostic approaches 67
    obstructive 65, 66, 67–8
    pancreatic cancer 59, 60
jaw thrust method 159, 160–1
jejunostomy, feeding 153, 154
juvenile polyps, colonic 36

Laerdel pocket mask 161
laparoscopic cholecystectomy,
        anaesthesia 136
laparotomy
    emergency
        postoperative hypoxia 167–8
        postoperative oliguria 186
        rapid sequence induction 137–8
    fluid regimes following a 145

large intestine
  malabsorptive syndromes 29, 30
  obstruction 44-6
laryngeal mask airway 161
left lower abdominal pain 33-4
leg pain with walking 97-8
leg ulceration, chronic 113-14, 117-19
limb ischaemia, acute 99, 100, 105-7
lipodermatosclerosis 114
lipolysis 154
liver 68
  benign tumours 70
  biopsy 69
  cirrhosis 68-70
  malignancies 70-2
  portal hypertension 70
  transplantation 69, 71
liver disease 127
Living Will 133
local anaesthesia 135, 140
  myocardial ischaemia/infarction risk
    178
  toxicity 140
lumpectomy 85
lumps
  in breast 81-6
  in neck 87-90
  in scrotum 73 5
  in thyroid gland 91-6
lymphadenopathy 87-8, 89-90
  thyroid carcinoma 91
lymphangioma 90
lymphatic disease 119-20
lymph nodes 87-8, 89-90
lymphoedema 119-20
lymphomas 15-16

magnetic resonance
  cholangiopancreatography 64, 67
malabsorption 28-30
malnutrition, preoperative chronic
    152-3
masks for airways management 161
mastalgia 81-2
mastectomy 85
mesenteric angiography 20-1, 27-8
mesenteric ischaemia 20, 21, 27-8
metabolic stress response to
    trauma/surgery 147
metastatic disease
  breast 83
  liver 70-1
microbial chronic gastritis 14
microdochectomy 82
midazolam 141
monoamine oxidase inhibitors 128
motility disorders in the oesophagus 4-5
  achalasia 5-6
  diffuse oesophageal spasm 6
  hypertensive peristaltic oesophagus 6
mucocele of the gall bladder 63

multinodular goitre 92, 94, 95, 96
multiorgan dysfunction syndrome
    186
Murphy's sign 62
muscle relaxants 140
myocardial infarction
  cardiogenic shock 163
  hypotension 174, 178-9
  hypoxia 169
  postoperative recovery 164
  preoperative assessment 125, 126
myocardial ischaemia
  hypotension 174, 175, 178, 179
  hypoxia 169, 178

nasogastric tube 154
nasojejunal tube 154
nausea, postoperative 144
neck lumps 88-9
  branchial cyst 90
  cystic hygroma 90
  lymph nodes 89-90
  midline swellings 89
  painless, and hoarseness 87-8
  salivary glands 90
neoplastic ulcers 118, 119
nerve end ischaemia 98
neurogenic shock 162, 164
neuropathic ulcers 118, 119
nutcracker oesophagus 6
nutrition, surgical 153, 156
  assessment of nutritional status 154
  postoperative 153
  preoperative 153
  preoperative chronic malnutrition
    152-3
  requirements 154
  specific surgical conditions 153
  support methods 154-5

obstructive jaundice 65, 66, 67-8
odynophagia 4
oesophageal cancer 2, 3, 6-8
oesophageal conditions
  cancer 6-8
  heartburn 1-2
  hiatus hernia 3-4
  motility disorders 4-6
    achalasia 5-6
    diffuse oesophageal spasm 6
    hypertensive peristaltic oesophagus
      6
  oesophagitis 3
  reflux 2, 3-4, 5
  swallowing difficulties 2
oesophageal spasm, diffuse 6
oesophageal stricture 2, 3, 4
oesophagitis 2, 3, 11
oesophagus 2-3
  corkscrew 6
  nutcracker 6

oliguria, postoperative 181, 183
  acute tubular necrosis 182-3
  aetiology 181-2
  following an emergency laparotomy
    179-81
  identification and quantification 182
  management 182
oophorectomy 85
oral contraceptive pill 128
oral nutritional support 154
osteomyelitis 108
ovarian cyst, ruptured 23
oxygen
  cascade 169
  delivery 169
  dissociation curve 170
  importance 168
  therapy
    hypotension 175, 177, 178
    hypoxia 172-3
    myocardial infarction risk
      reduction 179
    sepsis 185, 187

pain management, postoperative 143-4
pancreas 55
  acute pancreatitis 53 7, 58
  carcinoma of pancreas and ampulla of
    Vater 59-61
  chronic pancreatitis 57-9
  malabsorptive syndromes 29, 30
  severe upper central abdominal pain
    53-5
pancreatic necrosis 57
pancreaticoduodenectomy 60
pancreatitis
  acute 53-7, 58
  chronic 57-9
pancreatotomy 59, 60
panproctolectomy 40
papillary carcinoma 94
para-umbilical hernia 78
parenteral nutritional support 153, 154,
    155
  malabsorptive syndromes 30
parotid gland 90
patient-controlled analgesia (PCA) 144
PEG (percutaneous endoscopic
    gastrostomy) tube 154
pelvic abscess 187
peptic ulcer 8, 9, 11, 12-14
  malabsorptive syndromes following
    surgery 29
percutaneous endoscopic gastrostomy
    (PEG) tube 154
percutanous transhepatic
    cholangiography 60
perforated ulcer 13
perianal conditions 48, 51
  abscess 47, 48-9
  anal fissues 46-7, 50-1

perianal conditions – *continued*
  bleeding on painful defecation 46–7
  fistula-in-ano 47, 49
  haematoma 50, 51
  haemorrhoids 47, 48
  painful swelling 47–8
  painless bleeding on defecation 47
  pilonidal sinus and abscess 49–50
  rectal prolapse 50, 51
periductal mastitis 82
perioperative care
  anaesthesia and sedation 133–44
  consent issues 132–3
  fluid management 145–8
  nutrition 152–6
  preoperative assessment,
    investigation and premedication
    122–32
  transfusion and blood products
    148–52
perioperative fluid therapy 147
peripheral arterial aneurysms
  abdominal aortic aneurysm 110–12
  popliteal artery aneurysm 112
peripheral arterial occlusive disease 98,
  101–4
peripherally inserted central catheter
  (PICC) line 153, 155
peripheral vascular resistance 177
peritonitis
  acute upper abdominal pain 8, 9
  faecal 33, 42
  perforated ulcer 13
phlegmasia caerulae dolens (painful blue
  leg) 192
phlegmatic alba dolens (painful white
  leg) 192
pilonidal sinus and abscess 49–50
plasma volume 146
platelet concentrates 151
  bacterial contamination 152
pleomorphic adenomas 90
plicae circulares 24
pneumatic compression stockings 129
pneumoperitoneum 19
pneumothorax
  as complication of TPN 155
  hypotension 176
  hypoxia 170, 173
polyps, colonic 36
popliteal artery aneurysm 112
portal hypertension 69, 70
postdural puncture headache 136
posthepatic jaundice 67
postoperative care 142
  ABC patient assessment and
    resuscitation 158–64
  assessment of critically ill surgical
    patient 164–7
  blood transfusion 148–52
  collapse 158–9

deep vein thrombosis and pulmonary
  embolism 189–95
fluid management 145–8
hypotension and cardiac ischaemia
  173–9
hypoxia 167–73
nutrition 152–6
oliguria and electrolyte disturbance
  179–84
pain management 143–4
postoperative nausea and vomiting
  144
recovery 142–3
sepsis 184–9
prehepatic jaundice 67
premedication 128
  risk of aspiration of gastric contents
    128–9
preoperative assessment 125, 127–8
  cardiovascular disease 125–6
  respiratory disease 126–7
preoperative care 125
  assessment of patients 125–8
  consent issues 132–3
  elective cholecystectomy in a diabetic
    patient 123–4
  elective varicose vein surgery 122
  emergency appendicectomy 124–5
  hernia repair in an elderly man
    122–3
  premedication 128–9
  prophylaxis 129–32
preoperative chronic malnutrition 152–3
preoperative surgical nutrition 153
pressure sores, prevention of 131
pretibial ulcers 118
prophylaxis, preoperative 132
  antibiotics 130–1
  chest infection 131
  deep vein thrombosis/pulmonary
    embolism 129–30
  hepatitis B 131–2
  HIV 131–2
  pressure sores 131
propofol 141
pruritis 66, 67
pruritis ani 49
pulmonary embolism (PE) 192–2, 194
  hypotension 174, 176
  hypoxia 172
  identification 192
  investigation 192–3
  management 193–5
  preoperative prophylaxis 122,
    129–30
pulmonary oedema 172
pulmonary sepsis 172
pulse oximetry 170
puncture headache, postdural 136
pyloric stenosis 10–11
pyrexia, postoperative 184–5

rapid sequence induction for an
  emergency laparotomy 137–8
recovery 142–3
rectal cancer 31–3, 36–9
rectal prolapse 50, 51
rectum 36
  see also colorectal conditions
recurrent abdominal pain 19–20
red cell concentrates 150
reflux, gastro-oesophageal 1, 2, 3–4, 5
  preoperative assessment 127
regional anaesthesia 135, 140
  myocardial ischaemia/infarction risk
    178
  toxicity 140
renal aspects of metabolic response to
  injury 147
renal impairment 127
respiration
  inadequate 173
  manoeuvres to improve 173
respiratory disease 126–7
respiratory function tests 171
resuscitation, postoperative 158–60
  airways management 160–2
  monitoring and reporting 160
  secondary survey 160
  shock management 162–4
Rhesus system 150
rheumatoid arthritis 127
right lower abdominal pain 17–18
rolling hiatus hernia 3, 4

salivary glands 90
salpingitis 23
scleropathy 70
scrotal lumps 74, 75
  epididymal cyst 74
  hydrocele 74
  painless groin swelling 73–4
  testicular tumour 75
  varicocoele 74
sedation
  agitated or restless patient 141
  diagnostic procedures 141–2
  safe administration of intravenous
    sedation 142
  techniques 141
seminoma 75
sepsis, postoperative 184–6, 188–9
  and hypotension 177, 184
  identification 186–7
  management 187–8
  quantification 187
  systemic inflammatory response
    syndrome 186–7
septic shock 162, 163, 185, 186
shock 158–9, 162, 164
  anaphylactic 162, 163
    and blood transfusion 151
  cardiogenic 162, 163

hypotension 175
hypovolaemic 158-9, 160, 162-3
  neurogenic 162, 164
  septic 162, 163, 185, 186
sigmoid volvulus 43-4
sliding hernia 3, 4, 78
small bowel 21
  abdominal pain and weight loss
    20-1
  acute right lower abdominal pain
    17-18
  appendicitis 21-3
  Crohn's disease 25-7
  malabsorption 28-30
  mesenteric ischaemia 27-8
  obstruction 23-5
  recurrent abdominal pain 19-20
  vomiting and abdominal distension
    18-19
smokers, preoperative assessment 127
spermatocoele 74
sphincterectomy
  anal fissure 51
  choledocholithiasis 64
  gallstone disease 65, 66
spinal anaesthesia 139-40
  for an inguinal hernia repair 135-6
spirometry 171
splanchicectomy 59
splenomegaly, congestive 70
squamous cancer
  neoplastic ulcers 118
  oesophagus 6-7
stenosis 10-11
stomach 11-12
  acute upper abdominal pain 8-9
  haematemesis 11
  malabsorptive syndromes 29, 30
  vomiting and weight loss 10-11
  see also gastric entries
strangulation 76
  large bowel obstruction 45
  small bowel obstruction 23-4
stress-related acute gastritis 14
submandibular gland 90
subphrenic abscess 185, 187
suction, for airways management 162
superior mesenteric artery 27
supraclavicular lymphadenopathy 2
suxamethonium 140
swallowing difficulties (dysphagia) 1, 2
  gastro-oesophageal reflux 5
  motility disorders 4-5
  oesophageal cancer 7
systemic inflammatory response
    syndrome (SIRS) 185, 186

tachyarrhythmias
  hypotension 174-5, 176
  myocardial ischaemia 178
  sepsis 185
tachypnoea
  hypotension 174
  sepsis 185
tenesmus 31, 37
tension pneumothorax
  hypotension 176
  hypoxia 170, 173
teratoma 75
testicular cancer 74
testicular tumour 74, 75
thrombocytopenia, heparin-induced 194
thrombolysis 106, 193
thrombophilia 192
thrombophlebitis 113
thrombosis 105-6
thyroglossal cyst 89
thyroid cancer 91, 94, 95
thyroidectomy 92, 94, 96
thyroiditis, autoimmune (Hashimoto's
    thyroiditis) 94
thyroid lobectomy 91, 96
thyroid lymphoma 94
thyroid problems 94
  diffuse swelling 92
  hyperthyroidism (thyrotoxicosis)
    93-4, 95-6
  multinodular goitre 92, 94, 95, 96
  painless swelling 91
  solitary nodule 91, 94, 95, 96
  weight loss and irritability 93-4
thyrotoxicosis (hyperthyroidism) 93-4,
    95-6
total body water 146
total intravenous anaesthesia (TIVA) 138
total parenteral nutrition (TPN) 153, 154,
    155
  malabsorptive syndromes 30
transfusion see blood transfusion
transient ischaemic attack (TIA) 100, 109
transjugular intrahepatic portosystemic
    shunt (TIPSS) 70
traumatic ulcers 118
Trendelenberg's test 113, 115-16
Troisier's sign 90
T-tube cholangiography 64

ulcerative colitis 25, 32-3, 39-41
umbilical hernia 78
upper abdominal pain, acute 8-9
upper central abdominal pain 53-5
upper gastrointestinal haemorrhage 11,
    12

urea breath test 12
urinary retention, postoperative 136

valvulae coniventes 24
varicoele 74
varicose ulceration 118
varicose veins 112-13, 114, 115-16
  general anaesthesia 133-5
  preoperative elective surgery 122
vascular conditions
  abdominal aortic aneurysm 110-12
  chronic arterial occlusive disease
    97-110
  surgery, and risk of myocardial
    infarction 178
  venous disorders 112-20
venous disorders 115
  chronic leg ulceration 113-14,
    117-19
  lymphatic disease 119-20
  varicose veins 112-13, 115-16
venous gangrene 192
ventilation/perfusion (VQ) mismatching
    172
ventricular filling 176
villous polyps, colonic 36
Virchow's node 90
Virchow's triad 191
volvulus of the colon 43-4
vomiting
  and abdominal distension 18-19
  of blood 11
  faeculent 76
  postoperative 144
  small bowel obstruction 23
  stomach and duodenal conditions
    10-11
  and tender groin swelling 75-6
  and upper abdominal pain 61-3

warfarin, perioperative care 128
water, total body 146
water haemostasis 146
weight loss
  and abdominal pain 20-1
  hyperthyroidism 93-4
  oesophageal conditions 2, 3
  stomach and abdominal conditions
    10-11
Whippler's operation 60
Wilson's disease 69
wound infection, minimizing the risk of
    130-1

Zollinger-Ellison syndrome 12